A Practical Guide to Crew Resource Management for Healthcare Teams

A Practical Guide to Crew Resource Management for Healthcare Teams

By

William S. O'Keefe, Lacey L. Schmidt, Louis P. Halamek, Danny Castro and Sharon P. Pickering

Cambridge Scholars Publishing

A Practical Guide to Crew Resource Management for Healthcare Teams

By William S. O'Keefe, Lacey L. Schmidt, Louis P. Halamek, Danny Castro and Sharon P. Pickering

This book first published 2022

Cambridge Scholars Publishing

Lady Stephenson Library, Newcastle upon Tyne, NE6 2PA, UK

British Library Cataloguing in Publication Data
A catalogue record for this book is available from the British Library

ISBN (10): 1-5275-8285-X
ISBN (13): 978-1-5275-8285-9

"If you want to learn how to apply the wealth of knowledge on how to deliver effective CRM training to your organization--this is the book you must have and need. [It] will provide all the practical and insightful guidance you must follow. Get it! A gem of a book written by experienced CRM scientists and practitioners."
—Eduardo Salas, Ph.D.
Allyn R. and Gladys M. Cline Professor of Psychology, Rice University, USA

"[The book] is a wonderfully practical resource that covers the fundamentals of CRM for healthcare. Packed with clear examples, useful tips, and valuable tools, this book will be an essential tool to any individual or organization looking to improve safety and quality in healthcare delivery."
—David Michael Musson, MD, PhD
Assistant Professor, Department of Anesthesiology, McMaster University, Canada

"If crew resource management has loomed before you like an imposing monolith, this book is your guide to conquering it. The authors' brilliant tone lends toward a conversation between old colleagues rather than an instruction manual, making this a quintessential read for clinical leaders, new or old."
—Dexter Buelow, RRT-NPS
Respiratory Therapy Clinical Coordinator, Texas Children's Hospital

"[The book] delivers an invaluable guide for today's complex and increasingly interdisciplinary healthcare systems. Bite-size lessons combined with a concise chapter framework using real-life scenarios provided by physician co-authors will foster learning for healthcare teams, trainees, and organizations, creating a team environment and culture which is adaptable across many scenarios including the intermingling of team members which undoubtedly occurs in healthcare settings."
—Ruth L. Bush, MD, JD, MPH
Professor of Vascular Surgery, University of Houston

"[This is] required reading for any debriefing facilitator. Clear examples illustrate essential team dynamics required in the complex milieu of healthcare. Practical scenarios, tabular examples and summary boxes are perfect 'just in time' references."
—Jeanine Graf, MD, Professor
Pediatric Intensive Care, Chief Medical Officer, Texas Children's Hospital West Campus

"Read this superb, comprehensive book if you've experienced a near miss or serious adverse event; your hospital is considering CRM; or already has CRM but wants more from it!"
Andrew Gaffney, MD
Professor of Medicine (Emeritus), Vanderbilt University, USA

CONTENTS

PREFACE

The fact that you have this practical guide demonstrates that you are aware of Crew Resource Management (CRM), and you are interested in how it can support effective team interactions and help your team in your daily care of patients.

Extensive material on CRM for healthcare has been produced by organizations, consultancies, and research institutions. These existing materials apply one of the following themes. These themes are not exhaustive but are aimed to highlight limitations that may prevent CRM from being used by healthcare practitioners today. They include:

1. Adoption of Commercial Aviation-Style CRM into Healthcare.
   CRM techniques and tools that are employed by airlines provide examples from aviation to illustrate their use in the cockpit (or other aviation environments such as the air traffic control tower). This approach advocates for the adoption of aviation CRM into healthcare. However, this approach often fails to account for differences between the two professions, including environmental and cultural differences. This approach provides minimum transferability of this style of CRM into healthcare, which in turn receives limited acceptance by healthcare professionals.
2. Theoretical and Experimental Approaches.
   These approaches provide broad recommendations to adopt CRM based on research that is typically conducted in non-healthcare domains. They often fail to provide real-life examples and limit practical methods for CRM adoption into healthcare settings.
3. Tailored Approaches to Implementing CRM in Specific Healthcare Settings.
   These typically present a reasonable understanding of CRM applied to specific cultural aspects and processes. However, they limit transferability of CRM principles and practices to other healthcare settings, thereby diluting its effectiveness as well as its potential benefits.

4. Personal Approaches by Healthcare Professionals with Limited CRM Knowledge and/or Experience.
   The authors of such material are intimately familiar with the healthcare context and have successfully implemented at least some form of CRM in practice. However, their knowledge of CRM tends to be lacking in depth, without refined understanding or applied expertise. This results in the sporadic use of CRM in some healthcare settings, rather than a fully embedded approach across all situations in healthcare.

So, why is our practical guide different? This guide is written to eliminate the limitations highlighted in the above themes. We, the authors of this guide, collectively cover the theoretical expertise and the applied experience to inform healthcare professionals on how to adopt CRM in practice. The authors include: two intensive care physicians who are actively engaged in clinical practice at academic institutions; two research doctorates with broad and deep experience using scientific evidence to develop applied CRM programs for multiple industries; and one highly experienced CRM instructor who has designed and implemented CRM training for NASA astronauts and flight controllers, oil and gas drilling crews, emergency responders, and many other highly specialized teams. Collectively, we explain CRM in practical terms that are both evidence-based and directly applicable to daily healthcare practice. Given our united approach, we can provide references to real-life examples where healthcare teams have displayed good CRM and areas where they could improve. Therefore, we show concrete CRM techniques to show specific behaviors that can improve the quality of your interactions and positively impact patient safety.

This guide is unique because it combines research with professional and practical expertise in a personal, usable, and relevant format. The focus is to help you, as the professional, to embed a proactive approach to your team interactions. This is to ensure that good behaviors become natural and easy, making it less likely for situations to go wrong. This guide is not, however, intended to tell you how to perform your role. CRM training often attempts to direct the user on exact ways to do CRM. This is inappropriate. The authors recognize that how we think you perform your role and how you actually perform your role will be mismatched. There is frequently a disconnect between work-as-imagined by administrators, researchers etc. and work-as-done by practitioners, which must be understood to ensure that planned work and actual work align (Anderson, 2017). Therefore, the contents of this guide are designed to inform you on how to do good CRM, on a behavioral level, but it is up to you to effectively adopt CRM.

Throughout this guide, evidence-based CRM practices are presented as behaviors in the context of real-life healthcare scenarios. Modifying how CRM is labelled to match healthcare-specific personnel/use is not our intent. This guide is intended to be used by all healthcare professionals, and therefore a tailored approach to the terminology is impractical. The examples will reference many working environments, and the practical approach will bridge the gap between theory and real-world practice by presenting knowledge in context that can easily be understood. This is aimed to encourage you to reflect and imagine how you would apply CRM to your daily interactions in a healthcare setting. Presenting all types of behaviors in all types of scenarios is impossible; therefore, the contents of this guide will stimulate your thoughts regarding how you act. This practical approach to learning brings alive examples of what good looks like to motivate you to model these behaviors as your way of working. This guide leads you on the path to success through demonstrating how to continually practice CRM, empowering you with skills to inspire change, thereby ensuring that your own accountability for the safe delivery of healthcare is modeled and transferable in order to guide others in your organization.

This guide is structured so that each major part begins with a healthcare scenario that describes the efforts of multidisciplinary team members to save a life. The scenario is used to represent a complex and comprehensive situation in which our selected CRM model can be presented in an advanced context. The principles and practices of the CRM model are explained in the context of the scenarios. Additional examples are provided to demonstrate the transferability of the CRM model skills; these will support your understanding of how CRM can be effective in healthcare settings. This guide has three parts. The first part discusses CRM skills. The second part of the guide discusses tools to help you apply these skills successfully. To demonstrate how tools help you apply CRM skills, you will see that each chapter demonstrates two important tools: a briefing and a debriefing. We believe that a good briefing enables CRM by discussing what is happening, what success looks like, and what threats or errors are possible and how you plan to prevent, avoid, or mitigate them. We also believe a good debriefing, using open-ended questions, will encourage you to consider tangible actions to improve CRM in your team and organization. Hence, the repetitive nature is meant to embed these beliefs, as we anticipate that you will engage in this book on an irregular and/or intermittent basis. The third section discusses how to influence your organization to implement CRM and how to evaluate its implementation. In every chapter, we attempt to provide just enough material that you can read the chapter in 30 minutes for a high-level understanding. However, we recommend that you revisit each chapter for a deeper understanding of how to apply the skills in practice. Finally, there is a glossary. If you run across a term that you do not know or understand, check the glossary. The glossary contains terms and concepts that we believe are crucial to your understanding of CRM. If a term is in the glossary, you must understand its significance. If you understand every term in the glossary, you have made the first step in understanding CRM concepts. Conversely, if a term is not in the glossary, it is not crucial to your understanding of CRM.

A consistent theme will become apparent: CRM for healthcare is focused on effective team interactions. As a healthcare professional, you will experience many challenging situations, ranging from daily resourcing issues to unprecedented times such as a pandemic. This guide is intended to not just teach you how to react in situations when things are going wrong, it is also about empowering team performance. Our purpose is to expand how you think, how you act, and how your team interacts in all daily activities so that best practice simply becomes the way that you work together to prevent, avoid, and mitigate potential errors before they have the potential to result in patient harm.

As a professional adopting CRM, you have a multitude of factors that impact your performance. While many factors are seemingly out of your control, remember that adopting CRM as your way of working is directly within your control. This will significantly benefit your daily activities to provide optimum care, contribute to the adoption of CRM across healthcare, and save lives.

Reference

Anderson, Janet E., Alastair J. Ross, and Peter Jaye. "Modelling Resilience and Researching the Gap Between Work-as-Imagined and Work-as-Done." Essay. In Resilient Health Care: Reconciling Work-as Imagined and Work-as-Done 3, edited by Jeffrey Braithwaite, Erik Hollnagel, and Robert L. Wears, 3:133–41. London: CRC Press, 2015.

CHAPTER 1

MAKING THE CASE FOR CRM IN HEALTHCARE

Chapter Briefing[1]

I want to call a quick STAR (Stop-Think-Act-Review): that means get off your email, stop your side conversations, and turn off the television.[2] Here is what we will do in this chapter: we will discuss what Crew Resource Management (CRM) is and how it applies to healthcare. We will be successful if you can explain:

- what CRM is (Section 1.1);
- why CRM is essential to healthcare (Section 1.2); and
- how our CRM model works in healthcare (Section 1.3).

The primary threat that you might experience is the introduction of a large number of concepts and terms, some of which you may have never encountered, and some of which you may think about in a different sense. We will therefore explicitly define and differentiate each term and concept. We also realize how busy you are. We will make sure that the chapter is short enough to be read in approximately thirty minutes. Finally, we provide Summary Boxes. The Summary Boxes serve two functions. First, they emphasize the take-home points in each section, and you can use them to check your understanding of those take-home points. Second, you can use them to determine if you and your team are implementing those take-home points. If a Summary Box does not make sense to you or you do not understand one or more take-home points, then review the related material before continuing to the next section.

---

[1] You will see this chapter briefing format for every chapter. We believe that it is important to emphasize that a good briefing builds mental models by discussing what is happening, what success looks like, what threats or errors are possible, and, how you plan to prevent, avoid, or mitigate them.

[2] For information on STAR, see Chapters 11-15.

Did I miss anything? Any concerns? Any questions? (Pause) No? Then, let's get started.

List of Abbreviations

CRM	Crew Resource Management

This chapter will provide an overview of what Crew Resource Management (CRM) is (Section 1.1), why CRM is essential in daily healthcare practice (Section 1.2), and how our CRM model fits with the reality of delivering consistently safe healthcare (Section 1.3).

1.1 What is CRM?

The Federal Aviation Administration (FAA) considers CRM as a team that uses all human, hardware, and software resources to be safe and effective (FAA 2004). This definition encompasses a broad approach in order to exclude nothing, and this is difficult to understand and adopt in practice. Many complex definitions aim to explain CRM. Our simple and concise viewpoint places emphasis on the team aspect of CRM. In our perspective, CRM is a way of managing and optimizing team interactions to improve performance and positively impact safety. In our CRM model, the core skills are your interpersonal skills: Exchanging Information, Communicating, Leading and Following, and Mutually Supporting. These core skills will be explained later in this chapter and in much more detail in subsequent chapters.

Our concept of CRM describes behaviors. When these CRM core skills are represented as behaviors, they complement your technical skills and enable you to combine the technical skills of your team to improve your overall team performance, thereby producing safe and effective patient care. Behaviors will be described simply as good and bad, whereby good behaviors are those that enable effective team interactions, and bad behaviors inhibit them.

Our model has four core skills, or four collections of behaviors, that you can learn to adopt and use in your daily activities:

1. Exchanging Information: Exchanging Information is about determining what information to exchange to whom and when. Everyone within a team will need information from another team

member at some point. No single team member can have access to all the information he or she needs at all times. The purpose of Exchanging Information is to fill gaps in individuals' situation awareness[3] (i.e., what you think is happening) and mental models (i.e., why, and how you think it is happening). Exchanging Information is concerned with the transfer of elements of situation awareness and mental models between team members. The products of Exchanging Information are every team member has the situation awareness and mental models required to fulfil their responsibilities.

2. Communicating: Communicating, in this sense, is all about how to exchange information. The important behaviors are delivering information clearly and concisely through protocols (i.e., the format and terminology of information to be delivered), active listening in an effort to understand, followed by confirmation of that understanding. Communicating with skill ensures that information is received and understood in time to achieve your team's goals.
3. Leading and Following: Each team member is both a leader and a follower at various times and situations. Leaders enable CRM by setting up psychological safety, articulating CRM expectations, and then modeling and rewarding those behaviors. Followers enable CRM by inquiring when they do not understand the leader or the situation, and then advocating and even asserting a position when they believe that safety is at risk. As an outcome of active CRM Leading and Following behaviors, followers provide the leader with all the information and knowledge required to make safe and effective decisions.
4. Mutually Supporting: Mutually Supporting the team is about offering and accepting physical, cognitive, psychological, and emotional support as well as providing feedback on both technical and non-technical behaviors. The outcome of your skill in Mutually Supporting others is a reduction in the impacts of Performance Shaping Factors such as stress and fatigue, thereby supporting fewer errors and reduced risk, even in complex and extreme environments.

[3] Some researchers and practitioners use the term 'situational awareness'.

Summary Box 1.1
Our Approach to Crew Resource Management

Our approach to Crew Resource Management is…

- a way of managing and optimizing team interactions, to improve performance, and positively impact safety;
- based on observable behaviors; and includes:
  - Exchanging Information: determining what information to exchange to whom and when.
  - Communicating: how to exchange information.
  - Leading and Following:
    - Leading is setting up psychological safety, articulating CRM expectations and then modeling and rewarding those behaviors.
    - Following is inquiring when they do not understand the leader or the situation, and then advocating and even asserting a position when they believe that safety is at risk.
  - Mutually Supporting: offering and accepting physical, cognitive, psychological, and emotional support as well as providing feedback on both technical and non-technical behaviors.

1.2 Why CRM?

The fact that you have this practical guide demonstrates that you are aware of CRM and interested in how it can support you and your team in your daily care of patients. As a healthcare professional, your team's top priority is to consistently deliver safe healthcare to every single patient. Every patient has the right to experience the safest care, and, in order to achieve this, you and your team endeavor to perform at your optimum in every situation. However, even with the best of intentions, things still go wrong. Harm to patients through adverse events is not only distressing for them and their family, but it also has a personal impact on healthcare professionals themselves, as explained by the second victim syndrome (Scott 2009). Adverse events create varying levels of patient harm: at the catastrophic end, figures estimate that 1 in 10,000 patients die every year as a result of a preventable medical error (de Vries 2008) and the annual number of preventable deaths cited in publications is often cited as greater than 200,000. (Austin 2019). The healthcare system is a highly dynamic, multifaceted, complex safety-critical profession. As a healthcare professional, you represent a key element within a vast network of interdependent roles and responsibilities. You strive to ensure that things always go right in the areas that you influence. When CRM becomes standard practice, you and your team will behave in a manner that ensures that you are continually competent and responsible for achieving a safe and successful outcome.

CRM was founded in aviation and has over forty years of history of contributing to the efforts of ensuring that flying remains the safest mode of transportation. The aviation industry recognized that to reduce their accident rates, focusing on improving technical aspects alone was insufficient. Therefore, CRM was derived from the concept of team skills training to enable pilots in the cockpit to effectively manage their interactions.

CRM began as part of a collaboration between NASA and the airlines. CRM has evolved through five generations of research, operational validity, and continued refinement. As a result, research continues to inform the application of CRM. Throughout decades, CRM has been adapted for use in multiple safety critical environments including defense, rail, maritime, and many others. In each of these environments, CRM has been shown to demonstrate positive impacts on safety with associated benefits to team performance, efficiency, cost reductions, and job satisfaction. The use of CRM in healthcare is not new; CRM has been adopted from aviation and applied in healthcare for several decades. Typically, aviation terminology is often adopted and packaged for healthcare without acknowledging the fundamental differences between aviation and healthcare, such as organizational factors and culture. Therefore, aviation-style CRM cannot, and should not, be directly adopted in healthcare. Healthcare has unique organizational structures, cultures, goals, and contexts. Healthcare is delivered in many environments ranging from clinics, ambulances, hospitals, and so forth, and many roles function within these varied environments. That said, healthcare can certainly benefit from CRM. What CRM can offer healthcare professionals in all roles is its relevance for each and every daily team interaction in all work settings. CRM skills, however, currently receive varied attention in healthcare and are not valued the same as mandatory technical skills. Other industries such as aviation have made CRM training a mandatory and integrated part of their overall training needs. Even with the increasing awareness and acceptance of the importance of team skills, CRM training is often considered as an add-on course that only captures a snapshot of the breadth of skills required for a team to continually deliver safe care in practice. Waiting to learn about CRM as required on the job, or after a critical event, will be too late; lessons can be learned at this stage, but only after significant impacts and potential losses, which could include loss of life. A major incentive to adopt CRM is to avoid creating a problem in the first place. If a problem does occur, and you and your team are practiced in CRM, you will be equipped with not only the knowledge, but also the applied skills, to manage the situation in a successful and safe manner. Preparedness is key, and the best way to be prepared is to practice CRM in all situations. Working through CRM must become a habit that is a fully embedded natural part of your normal practices.

CRM may offer a multitude of benefits relevant to healthcare. Benefits include, but are not limited to, the following:

- Efficient team interactions, with less time required to orient all team members.
- Adaptive team interactions with clearer and more accurate communication, even through extreme and evolving circumstances.
- Reduction in the frequency of partial information, increasing the quality of communication, individual performance, and team performance.
- Effective conflict resolution.
- Reduction in both potential and actual error rates.
- Fewer risks and liability.
- Reduced operating costs due to a high performing workplace.
- Increased personal satisfaction and job satisfaction.
- Improved safety by limiting the psychological impacts of causing harm.
- Established resilience.

CRM must be adopted at the individual, team, and organizational levels to be effective. Teams are comprised of individuals with a common goal, and teams operate within broader complex organizational structures. Many factors influence individual behaviors, and a breakdown in team performance can dramatically impact the outcome of a situation. Research has demonstrated that CRM training in healthcare has positive impacts on reducing the number of adverse events and errors while improving training participants' knowledge and performance behaviors (O'Connor, O'Dea, & Keogh 2013). For example, O'Connor and colleagues (2013) completed a meta-analysis on CRM training in healthcare and found that all of the included fourteen studies resulted in significant reductions both in the number of errors as well as the time needed to complete clinical tasks. CRM training may be considered costly; however, given the reported reductions in adverse events and their related costs, economic benefits have been demonstrated (Moffatt-Bruce, Hefner, Mekhijian 2017).

Summary Box 1.2
Why CRM is Important to Healthcare

- You and your team will behave in a manner that ensures that you are continually competent, and responsible for, achieving a safe and successful outcome.
- Adopting CRM in your daily practice will avoid creating a problem in the first place.
- If a problem does occur, you and your team will be equipped with the knowledge and skills to manage the situation in a successful and safe manner.

1.3 How our CRM Model Fits with the Reality of Delivering Consistently Safe Healthcare

The CRM model that we present for adoption in healthcare are modified versions of the TeamSTEPPS and Team Dimensional Training CRM models (Smith-Jentsch 1998). These models were selected for their ease of understanding, transferability to healthcare settings, and the overall benefits to healthcare.

What characteristics of our CRM model make it effective in healthcare?

- Our CRM model is evidence-based and/or grounded in science: there must be evidence that the skills improve safety. Further, the basis of the CRM model presented in this guide is well researched, validated, and used by many national organizations, including the U.S. Navy, NASA, Agency for Healthcare Research and Quality (AHRQ), and several regionally-based firefighting and healthcare organizations.
- Our CRM model is valid: a valid CRM model in healthcare must specify behaviors and best practices used in that profession. Skills must be articulated to match the actual tasks, culture, and terminology of the profession in which they are used.
- Our CRM model has a high level of usability: the specific core skills must be easy to recall and apply. The CRM model must be

able to be employed by team members without constant reference to documentation.

- Our CRM model is focused on team interactions: Exchanging Information refers to the team interactions when a team member needs to determine what information to pass to whom and when. Communicating involves the team determining how they will interact to exchange that information. Leading and Following pertain specifically to sustaining efforts to obtain all the information that the leaders need to make good decisions. Mutually Supporting concerns how team members interact to proactively prevent or mitigate errors.
- The core skills in our CRM model are discernible by observable behaviors: a team member can provide feedback utilizing actual acts or verbal examples of behaviors. This prevents ambiguous feedback based on subjective impressions or personal conclusions.

By contrast, any CRM model for healthcare cannot be any of the following…

- a process: defining a sequence of steps (e.g., first develop situation awareness, then communicate situation awareness, then …). Rather, all CRM skills must be done continuously and must be fully integrated with technical skills for all tasks. All core team skills, both technical and CRM, must therefore be integrated and performed simultaneously for a functional and effective team.
- a tool: the CRM model we will present contains tools such as Stop-Think-Act-Review (STAR), briefings, and debriefings, among others. Tools are critical in doing good CRM, but tools themselves are not CRM skills.
- individual skills that do not require interaction with another individual (e.g., time management and personal stress management): CRM is about fluid and dynamic interactions between team members. If a skill can be performed alone, then this is not CRM.
- unobservable characteristics (e.g., attitudes): if no categorized observable behavior occurs, it is not CRM. While an appropriate attitude is critical to the success of doing good CRM, it is only one of the motivating reasons to practice the good behaviors that comprise CRM skills.
- pre-existing conditions: any condition that exists before a team interaction is a pre-existing condition. Examples include whether

an organization's CRM training is strong or weak, or whether CRM is or is not embedded into policies and procedures. The team needs to be aware that a pre-existing condition might enable CRM or disable CRM. They can take advantage of an enabler--and work through a disabler--using core CRM skills.

- another skill or competency that may be enabled by CRM (e.g., adaptability, decision-making, or mission-planning). By nature, all competencies are interrelated, but the main reason for adopting the core skills is to provide you and your team with the fundamental team skills to enable you to be adaptable, make appropriate decisions, and plan accordingly, even when members of a team are unfamiliar with each other.

Summary Box 1.3
How our CRM Model Fits with the Reality of Delivering Consistently Safe Healthcare

Our CRM model…
• is evidence-based and/or grounded in science.
• specifies behaviors and best practices valid for healthcare.
• focuses of team skills usable by healthcare teams.
• focuses on observable behaviors applicable to healthcare teams.

Let us start looking at each skill in more detail, starting with examining how Exchanging Information helps teams have the situation awareness they need to be safe and effective.

Chapter Debriefing

I want to call a quick STAR (Stop-Think-Act-Review): get off your email, stop your side conversations, and turn off the television. [4] Let's see if you can expand upon these statements:

Our version of Crew Resource Management (CRM) is:

- a way of managing and optimizing team interactions, to improve performance, and positively impact safety.
- based on observable behaviors.

[4] See Chapters 11-15 for information on STAR.

- includes
  - Exchanging Information: determining what information to exchange with whom and when.
  - Communicating: how to exchange information.
  - Leading and Following:
    - Leading is setting up psychological safety, articulating CRM expectations and then modeling and rewarding those behaviors.
    - Following is inquiring when they do not understand the leader or the situation, and then advocating and even asserting a position when they believe that safety is at risk.
  - Mutually Supporting: offering and accepting physical, cognitive, psychological, and emotional support as well as providing feedback on both technical and non-technical behaviors.

CRM is important to healthcare because:

- you and your team will behave in a way that ensures that you are continually competent and responsible for achieving a safe and successful outcome.
- adopting CRM will avoid creating a problem in the first place.
- in the event that a problem does occur, you and your team will be equipped with the knowledge and skills to manage the situation in a successful and safe manner.

Our model:

- is evidence-based and/or grounded in science.
- specifies behaviors and best practices valid for healthcare.
- focuses of team skills usable by healthcare teams.
- focuses on observable behaviors applicable to healthcare teams.

If this was an actual debriefing, we would ask you to expand further on each of these statements. Depending on your response, we would ask open-ended follow-up questions until we were sure you understood the material and had a plan to implement one or more best practices. We might ask, "Why has CRM not been adopted by your organization?" We would not be satisfied if you said, "We have too many people who resist using CRM." Again, we would ask open-ended follow-up questions until you might say,

"We have a problem with team members who believe that CRM is not applicable to their organization." We would then ask, "What can you do to fix that problem on your next shift?" You might say, "I can start introducing CRM to my team in my briefing, showing them how CRM helps them be safer and more effective. I can also discuss CRM in the debriefing to show them how CRM helped us avoid an error." We would then ask, "That helps convince your team, but what about the organization?" We would then continue to ask open-ended follow-up questions until you might say, "We need to develop a briefing to give to every member of our organization so that each team member knows what CRM is, why CRM is important to healthcare and how to apply our model."

The following chapters will describe how our CRM model can be applied, and how you can empower your team members to adopt CRM into their daily practice.

References

Austin, Matt, and Jordan Derk. "Lives Lost, Lives Saved: An Updated Comparative Analysis of Avoidable Deaths at Hospitals Graded by the Leapfrog Group." Armstrong Institute for Patient Safety and Quality, Johns Hopkins Medicine, 2019. https://www.hospitalsafetygrade.org/media/file/Lives-Saved-White-Paper-FINAL.pdf.

de Vries, Eefje N., Maya A. Ramrattan, Susanne M. Smorenburg, Dirk J. Gouma, and Marja A. Boermeester. "The Incidence and Nature of In-Hospital Adverse Events: A Systematic Review." Quality & Safety in Health Care. U.S. National Library of Medicine. Accessed October 30, 2021. https://pubmed.ncbi.nlm.nih.gov/18519629/.

Moffatt-Bruce, Susan D., Jennifer L. Hefner, Hagop Mekhjian, John S. McAlearney, Tina Latimer, Chris Ellison, and Ann Scheck McAlearney. "What Is the Return on Investment for Implementation of a Crew Resource Management Program at an Academic Medical Center?" American Journal of Medical Quality 32, no. 1 (2016): 5–11. https://doi.org/10.1177/1062860615608938.

O'Connor, Paul, Angela O'Dea, and Ivan Keogh. "Is Crew Resource Management Training Effective in Healthcare Settings?" Proceedings of the International Symposium on Human Factors and Ergonomics in Health Care 2, no. 1 (June 2012): 105–7. https://doi.org/10.1177/2327857913021020.

Scott, Susan D., Laura E. Hirschinger, Karen R. Cox, Myra McCoig, Julie Brandt, and Leslie W Hall. "The Natural History of Recovery for the Healthcare Provider 'Second Victim' after Adverse Patient Events." Quality and Safety in Health Care 18, no. 5 (2009): 325–30. https://doi.org/10.1136/qshc.2009.032870.

McPherson, James A., Rhonda L. Zeisig, and Kimberley A. Smith-Jentsch. "Team Dimensional Training: A Strategy for Guided Team Self-Correction." Essay. In Making Decisions Under Stress: Implications for Individual and Team Training, edited by Janis A. Cannon-Bowers and Eduardo Salas, 271–96. Washington, D.C.: American Psychological Association, 1998.

"Online Resource - Resources for Pilots." FAA. Accessed October 30, 2021. https://preprod.faasafety.gov/gslac/onlineresources.aspx?categoryId=27&masterId=1.

Part 1.

Crew Resource Management Skills

PART 1A.

EXCHANGING INFORMATION

Briefing[5]

I want to call a quick STAR (Stop-Think-Act-Review): that means, get off your email, stop your side conversations, and turn off the television.[6] Here is what we will do in the next six chapters: we will discuss how team members build their situation awareness and mental models, and then use the CRM skill of Exchanging Information to ensure that everyone has situation awareness and mental models despite team, organizational and environmental barriers. We will be successful if you can describe:

- what situation awareness is and how you can develop it (Chapter 2);
- how team members use the CRM skill called Exchanging Information to ensure everyone has situation awareness and mental models (Chapter 3);
- what information to exchange during handovers (Chapter 4);
- various Situation Awareness and Exchanging Information Demons (Chapter 5);
- Situation Awareness and Exchanging Information best practices (Chapter 6); and
- how a leader improves situation awareness through mental models (Chapter 7).

---

[5] We will use the chapter briefing format throughout the book. You may feel the repeated use is redundant. However, we believe that it is important to continue to emphasize that a good briefing builds mental models by discussing what is happening, what success looks like, and what threats or errors are possible and how you plan to prevent, avoid, or mitigate them. Hence, the repetitive nature is meant to cement this belief with an understanding that you will also immerse yourself in this book on an irregular and/or intermittent basis. For more information on briefings and how this briefing embeds CRM concepts, see Section 14.2.

[6] For more information on STAR, see Chapters 11-15.

The primary threat that you might experience is the introduction of a large number of concepts and terms, some of which you may have never encountered, and some of which you may think about in a different sense. We will therefore explicitly define and differentiate each term and concept. We also realize how busy you are. We will make sure that the chapter is short enough to be read in approximately thirty minutes. Finally, we provide Summary Boxes. The Summary Boxes serve two functions. First, they emphasize the take-home points in each section, and you can use them to check your understanding of those take-home points. Second, you can use them to determine if you and your team are implementing those take-home points. If a Summary Box does not make sense to you or you do not understand one or more take-home points, then review the related material before continuing to the next section.

Did I miss anything? Any concerns? Any questions? (Pause) No? Then, let's get started.

Let us start with a scenario that will show good (effective) and bad (ineffective) examples of the Exchanging Information skill.[7] We will use this scenario as we discuss Exchanging Information further, in Chapters 2-7.

Abbreviations

COPD	Chronic Obstructive Pulmonary Disease
CXR	Chest X-Ray
DOC	Physician
ED	Emergency Department
ICU	Intensive Care Unit
MVA	Multiple Vehicle Accident
NUR	Nurse
PEEP	Positive End-Expiratory Pressure
PIP	Peak Inspiratory Pressure

[7] Here, we need to differentiate between the CRM skills of Exchanging Information and Communicating. Every team member must realize that he or she has information that other team members need, or other team members have information that he or she needs. Exchanging Information requires each team member to figure out what specific information each team member needs or has. Exchanging Information is about the what, who and when. Communicating is the process of passing information, or, about the how. Both Exchanging Information and Communicating have their own threats and errors, as well as best practices.

RT	Respiratory Therapist
TBI	Traumatic Brain Injury

Personnel Involved in Scenario

Emergency Department: ED DOC #1, ED DOC #2, ED NUR, ED charge nurse

Intensive Care Unit: ICU charge nurse, ICU DOC #1, ICU DOC #2, ICU NUR #1, ICU NUR #2, ICU NUR #3, ICU NUR #4, RT #1, RT #2

It has been a busy shift in the emergency department (ED) of the community hospital which is exemplified by the arrival of motor vehicle accident (MVA) victims. Cardiopulmonary resuscitation (CPR) is ongoing in one trauma room while, in another, an intubation is being performed because one of the victims has developed severe traumatic brain injury (TBI). ED DOC #1 just finished the intubation on Mrs. Smith. Although coming to the end of the shift, ED DOC #1 has some time to see another patient. Mr. Lopez is a 52-year-old male with chronic obstructive pulmonary disease (COPD), diabetes and hypertension who came to the ED because of difficulty breathing for the past 2 days. ED DOC #1 picks up Mr. Lopez's chart, quickly reviews it, and then goes to see him. By the end of this interaction, ED DOC #1's shift has ended, and ED DOC#2 has come to replace ED DOC #1, so they perform a handoff.

> ED DOC #1: "Mrs. Smith is a 35-year-old female who was intubated after an MVA for severe TBI. She has a bed ready in the ICU, and I will transport her myself before I leave. Next is Mr. Lopez, a 52-year-old male who presented to the ED for respiratory distress. He reported a 2-day history of shortness of breath and productive cough. Overall, he looked good when I saw him, but he was mildly hypoxemic, so I placed him on 2 liters of oxygen via nasal cannula and ordered a chest x-ray (CXR) and blood gas that you will need to follow up on. Any questions?"
>
> ED DOC #2: "Do you think the cause of his respiratory symptoms could be due to an infectious process? Were antibiotics started?"
>
> ED DOC #1: "I am not sure, possibly. I didn't ask about fever, rhinorrhea, or recent sick contacts. I was waiting for the CXR to be done before starting antibiotics."[8]

[8] Rhinorrhea= runny nose.

ED DOC #2: "Okay, thanks. I'll transfer Mrs. Smith to the ICU for you. Go get some rest. You've had an eventful shift."

ED DOC #1: "I sure did. Thanks."

After the handoff, ED DOC#2 goes to examine Mr. Lopez and then speaks with his nurse.

ED DOC #2 (to ED NUR): "I just saw Mr. Lopez, and he doesn't look good. His CXR and blood gas look fine, but he is laboring to breathe, as he could not complete a full sentence. He is also breathing fast and has a rapid heart rate. Upon speaking further with his wife, I discovered he has diabetes, hypertension, and COPD for which he is on chronic medications. The COPD history is of particular significance to his current presenting symptoms. We need to start non-invasive ventilation (NIV) as soon as possible, but we should prepare for intubation in case he doesn't improve with NIV. Can you call the Respiratory Therapist (RT)? I'll notify the ED charge nurse to arrange for an ICU bed."

ED NUR: "Yes, of course. The nurse from the previous shift mentioned that he was worried about Mr. Lopez but there was so much going on after the MVA, that he didn't have a chance to tell ER DOC #1."

ED DOC #2: "Oh, really? ER DOC #1 told me he looked fine."

ED NUR: "Hmm…not sure where the disconnect was. After you speak with the ED charge nurse, let me know what medications you would like in case intubation is needed."

ED DOC #2: "Okay."

Meanwhile, it is a usual morning in the Intensive Care Unit (ICU). The physician team is conducting patient care rounds, consulting teams are also seeing patients, and bedside nurses and RTs are doing their routine daily assessments.

The ICU charge nurse hangs up the phone and then speaks with the physician team, which just finished rounding.

ICU charge nurse (to ICU DOC #1 and ICU NUR #1): "A 52-year-old male with COPD, diabetes and hypertension who presented to the ED for respiratory distress is coming and will either be on non-invasive ventilation or be intubated. The ED team is in the process of figuring it out."

ICU DOC #1 (to ICU charge nurse): "Okay, thanks." (to physician team): "Let's tend to our other patients and tasks in order to free ourselves up should this patient arrive and require our immediate attention."

An hour later, the ED team arrives in the ICU, where they are met by the ICU physicians, nurses, and RTs. The patient is on non-invasive ventilation. The ED and ICU RTs transition the patient to the ICU set up and perform their individual handoffs. The ED and bedside nurses conduct a handoff, as other nurses help the patient transition to his ICU bed and place him on monitors. ED DOC #2 and the ICU DOC #1 also handoff during this process.

ER DOC #2: "Mr. Lopez is a 52-year-old male who presented to the ED for respiratory distress. He reported a 2-day history of shortness of breath and productive cough. Mr. Lopez has a history of COPD, diabetes, and hypertension. When I examined him, Mr. Lopez was laboring to breathe, as he could not complete a full sentence, and had a rapid heart rate and breathing rate. I think Mr. Lopez is having a COPD exacerbation and I was concerned that he may need intubation. His oxygen saturation, CXR, and blood gas were reassuring so we tried non-invasive ventilation which seemed to alleviate his symptoms. Any questions?"

ICU DOC #1: "Do you think he could have a concurrent infection that is causing an exacerbation of his COPD?"

ER DOC#2: "I had a similar thought and started antibiotics although he did not report fever, rhinorrhea, or recent sick contacts. However, we did not send for any additional diagnostic studies or cultures."

ICU DOC#1: "Okay, thanks."

Shortly after the ICU and ED team leave the bedside, Mr. Lopez's wife tells the ICU Nurse #1 that he is very sleepy, which is a sudden change. The nurse tries to arouse Mr. Lopez, but he only responds by moaning.

ICU NUR #1 (dials ICU DOC#1 on the phone): "Doctor, I am calling about Mr. Lopez in Bed 905. His wife informed me that he was suddenly very sleepy and, when I went to assess him, he would only moan when I tried to arouse him. Can you come to the bedside to check him out?"

ICU DOC #1 (to ICU NUR #1): "Sure, my colleague and I will be right over."

ICU DOC #1 arrives with ICU DOC #2, examines Mr. Lopez, and notes that he is sleepy, and that his breathing is shallow. During the exam, ICU DOC #1 also notices that his heart rate has gradually increased to 120 beats per minute (bpm) from 80 bpm, and his oxygen saturation has also drifted to 80%.

ICU DOC #1 (to ICU NUR #1): "Prepare to intubate!"

ICU NUR #1 hits the code button, and several nurses, RTs and physicians arrive.

ICU DOC #1 (to ICU DOC #2): "Go ahead and intubate."

Hearing this, the rest of the team prepares for intubation. The intubation is performed and, immediately after, the oxygen saturation and heart rate normalize briefly, and then gradually decline, from 100% to 70% and 100 bpm to 50 bpm, respectively.

ICU DOC #1 (to no one in particular): "What's his blood pressure? Does he have a pulse?"

The nurse (ICU NUR #2) nearest the monitor checks for the blood pressure and 2 other nurses (ICU NUR#3 and #4), on opposite sides of the bed, check for a pulse.

ICU NUR #2: "Blood pressure is 130 over 75."

ICU NUR #3: "He has a femoral pulse."

ICU NUR #4: "He has a femoral pulse."

ICU DOC #1 (to ICU DOC #2): "Are we in?"

ICU DOC #2: "I think so, I saw the tube go through the cords."

ICU DOC #1 (to RT #1): "What PIP are we bagging with? And what is our PEEP valve set at?"

RT #1 (to ICU DOC #1): "PIP of 20 cm H20 and PEEP valve is set at 5 cm H20."

ICU DOC#1 (to RT#1): "Bag to a PIP of 30 cm H20 and increase the PEEP to 10 cm H20."

RT #1 (to no one in particular): "Can someone listen for breath sounds? The tube may not be in."

ICU DOC #2 (to RT #1 and ICU DOC #1): "I saw the tube go through the cords, there's mist in the tube, and there is color change in the end-tidal CO2 detector."

ICU DOC #1 (at the foot of the bed to ICU DOC#2): "Also looks like symmetrical chest rise from here."

ICU DOC #2 (at the head of the bed to ICU DOC#1): "Actually, I see asymmetrical chest rise from here. I think we may be in the right mainstem bronchus."

RT #2 (auscultating): "I hear good breath sounds on the right and diminished breath sounds on the left."

ICU DOC #1 (to ICU DOC#2): "I think you're right! This is a right mainstem intubation."
(to RT#1) "Pull back on his tube."
(to RT#2) "Auscultate and let us know when you hear equal breath sounds on both the right and left sides."
(to RT #1) "At which point, you can stop pulling back and then secure the tube in place."

RT #1 (to ICU DOC #1): "Okay, will do."
(to ICU NUR #2): "Can you take over bagging?"

ICU NUR #2 (to RT#1): "Yes, I'll take over."

The endotracheal tube was successfully repositioned, and Mr. Lopez's oxygen saturation and heart rate normalized. Routine post-intubation care ensued. This brought the team to the end of their shift, so they handed off to their respective counterparts and headed home.

CHAPTER 2

DEFINING SITUATION AWARENESS

Chapter Briefing[9]

I want to call a quick STAR (Stop-Think-Act-Review): get off your email, stop your side conversations, and turn off the television.[10] In this chapter we will discuss situation awareness. We will be successful if you can:

- define situation awareness (Section 2.1);
- explain problems in developing situation awareness and how to remedy them (Section 2.2);
- explain the role of mental models in developing situation awareness (Section 2.3); and
- explain how the mnemonic tool known as STEP helps you get Total Situation Awareness (Section 2.4).

The primary threat that you might experience is the introduction of a large number of concepts and terms, some of which you may have never encountered, and some of which you may think about in a different sense. We will therefore explicitly define and differentiate each term and concept. We also realize how busy you are. We will make sure that the chapter is short enough to be read in approximately thirty minutes. Finally, we provide Summary Boxes. The Summary Boxes serve two functions. First, they emphasize the take-home points in each section, and you can use them to check your understanding of those take-home points. Second, you can use

---

[9] By now, you may feel that repeated use of the chapter briefing format is redundant. However, we believe that it is important to continue to emphasize that a good briefing builds mental models by discussing what is happening, what success looks like, and what threats or errors are possible and how you plan to prevent, avoid, or mitigate them. Hence, the repetitive nature is meant to cement this belief with an understanding that you will also immerse yourself in this book on an irregular and/or intermittent basis.

[10] For more information on STAR, see Chapters 11-15.

them to determine if you and your team are implementing those take-home points. If a Summary Box does not make sense to you or you do not understand one or more take-home points, then review the related material before continuing to the next section.

Did I miss anything? Any concerns? Any questions? (Pause) No? Then, let's get started.

List of Abbreviations

COPD	Chronic Obstructive Pulmonary Disease
CRM	Crew Resource Management
DOC	Physician
ED	Emergency Department
ICU	Intensive Care Unit
NASA	National Aeronautics and Space Administration
RT	Respiratory Therapist
STEP	Status-Team-Environment-Progress
TeamSTEPPS	Team Strategies and Tools to Enhance Performance and Patient Safety

The first skill in our Crew Resource Management (CRM) model is Exchanging Information, or passing the right information to the right person at the right time. How will you know what is the right information? Who is the right person? What is the right time? Your situation awareness will give you all those answers. In this chapter, you will learn what situation awareness is (Section 2.1), and what you must do to get and keep it despite adverse organizational, cultural, and environmental conditions (Section 2.2). We will introduce the concept of mental models and the role they play in developing situation awareness (Section 2.3), as well as a mnemonic tool, called STEP, to help you have all the elements of situation awareness (Section 2.4).

2.1 Definition of Situation Awareness

The most cited definition of situation awareness is "the perception of the elements in the environment within a volume of time and space, comprehension of their meaning and the projection of their status in the near future." (Endsley 1997, 207)

Fig. 2-1
Levels of Situation Awareness

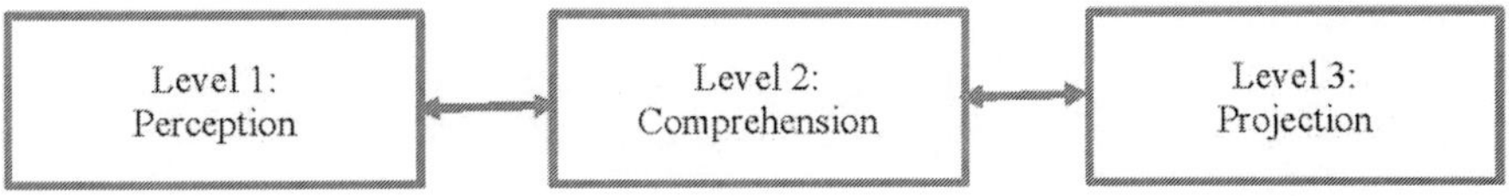

Situation awareness is built by someone perceiving what is happening (i.e., seeing, hearing, feeling, tasting, or touching the environment). We will define that as Level 1 Situation Awareness (or Perception). An individual uses Level 1 Situation Awareness as inputs to determine the significance of what is happening, what it means now and in the near future. We will define that as Level 2 Situation Awareness (Comprehension) and Level 3 Situation Awareness (Projection). An example of good (but not Total) situation awareness occurs when the physician in the preceding scenario (ICU DOC #1) observes that the patient was lethargic, breathing shallowly, and had increased heart rate and declining oxygen saturation (Level 1 Situation Awareness). ICU DOC #1 knew that meant that the patient was in severe respiratory distress (Level 2 Situation Awareness), and his condition would continue to deteriorate without an intubation (Level 3 Situation Awareness).[11] An example of bad Level 1 Situation Awareness was exhibited by ED DOC #1 by not checking for other symptoms (e.g., rhinorrhea and fever) to get enough information to develop Level 2 Situation Awareness.

According to TeamSTEPPS, to gain situation awareness, you need to monitor the situation.[12] Situation monitoring is "the process of continually scanning and assessing what is going on around you to maintain situation awareness" (TeamSTEPPS Pocket Guide 2013, 20). Linking their definition of situation monitoring to our definition of situation awareness, "scanning" is perceiving, and "assessing" is comprehending and projecting. By monitoring the situation, each team member is trying to determine what is happening, and what it means now and in the near future. In this context, situation awareness is the product of situation monitoring.

---

[11] See Section 2.4 for more information on Total Situation Awareness.

[12] TeamSTEPPS®, or Team Strategies and Tools to Enhance Performance and Patient Safety, is a teamwork system developed jointly by the Department of Defense (DoD) and the Agency for Healthcare Research and Quality (AHRQ) to improve institutional collaboration and communication relating to patient safety.

Summary Box 2.1
The Three Levels of Situation Awareness

Do your team members develop situation awareness by perceiving what is going on (Level 1 Situation Awareness), comprehending its significance (Level 2 Situation Awareness), and projecting its effect into the future (Level 3 Situation Awareness)?

2.2 Problems Developing Situation Awareness (and Remedies)

Dissecting the three levels of situation awareness, Level 1 Situation Awareness/Perception is all about keeping your eyes and ears open. What could be easier? Unfortunately, 76% of errors in situation awareness are Level 1 errors. (Endsley and Jones 1996) Why would people not see what they are supposed to see, or not hear what they are supposed to hear? Someone might not perceive something because it is too dark or too loud, or those involved are stressed, busy, or distracted. Pertinent examples of this from the preceding scenario include an ED that is stressed from working a difficult shift; an ED physician who was too distracted to read the patient chart in enough detail to detect important pre-existing conditions (i.e., COPD, diabetes, and hypertension); and an ED nurse who was too busy to inform the ED physician of the patient's worsening condition. Other reasons why someone might not see or hear something include use of a display that does not portray important patient information in a user-friendly format, or inadequate training that fails to prepare a healthcare professional to accurately perceive key information. Errors in Level 2/Comprehension and Level 3/Projection make up 20% and 4% of the situation awareness errors, respectively. (Endsley and Jones 1996) Why would people not understand the significance of what is happening and how it will affect the future? The main causes of these errors are similar to Level 1 where stress, workload, distractions, interruptions, and multitasking do not allow the time or cognitive resources to comprehend or project. It is also possible that those involved were never trained and had no experience in how to comprehend or project, or that the effect of training waned over time.

Some of the factors that limit an individual's ability to have situation awareness are outside the control of the individual, even a leader, during his or her shift and the team just has to deal with them.[13] Examples of this include poorly designed displays or lack of appropriate training. The factors that a leader can manage are stress, workload, distractions, interruptions, and multitasking. What should you as a leader do when you know that an individual is too overwhelmed to have the luxury of perceiving, comprehending, or projecting? The number one way you can improve an individual's ability to have situation awareness is to give the team member the time, confidence, and ideas of where and what to perceive, comprehend, and project. Reducing their workload, distractions, interruptions, and multitasking; removing or delaying tasks; or assigning additional personnel are strategies for giving a person the time. For example, in our scenario, workload was handled by dividing up tasks between two physicians, four nurses, and two respiratory therapists. Reducing stress is a strategy to increase a team member's confidence. For example, the briefing could mention, "We may be very busy, possibly handling a new patient in respiratory distress. But we can tend to our other patients and prep the room and equipment ahead of time. That will give us the time and resources to handle that new patient." The task or shift briefing is another tool to help team members know what information to look for and where, and what that information means now and what it will mean in the future.[14] You can also use tools such as procedures, displays, algorithms, and even pen-and-paper notes to augment your situation awareness.

Summary Box 2.2
How to Deal with Problems Developing Situation Awareness

Do you and your team members develop all levels of situation awareness by…

- controlling workload, distractions, interruptions, and multitasking?
- using tools (e.g., hardware, software, documentation, etc.) to assist you?
- dealing with lack of training or experience by briefing where and what to perceive and what it means?

---

[13] In this context, "leader" is defined as anyone who steps up to address team issues. When we are referring to the formal designated leader, we will use the term "team leader".

[14] For more information on briefings, go to Chapter 14.2

2.3 Mental Models Turn Level 1 Situation Awareness Into Levels 2 and 3 Situation Awareness

To properly understand how Level 1 Situation Awareness (Perception) gets turned into Level 2 (Comprehension) and Level 3 (Projection), you have to understand mental models. A mental model is how you believe something works (Forrester 1971). The Emergency Department (ED) physician has a mental model regarding how a patient should react to a non-invasive ventilation. The Intensive Care Unit (ICU) physician has a mental model related to how a patient should react to a successful intubation. How is a mental model linked to situation awareness? A mental model is like a recipe. Where a recipe turns raw ingredients into a rich meal, a mental model allows you to turn your raw perceptions into rich comprehension and projections. In other words, what you see, hear, and so forth as part of Level 1 Situation Awareness are inputs into your mental model, and the outputs are your comprehension of the present significance (Level 2 Situation Awareness) and a projection into the future (Level 3 Situation Awareness).

Fig. 2-2
How Mental Models Turn Perception Into Comprehension and Projection

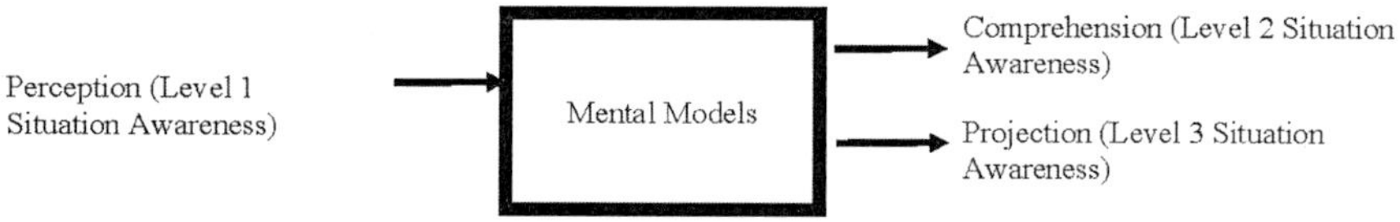

The more complete and accurate your mental model, the better your comprehension and projection. If you predict that something bad might happen, then your mental model will help you decide what things to look for to determine if something bad is happening. So, in Figure 2-2 above, a more detailed illustration would include feedback loops from Comprehension and Projection, back to Perception. The best mental models will also include what to perceive to determine whether your projection is correct or incorrect. Hearing during the handover that the patient was on non-invasive ventilation, the physician expected to see fairly normal breathing, heart rates, and oxygen saturation. When the physician saw that the patient was lethargic, heart rate of 120, and oxygen saturation was 80%, the physician knew the ventilation was inadequate. This interplay between projection and subsequent perception functions as a feedback loop, allowing continuous refinement of situation awareness during rapidly evolving circumstances.

The good news is that with more knowledge and more diverse experience, the more complete your mental model will become. Your mental model is constantly changing. As you learn and experience more, your mental model should improve. The bad news is that no matter how much knowledge and experience you have, everyone has holes or gaps in their mental model when dealing with complex systems (e.g., a human being) in complex situations (e.g., a premature birth). We will discuss how teams help overcome gaps in your situation awareness and mental models in Chapter 3.

2.4 STEP and Mental Models

A person activates several mental models at a time. The number and type of mental models are fluid between professions, organizations, teams, and even tasks (Druskat and Pescosolido 2002). To determine what mental models a team member must have, we are going to use a modified form of a TeamSTEPPS mnemonic, called STEP (some readers may already be familiar with it). [15] STEP stands for Status, Team, Environment and Progress. Each letter represents one or more mental models required to have Total Situation Awareness, or having situation awareness in all the necessary areas.

2.4.1 S = Status Mental Models

S stands for Status. In healthcare, Status includes the Patient and the Tasks to be performed on behalf of the patient. [16] Besides knowing the normal oxygen saturation of a 52-year-old male, you also need to know how an intubation should affect that saturation. You also need to know how your task might affect what other team members are doing (e.g., does your task affect or is affected by what other team members are doing)? You need to know what threats might affect your task, such as the potential for a mainstem intubation. You also need to know that today you are working with the *X* even though you are used to working with a *Y* (e.g., use of a curved versus straight laryngoscope blade or an incandescent versus

---

[15] TeamSTEPPS®, or Team Strategies and Tools to Enhance Performance and Patient Safety, is a teamwork system developed jointly by the Department of Defense and the Agency for Healthcare Research and Quality to improve institutional collaboration and communication relating to patient safety.

[16] Another way to look at the first part of Status is as an operand, or what your team is operating on. For NASA teams, it would be the spacecraft; for drillers, the formation; for firefighters, the fire.

fiberoptic laryngoscope light bulb). How do the differences between these two devices affect your task?

2.4.2 T = Team Mental Models

T stands for Team, which includes Teamwork and Team Members. Teamwork is how you expect the team to operate. This is where many teams come up short, as different team members may have different thoughts on how they should work with each other. If you have ever heard "I assumed you were…" or, much worse, "It didn't look right, but I…", then you have teamwork issues. This is where CRM proves useful because CRM is a Teamwork Mental Model.

Team Members refers to more than just who is or could be on your team. It is also about their roles and responsibilities (who is doing what), knowledge and skills (who knows and can do what), strengths and weaknesses (who can help or needs help), goals (who wants what), and ability to work as a team (who is good or bad in a team environment).[17] You know that Jody is one of the nurses, but have you worked with Jody before, or does your organization have strong Standard Operating Procedures? If the answer is "no" to both questions, you will need to talk to Jody to make sure that you both understand what you need from Jody and what Jody needs from you. You also need to know if Jody is inexperienced, or highly experienced, but until recently worked at another hospital. Either of those conditions might affect how you interact with Jody. You also need to know what errors other teams have made, how they have handled past threats, and, if you are having trouble, who can help you as well as who you can help, and how. Finally, who is on your team changes with the situation. You may have to call upon people with additional knowledge, skills, or experiences outside the core team when an unusual situation arises.

2.4.3 E = Environment Mental Models

E stands for Environment, or the context or conditions in which you are undertaking a task. It could be your organization's philosophies, policies, procedures, and practices, or that you are operating in an unfamiliar setting.

[17]What is the goal of patient safety: is it doing no harm, healing, curing, or crafting a dignified end of life for a patient? Each expert may have a different opinion on what success is, but even if they agree on that, they may disagree on why, or how to achieve it. You will need Situation Awareness on what patient care standards each team member intends to apply for this situation.

Environment also includes its own set of threats and errors. Bad timing is a common example of an environmental threat. You cannot control when an ambulance arrives from a motor vehicle accident, but you will nevertheless have to respond. Weather is another environmental threat. You can discuss the threats with your team with as little as "Snow and freezing ice are predicted tonight. We should expect more motor vehicle accidents." You also should discuss the most likely errors. Examples might be, "I know we are in a stressful situation working multiple accidents. What I am most worried about is …"

Finally, Environment includes the past: past illnesses, past medication, past healthcare decisions, past family decisions, and so forth. In the scenario, the past covers a patient with diabetes, hypertension, and COPD, for which he is on chronic medications. All of these affect how your team will work today.

2.4.4 P = Progress Mental Models

P stands for Progress, or progress toward a shared and valued goal. [18] It is both your progress and the progress of everyone else who affects you and is affected by you. Think of it as progress against your schedule. If you are having problems with your task and behind schedule, who do you need to tell? To understand progress, you also have to understand time-to-effect, or how long before something needs to be done or something bad happens (also called the "no kidding, drop-dead, deadline"). Did the ED team decide that if the oxygen saturation did not respond to non-invasive ventilation within *X* minutes, they would do an intubation? How long has it been since you started ventilation? Who is monitoring that time? Keeping track of time can be especially difficult when working under time pressure, or when fixated on a task. For example, a patient died when physicians spent too much time trying to intubate after losing track of how long the patient was without oxygen (McClelland and Smith 2016). To remedy this type of failure, NASA flight controllers explicitly define time-to-effect (e.g., a system will fail in 45 minutes [relative time] or at 0923 [absolute time]) and have a countdown clock displayed on a large screen in the front of the Mission Control Center, where everyone can see the countdown to the deadline. [19]

---

[18] "Shared" means that everyone is working to the same goal. "Valued" means everyone is willing to put forth a maximum effort to accomplish it.

[19] Absolute time is a better time reference. With relative time, you must remember relative to what: 45 minutes from when?

Closely related to time-to-effect is margin, or how far is a critical data parameter from reaching a point at which you must go to a contingency plan? In the case of the intubation, if the oxygen level reached 80%, regardless of time, you would need to do something else. How close are you to 80%? Who is monitoring that parameter?

You can use your briefing to make sure each team member will activate the right mental models for Status, Team, Environment and Progress.[20] One of the authors of this book hands out index cards that ensure the team activates the right Status-Patient, Status-Task and Team Mental Models.[21] In your briefing, you can also explain what your team should see or hear, what each perception means now, and project what it is likely to mean in the future. For example, if the ICU physician had known that the ED physician had not checked for fever, rhinorrhea, or recent sick contacts, the ICU physician could have briefed, "If we see fever, rhinorrhea, or learn about recent sick contacts, we will assume ... and we will do .... If we don't, we will assume ... and we will do ..."

---

[20] See Section 14.2 for more information on how briefings improve mental models. See Chapter 7.2.1 for more information on how to activate the right mental models.
[21] See Appendix C for more information on the index card.

Table 2-1
Type of Mental Models using Status-Team-Environment-Progress (STEP)

Type of mental model	Description of mental model/how you believe	Example of mental model
Status: Patient and Task	Patient: how the human body works: physiology and anatomy, and how various conditions (e.g., pregnancy, trauma, disease, etc.) affect it. Task: how interventions affect the patient and how they affect other tasks, and vice versa. Includes how to use hardware, software, execute procedures, and manage threats.	Patient: What are normal breathing, heart rate, and oxygen saturation levels for a 52-year-old male? What could go wrong (threats)? What are the indications of each threat? Task: What are the indications of a successful intubation? How do your tasks during an intubation impact the nurses' tasks? How do the nurses' tasks impact your delivery of intubation? What threats exist to the effective use of intubation?
Team: Teamwork and Team Members	Teamwork: how to work as a team. CRM is a Teamwork Mental Model. Team Members: how the roles and responsibilities, knowledge and skills, and strengths and weaknesses of each team member will affect the team, and who else you can include and what they bring.	Teamwork: the why, what, how and when to exchange information, communicate, lead and follow, and mutually support. Team members: The roles and responsibilities, knowledge and skills, and strengths and weaknesses of the physicians, nurses and respiratory therapists on your team.

Environment	This is the context of the situation: How the time, place, organizational philosophies, policies, procedures and practices, and any previous conditions, actions or decisions might affect you and your team.	How do the other patients impact your ability to treat the 52-year-old patient? How does the fact that this is the first or last hour of your shift impact you? What are your hospital's policies and procedures on how to handle this situation? What medication did the patient take earlier?
Progress: Schedule, Time-to-effect and Margin	Schedule: The extent to which you and your colleagues are accomplishing your tasks. Time-to-effect: How much time can elapse before you see whether your efforts are successful or not. Margin: How much can a critical data parameter increase or decrease before you must go to a contingency plan?	Schedule: What task is the team supposed to be working on now? Are all previously scheduled tasks done? Time-to-effect: How long can you wait to see if intubation is working before you go to Plan B? Who is keeping track of time? Margin: If blood oxygen level reaches 80%, regardless of time, you must intubate. Who is keeping track of the oxygen level?

Summary Box 2.3
Mental Models and Status-Team-Environment-Progress (STEP)

Do your team members… • have the mental models to turn Level 1 (Perception) into Level 2 (Comprehension) and Level 3 (Projection)? • have multiple mental models: Status (Patient and Task), Team (Teamwork and Team Members), Environment and Progress (Schedule, Time-to-Effect and Margin)? • use the briefing to help develop mental models?

Now you can take all your Level 1 Situation Awareness (Perception)--what you are seeing and hearing--and input them into your STEP mental models to get Total Situation Awareness. There are two requirements to getting Total Situation Awareness. First, having Total Situation Awareness requires you to have situation awareness in all the areas that you affect and that affect you[22]. Second, you must integrate the situation awareness from all the areas. For example, the attending physician needs to know that a patient might require an intubation (Status), but also that the resident may be fatigued (Team) due to the organization policy that residents work for three nights (Environment) and might miss tracking how long the patient has been at low oxygen saturations (Progress). Total Situation Awareness is the "Big Picture", assuming the Big Picture is an integration of all the elements of STEP. Some instances of Total Situation Awareness are unique (i.e., only one team member sees or knows some information, therefore that team member is responsible to pass on that information). Some instances of Total Situation Awareness are common (i.e., other team members should be seeing and knowing it too, but each team member is responsible for checking to see that other team members do have that information).

Here is another example.[23]

- You see that a ventilated patient is showing a marked increase in respiratory rate (Level 1 Situation Awareness). Your Patient Mental Model says that increase in respiratory rate might indicate an increased level of pain (Level 2 Situation Awareness) that will

[22] Total Situation Awareness can also be thought of Systems Thinking or Holistic Thinking. STEP is the mnemonic to remind you what you must consider to be Systems or Holistic Thinking.
[23] Modified from an example used in TeamSTEPPS.

increase with time if left untreated (Level 3 Situation Awareness. Only you have that information (i.e., unique situation awareness), therefore you are responsible to pass on this information.

- You read that it has been three hours since the last pain medication (Level 1 Situation Awareness). Your Schedule Mental Model says that the patient should have been given medication within the last 15 minutes (Level 2 Situation Awareness). Others should know about the medication schedule (i.e., common situation awareness), therefore you are responsible for passing on the information only if it seems a team member does not know this information.
- You see a nurse is busy helping another patient (Level 1 Situation Awareness). Your Team Member Mental Model says that she is the patient's nurse (Level 2 Situation Awareness) and will be too busy to give the medication (Level 3 Situation Awareness). Only you have that information (i.e., unique situation awareness), therefore you are responsible to pass on this information to possibly another nurse.
- You hear other people talking in your vicinity (Level 1 Situation Awareness). Your Schedule Mental Model tells you that a shift change is occurring, and you can tell the on-coming nurse to give the medication (Level 2 Situation Awareness). Others should know about the shift schedule (i.e., common situation awareness), therefore you are responsible for passing on the information only if it seems a team member does not know this information.

If you have this level of awareness in all of the areas that you affect and those that affect you, then you have Total Situation Awareness.

Summary Box 2.4
Total Situation Awareness

Do your team members have Total Situation Awareness? Does each team member know…

- the status of the patient, and how his or her tasks are affecting the patient as well as the other team members?
- the roles, strengths, and weaknesses of each team member, who knows what, and who can do what?
- how the environment is affecting the team?
- how they are progressing against the schedule, times-to-effect, and margin?

Without Total Situation Awareness, you are missing crucial knowledge.

Now, you need to get your Total Situation Awareness out of your head and into the heads of the members of your team. Which parts of your Total Situation Awareness need to be imparted? To whom? When?[24] In other words, team members need to exchange information to ensure every team member has situation awareness and mental models. All of these details will be covered in the next chapter.

Chapter Debriefing

I want to call a quick STAR (Stop-Think-Act-Review): get off your email, stop your side conversations, and turn off the television.[25] Let's see if you can expand upon these statements:

- Situation awareness requires that you perceive what is happening around you, and to comprehend and project its significance.
- Build situation awareness by controlling workload and distractions.
- Help your team members build their situation awareness via an effective briefing.
- Mental models are required to turn Perception into Comprehension and Projection.
- Mental models must include the Status, Team, Environment and Progress (STEP).
- CRM is a Team/Teamwork Mental Model.
- To have Total Situation Awareness, you need to integrate all the areas of situation awareness (Status, Team, Environment and Progress), and all Levels (Perception, Comprehension and Projection).

If this was an actual debriefing, we would ask you to expand further on each of these statements. Depending on your response, we would ask open-ended follow-up questions until we were sure you understood the material and had a plan to implement one or more best practices. We might ask, "What is a specific situation awareness problem that you experience on your job?" We would not be satisfied if you said, "My situation awareness isn't as good as I need it to be." Again, we would ask open-ended follow-up questions until you might say, "I have a problem with getting and keeping the Big Picture." We would then ask, "Why do you miss parts of the Big Picture?" We would then continue to ask open-ended follow-up questions

[24] "How" to exchange information will be covered in the Communicating chapter, Chapter 8.
[25] See Chapters 11-15 for information on STAR.

until you might say, "I need to consider all of the STEP elements." We would then ask, "How are you going to do that?" We would continue doing this until you came up with a concrete action you could take to improve your Total Situation Awareness. We might even ask, "That helps you, but what can you do to help others in your organization get the Big Picture". Again, more open-ended questions until you say, "I can work with management to change our training to specifically address STEP."

References

Druskat, Vanessa Urch, and Anthony T. Pescosolido. "The Content of Effective Teamwork Mental Models in Self-Managing Teams: Ownership, Learning and Heedful Interrelating." Human Relations 55, no. 3 (2002): 283–314. https://doi.org/10.1177/0018726702553001.

Endsley, Mica. "The Role of Situation Awareness in Naturalistic Decision Making." Essay. In Naturalistic Decision Making, 269–83. New York, NY: Psychology Press, 1997.

Forrester, Jay. "Counterintuitive Behavior of Social Systems." Technology Review 73, no. 3 (January 1971): 52-68.

Endsley, Mica, and Debra Jones. "Sources of Situation Awareness Errors in Aviation." Aviation, Space and Environmental Medicine 67, no. 6 (June 1995): 507-512.

McClelland, Guy, and Matthew Smith. "Just a Routine Operation: A Critical Discussion." Journal of Perioperative Practice 26, no. 5 (2016): 114–17. https://doi.org/10.1177/175045891602600504.

TeamSTEPPS: Pocket Guide: Strategies & Tools to Enhance Performance and Patient Safety. Bethesda, MD: U.S. Dept. of Health and Human Services, Agency for Healthcare Research and Quality, 2006.

CHAPTER 3

EXCHANGING INFORMATION TO ENSURE SITUATION AWARENESS AND MENTAL MODELS

Chapter Briefing[26]

I want to call a quick STAR (Stop-Think-Act-Review): that means, get off your email, stop your side conversations, and turn off the television.[27] In this chapter, we will discuss how team members use the CRM skill called Exchanging Information to ensure every team member has Total Situation Awareness and STEP Mental Models. We will be successful if you can:

- explain how Exchanging Information ensures that every team member has Total Situation Awareness and STEP Mental Models (Section 3.1);
- explain how team members determine what information to exchange (Section 3.2);
- explain why Exchanging Information requires more than just pushing and pulling information (Section 3.3); and
- explain what you should do if your situation awareness or mental model does not match the situation awareness or mental model of your team members (Section 3.4).

---

[26] By now, you may feel that repeated use of the chapter briefing format is redundant. However, we believe that it is important to continue to emphasize that a good briefing builds mental models by discussing what is happening, what success looks like, and what threats or errors are possible and how you plan to prevent, avoid or mitigate them. Hence, the repetitive nature is meant to cement this belief with an understanding that you will also immerse yourself in this book on an irregular and/or intermittent basis.

[27] For more information on STAR, see Chapters 11-15.

The primary threat that you might experience is the introduction of a large number of concepts and terms, some of which you may have never encountered, and some of which you may think about in a different sense. We will therefore explicitly define and differentiate each term and concept. We also realize how busy you are. We will make sure that the chapter is short enough to be read in approximately thirty minutes. Finally, we provide Summary Boxes. The Summary Boxes serve two functions. First, they emphasize the take-home points in each section, and you can use them to check your understanding of those take-home points. Second, you can use them to determine if you and your team are implementing those take-home points. If a Summary Box does not make sense to you or you do not understand one or more take-home points, then review the related material before continuing to the next section.

Did I miss anything? Any concerns? Any questions? (Pause) No? Then, let's get started.

List of Abbreviations

CRM	Crew Resource Management
DOC	Physician
ED	Emergency Department
ICU	Intensive Care Unit
NUR	Nurse
PEEP	Positive End-Expiratory Pressure
PIP	Peak Inspiratory Pressure
STEP	Status-Team-Environment-Progress

The goal of CRM is a team that is safe and effective, but how does CRM achieve that? To accomplish that goal, every team member must have the Total Situation Awareness and STEP Mental Models required to meet his or her responsibilities. In this chapter, you will learn more about how Exchanging Information ensures every team member has Total Situation Awareness and STEP Mental Models (Section 3.1), how team members work together to exchange information (Section 3.2), why Exchanging Information is more than the simple addition of the situation awareness of all team members (Section 3.3), and what your responsibility is if your situation awareness does not match the situation awareness or mental models of your team members (Section 3.4).

3.1 Exchanging Information Ensures Every Team Member has Total Situation Awareness and STEP Mental Models

Simply put, making your team safe and effective requires that every team member has the STEP Mental Models to turn their perceptions into the Total Situation Awareness needed to meet his or her responsibilities. But in today's sophisticated healthcare system and, during complex situations, no one person can see or hear everything (Level 1 Situation Awareness) without help from other team members. Also, no one person can have all the knowledge and experience (complete and accurate mental models) to comprehend and project significance (Levels 2 and 3 Situation Awareness) to achieve Total Situation Awareness without help. Another way to put it is that the nurse sees and knows something that the physician needs, and vice versa. Every team member has information that needs to be exchanged. Only together can every team member have Total Situation Awareness and STEP Mental Models. The team members' Total Situation Awareness and STEP Mental Models, however, are not the same, because their tasks, roles, and responsibilities are different. The Total Situation Awareness and STEP Mental Models of every team member must, however, complement each other for the team to achieve its goals.[28] For example, the ED physician will have a different situation awareness and mental models than will the ED nurse. Although the nurse saw that the patient was experiencing respiratory distress, the nurse's mental model did not tell her that the distress was significant enough to override her tasks with the patients from the motor vehicle accident and tell the physician about her concerns. If the physician had heard that information, the physician's mental model would have led to comprehension that the level of respiratory distress requires a more aggressive intervention. The situation awareness and mental model of the ED physician and nurse must complement each other for both to have their required Total Situation Awareness and STEP Mental Models.

[28] See Section 7.1.2 for more information on complementary situation awareness and mental models.

Summary Box 3.1
Exchanging Information Builds Total Situation Awareness and STEP Mental Models

> Do your team members realize that…
> - for a team to be safe and effective, every team member must have Total Situation Awareness and STEP Mental Models?
> - they must exchange information that others need to have Total Situation Awareness and STEP Mental Models?
> - although each team member has different Total Situation Awareness and STEP Mental Models, they must complement each other?

3.2 The CRM Skill of Exchanging Information

Since you know that you have information that others need to build their Total Situation Awareness and STEP Mental Models, you could just broadcast all your knowledge and hope each team member figures out what portions he or she needs. Or you could recognize that you have knowledge, different parts of which must be passed up to your leader, down to your team, and, horizontally, to other teams. Determining the right information to the right person at the right time is the CRM skill of Exchanging Information.

To define Exchanging Information, we started with Team Dimensional Training's definition of Information Exchange:

> "Information exchange involves pushing and pulling information to and from the right people at the right time. Specifically, crew members are expected to fully utilize all possible sources of information, to pass information proactively to others, and to integrate information to provide teammates with situational updates." (Smith-Jentsch 2015, 17)

Our definition of Exchanging Information modifies Team Dimensional Training's definition to: Exchanging Information involves pushing and pulling the right information to and from the right people, at the right time, to integrate information and therefore to allow everyone to have Total Situation Awareness and STEP Mental Models.

The first part of that definition of Exchanging Information requires determining the right information, the right people, and the right time. To do that, each team member must use his or her STEP Mental Models: Patient and Task Mental Models determine the right information, Team Member

Mental Model determines the right person, and Progress Mental Model determines the right time.

Because the ED physician knew what tasks needed to be done for the patient (Patient and Task Mental Models), and by whom (Team Member Mental Model), the physician knew that he had information that had to be passed to the ED nurses, and other information that needed to be passed to the ICU team. The physician used those same mental models to determine what information was needed from the nurses. The physician's Progress Mental Model determined when to pass that information. Unfortunately, in our example, the physician's Status Mental Model was incomplete when, due to workload, he could not get information on fever, rhinorrhea or recent sick contacts.

Your first part of Exchanging Information is complete when you give the required information to all the team members who need it from you, and all the team members give you the information that you need. The team's first part of Exchanging Information is complete when every team member exchanges his or her information. What information to pass to whom and when can change, either due to a different situation or as a specific situation evolves. A good briefing by the leader can help the team anticipate those changes and react appropriately.

Summary Box 3.2
The First Part of Exchanging Information is Exchanging the Right Information with the Right Team Member(s) at the Right Time

> Do your team members use their Total Situation Awareness (i.e., situation awareness in all areas of Status-Team-Environment-Progress [STEP]) to determine who needs what information and when, and who has information they need?
> If every team member exchanges (gives and gets) the right information to/from the right person at the right time, the team has accomplished the first part of Exchanging Information.

3.3 Exchanging Information Requires More Than Just Pushing and Pulling Information

The goal of Exchanging Information is to give everyone the information they need to build Total Situation Awareness and STEP Mental Models. That goal cannot be achieved by the simple addition of information exchanged between team members. The second portion of our definition of Exchanging Information requires the integration of the information. The integration of the situation awareness and mental models of all team members achieves Total Situation Awareness and STEP Mental Models that are more comprehensive than the initial situation awareness and mental models of each individual team member (Stanton, Stewart, Harris, Houghton, Barber, et al 2006). Another way to say that is everyone exchanges information based on their current Total Situation Awareness and STEP Mental Models, but the result of that integration is improved Total Situation Awareness and STEP Mental Models. To illustrate, think of the story of the six blindfolded team members.[29] Imagine a few days later as part of continuation training, the ED and ICU teams are blindfolded, taken to a place and asked what they perceived and what it meant. The ED physician feels something pointed (Level 1 Situation Awareness). He determines that it is a spear (Level 2 Situation Awareness: what to exchange). He determines everyone (who) needs to know that it is a spear, and they need to know it now (when). He believes that he has the Total Situation Awareness and the mental model he needs. He says, "I felt a spear."

The other five team members say,

"I felt a snake."
"I felt a wall."
"I felt a tree."
"I felt a fan."
"I felt a rope."

If they only add the situation awareness of the six individuals, they all felt six different things, except the instructor then tells them that they all felt parts of the same thing. The ED physician now knows that his mental model may be incorrect: pointed might not mean a spear. The other five team members realize that their mental models may also be incorrect. The six

[29] https://en.wikipedia.org/wiki/Blind_men_and_an_elephant

people need to figure out a mental model where spear, snake, wall, tree, fan and rope all make sense simultaneously. They start brainstorming possibilities, none of which covers everything, until one ICU nurse says “elephant?”. With that new mental model, spear = tusk, snake = trunk, wall = body, tree = leg, fan = ear and rope = tail. The team went to the zoo and felt an elephant.

What should you derive from that story?

1. Simply passing the right information to the right team member at the right time might not give you complete Total Situation Awareness (what is happening) or STEP Mental Model (why and how it is happening). It requires integration.
2. Integration can result in emergent knowledge: something that no one individual could know on one’s own but results from the integration of everyone’s situation awareness and mental model (i.e., it is an elephant).
3. Integration will also provide context to the situation awareness of each individual (i.e., the spear is really a tusk).
4. Integration may improve each team member’s situation awareness or mental models. Suppose the “fan” that the ICU physician felt was only a foot or so across. She thinks that an elephant’s ear would be bigger than that. The ED nurse says that an African elephant’s ears are bigger than that, but an Asian elephant’s ears are smaller, so a foot or so would be right for an Asian elephant. The ICU physician’s mental model on elephants and their ears is now more complete.
5. A team, and specifically a leader, should ensure that integration is achieved.[30] A leader should be forcing the team to ensure that they are not missing something or coming to the wrong conclusion. A nurse might ask: “Did anyone smell anything? Did anyone hear anything? Was anything moving?” Everyone shakes their heads. Someone suggests an elephant replica on exhibit. Another nurse asks if anyone has any information that would challenge that conclusion. Everyone shakes their heads. Until further information causes them to review it, they conclude that they went to the Asia exhibit at the Museum of Natural Science.

[30] By “leader”, we mean the situational leader, or whomever steps up to ensure everyone has situation awareness and mental models.

The intubation scenario provides another example. Each physician, nurse, and respiratory therapist had information that, by itself, was insufficient to determine if the intubation was successful or not. Integrating their information allows them to determine whether intubation was successful.

Summary Box 3.3
The Second Portion of Exchanging Information is Integration

If done properly, the integration yields… • emergent knowledge; • context; and • improved Total Situation Awareness and STEP Mental Models. It is every team member's responsibility to ensure integration.

There are two important things to note: firstly, no single individual will have The Situation Awareness or The Mental Model. The team leader, however, may have the broadest, but not necessarily the deepest, situation awareness and mental model since the team leader usually has the most interactions with the most team members. The team leader has a responsibility to pass on knowledge of goals, changes in situation, changes in roles and responsibilities, and so forth, to the team members so that they can modify their situation awareness and mental models accordingly. Those modified situation awareness and mental models may change what is the right information, the right team member, or the right time. Everyone has the responsibility to be a situational leader to make sure that all team members have the Total Situation Awareness and STEP Mental Models needed to fulfil their responsibilities. Secondly, and hopefully this is not a surprise, CRM is a tool to build every team member's Total Situation Awareness and STEP Mental Models.

One more important aspect about integrating situation awareness and mental models--since integration is much different and more difficult to do than simply adding them--is that integration requires the "Power of And", which is another way of saying, how might your situation awareness or mental model be correct, And the situation awareness or mental model of a team member be correct too?[31] Is your team member's different situation awareness or mental model related to a gap or error in your situation

[31] See the discussion on Active Listening in Section 8.5 for a needed tool to integrate situation awareness and mental models.

awareness or mental model, or is he or she considering something entirely new to the team? The quality of your Total Situation Awareness and STEP Mental Models might be determined by how you treat the "dumb question" from the newest member of your team, or "that is not what I am seeing…" by the person from another organization, or "that is not what I think will happen…" by the person who does not understand how you operate. Do you ignore, or do you integrate? You may be unwittingly dismissing information that you need to achieve better Total Situation Awareness and STEP Mental Models. The "Power of And" should result in broader, deeper and more refined situation awareness and mental models than the initial situation awareness or mental models of the team members and should more completely explain what all team members think is happening, how, and why.

3.4 What Do You Do When Your Situation Awareness or Mental Model Does Not Match The Rest of the Team?

What do you do if you think what you are seeing or doing does not match what others are seeing or doing (i.e., your perceptions or tasks are incongruous with the perceptions or tasks of others)? A team must find ways to make sure that every team member's situation awareness and mental models adequately represent the situation. In our example, the Intensive Care Unit (ICU) physician announced the decision to change the PIP and PEEP, which allowed the nurses to decide if their situation awareness or mental model agreed with that assessment and decision. If they disagree, then team members must discuss any differences until they figure out who or what is incorrect. The physician also announced that she was not sure that the intubation was successful. This prompted the other members of the team to check their situation awareness and mental models, to confirm or refute a successful intubation.

Let us look at the dialog in the scenario:

ICU DOC #1: "Is it (the intubation tube) in?"

ICU DOC #2: "I think so, I saw the tube go through the (vocal) cords."

ICU DOC #1: "Can someone auscultate (listen for sounds using a stethoscope)? I am not sure that the tube is in."

> ICU DOC #2: “The tube went through the cords. Plus, we have color change on the end tidal detector and mist in the tube.”
>
> ICU DOC #1: “Also looks like symmetrical chest rise from here.”
>
> ICU DOC #2: “Actually, I see asymmetrical chest rise from here. I think we are mainstemmed.”
>
> RT #2: “I hear good breath sounds on the right and diminished breath sounds on the left.”

This dialog shows that ICU DOC #1 is initially concerned whether the intubation tube is properly inserted when oxygen saturation and heart rate do not stay within normal ranges. ICU DOC #2 sounds unsure about the intubation when she uses the verbal caveat “I think so…” but has confirming information that it is inserted properly: past the vocal cords, color change on the detector and mist in the tube. Then ICU DOC #1 sees another confirming cue: symmetric chest rise. In too many cases, their analysis would stop there, at least until the situation worsens significantly, and forces them to reexamine. In an extreme example of fighting Confirmation and Expectation biases, ICU DOC #2 went against her own situation awareness to recognize asymmetrical chest rise. She then used that new Level 1 Situation Awareness and her mental model to realize that there is a mainstem intubation, confirmed by the respiratory therapist. Too bad all of us are not as willing to challenge our situation awareness as ICU DOC#2.

One responsibility of every team member is to speak up if his or her situation awareness or mental model does not seem to match the situation awareness or mental model of other team members. ICU DOC #2 saw signs of asymmetric chest rise that did not match the situation awareness of other team members of a successful intubation. She was required to speak up until this difference between her situation awareness and the situation awareness of the other team members were resolved.

Summary Box 3.4
If Your Situation Awareness Does Not Match the Situation Awareness of Others, Inquire

Does your team…
- find ways to compare situation awareness and mental models?
- feel comfortable asking questions if there is a difference between an individual's situation awareness or mental models and the situation awareness or mental models of the rest of the team?
- figure out why there is a difference, and if required, use the "Power of And" to achieve a broader, deeper and more refined Total Situation Awareness and STEP Mental Models?

Now that your team has exchanged information to build the Total Situation Awareness and STEP Mental Models of your team members, how do you exchange information to build the Total Situation Awareness and STEP Mental Models of the members of the next team? This is covered in the next chapter.

Chapter Debriefing

I want to call a quick STAR (Stop-Think-Act-Review): get off your email, stop your side conversations, and turn off the television. Let's see if you can expand upon these statements:

- For a team to be safe and effective, everyone must have Total Situation Awareness and STEP Mental Models. But everyone has information that someone else needs, or needs information from someone else, to improve their Total Situation Awareness and STEP Mental Models (i.e., they must exchange information).
- The improved Total Situation Awareness and STEP Mental Models result in emergent knowledge and context.
- Exchanging Information requires everyone to have complementary Task, Team and Progress Situation Awareness/Mental Models. Complementary Task Situation Awareness/Mental Models refer to how your task affects and is affected by other tasks and determines what information must be exchanged. Similarly, complementary Team Situation Awareness/Mental Models refer to who needs to exchange with whom, and complementary Progress Situation Awareness/Mental Models determine when to exchange information.

- The improved Total Situation Awareness requires integration and the "Power of And".
- Everyone has a responsibility to inquire if their situation awareness or mental model does not match the situation awareness or mental models of other team members.

If this was an actual debriefing, we would ask you to expand further on each of these statements. Depending on your response, we would ask open-ended follow-up questions until we were sure you understood the material and had a plan to implement one or more best practices. We might ask, "What is a specific situation awareness problem that your team experiences on the job?" We would not be satisfied if you said, "The situation awareness of our team members isn't as good as we need." Again, we would ask open-ended follow-up questions until you might say, "We have a problem with team members not having the information they need." We would then ask, "What can you do to fix that problem on your next shift?" You might say, "I can discuss who needs what information in the briefing, provide immediate feedback during the shift if a team member is not passing the right information in the right format, and debrief any Exchanging Information problems." We might then ask, "That helps your team. What can you do to help other teams?" We would then continue to ask open-ended follow-up questions until you might say, "We need to modify our briefing guide to discuss who needs what information when."

References

Endsley, Mica R. "Toward a Theory of Situation Awareness in Dynamic Systems." Human Factors: The Journal of the Human Factors and Ergonomics Society 37, no. 1 (1995): 32–64. https://doi.org/10.1518/001872095779049543.

Smith-Jentsch, Kimberley. "On Shifting from Autonomous to Interdependent Work." NASA Johnson Space Center, February 2014. https://www.researchgate.net/publication/292783480_On_Shifting_from_Autonomous_to_Interdependent_Work. NASA/TM-2015-218563

Stanton, N. A., R. Stewart, D. Harris, R. J. Houghton, C. Baber, R. McMaster, P. Salmon, et al. "Distributed Situation Awareness in Dynamic Systems: Theoretical Development and Application of an Ergonomics Methodology." Ergonomics 49, no. 12-13 (2006): 1288–1311. https://doi.org/10.1080/00140130600612762.

CHAPTER 4

EXCHANGING INFORMATION DURING HANDOVERS

Chapter Briefing[32]

I want to call a quick STAR (Stop-Think-Act-Review): that means, get off your email, stop your side conversations, and turn off the television.[33] In this chapter we will discuss how to hand over your Total Situation Awareness and STEP Mental Models. We will be successful if you can:

- define Exchanging Information during a handover (Section 4.1);
- explain the information required for a good handover (Section 4.2); and
- explain how the NASA example ensures a check of integration and quality (Section 4.3).

The primary threat that you might experience is the introduction of a large number of concepts and terms, some of which you may have never encountered, and some of which you may think about in a different sense. We will therefore explicitly define and differentiate each term and concept. We also realize how busy you are. We will make sure that the chapter is short enough to be read in approximately thirty minutes. Finally, we provide Summary Boxes. The Summary Boxes serve two functions. First, they emphasize the take-home points in each section, and you can use them to check your understanding of those take-home points. Second, you can use

[32]By now, you may feel that repeated use of the chapter briefing format is redundant. However, we believe that it is important to continue to emphasize that a good briefing builds mental models by discussing what is happening, what success looks like, and what threats or errors are possible and how you plan to prevent, avoid or mitigate them. Hence, the repetitive nature is meant to cement this belief with an understanding that you will also immerse yourself in this book on an irregular and/or intermittent basis.

[33] For more information on STAR, see Chapters 11-15.

them to determine if you and your team are implementing those take-home points. If a Summary Box does not make sense to you or you do not understand one or more take-home points, then review the related material before continuing to the next section.

Did I miss anything? Any concerns? Any questions? (Pause) No? Then, let's get started.

List of Abbreviations

COPD	Chronic Obstructive Pulmonary Disease
CRM	Crew Resource Management
CXR	Chest X-ray
DOC	Physician
ED	Emergency Department
ICU	Intensive Care Unit
NASA	National Aeronautics and Space Administration
SBAR	Situation-Background-Assessment-Recommendation
STEP	Status-Team-Environment-Progress
TeamSTEPPS	Team Strategies and Tools to Enhance Performance and Patient Safety

Even if all of your team members have Total Situation Awareness and STEP Mental Models, you may eventually need to pass that situation awareness and mental models to a new team (e.g., the next shift). Research shows that if a new team is going to make an error due to poor situation awareness, it is most likely to happen in the first 1-2 hours when the team is still trying to fully build their own situation awareness (Endsley 2006). A good handover can lessen that period of vulnerability by properly and fully passing your situation awareness and mental models to the incoming team. In this chapter, you will learn what is a good handover (Section 4.1), and what goes in a good handover (Section 4.2). We will provide an example of how one team ensures a good handover (Section 4.3).

4.1 Definition of Exchanging Information During a Handover

Exchanging Information during a handover is defined as passing on the facts, the context, and the mental model for all areas, while also ensuring integration and quality. Facts, context, and mental models in all areas are the correct content of Exchanging Information.[34]

In too many industries and professions, a handover consists of data (facts) such as the temperature is *X*, the pressure is *Y*, we are on Step 3, and so on, or, in the scenario: the ED physician stated that the patient reported a 2-day history of shortness of breath and productive cough. We consider this a handover of Level 1 Situation Awareness, or a handover of information that could be gleaned as easily by looking at the patient, displays, or logs. Such a handover helps the incoming team know the present state of the patient, but does not provide, support, or allow a comparison of Level 2 (Comprehension) and Level 3 (Projection Situation Awareness), and the mental model. Such a handover is too shallow, and consequently not a good handover.

Other handovers provide enough information to offer a comparison of Level 2 and 3 Situation Awareness but only at the patient level. One format to pass all situation awareness levels is SBAR, or Situation-Background-Assessment-Recommendation, where S is Level 1 Situation Awareness (facts), B is context, A supports and allows comparison of Levels 2 and 3 Situation Awareness, and R supports and encourages the comparison of mental models. The problem with those handovers is the handover is only at the patient level or only the Status in STEP. In our scenario, the handover between the ED physician and the Intensive Care Unit (ICU) physician did not cover all areas of STEP, such as the previous team was very busy (Team) dealing with a motor vehicle accident with multiple patients (Environment) at the end of their shift (Progress). Therefore, their handover was too narrow, and thus inadequate.

---

[34] The right person is the person to whom you are handing over. The right time is during the handover, hopefully during a lull in the action where both people have the cognitive resources to perform 3-way communication and active listening (see Section 8.4).

4.2 What Is a Good Handover?

A good handover should include all levels (Perception, Comprehension and Projection) and all areas (Status, Team, Environment and Progress) of situation awareness. The goal of a handover is to not only pass along all needed information but also to provide the incoming team an opportunity to check their situation awareness and mental models against those of the off-going team.

Some organizations have developed approved formats to assist team members to remember what information to include in a handover. Do not confuse the format that SBAR recommends with the content that SBAR requires. [35] Emphasizing the format without fully understanding what information is required, and why, can be counterproductive. It can lead to a fill-in-the-blank mentality that is procedurally correct, but it does not transfer situation awareness. SBAR, a list of required information, allows the next shift a chance to see if their situation awareness and mental models matches yours. Besides SBAR, there are other formats that provide all areas and all levels of situation awareness and allow for situation awareness and mental model comparison. NASA's International Space Station flight controllers use F-I-W, or Failure, Impact and Workaround. [36] Another TeamSTEPPS format is I PASS the BATON, or Introductions, Patient, Assessment, Situation, Safety, Background, Actions, Timing, Ownership and Next.[37] Again, we are not advocating a specific format. We are simply emphasizing that whatever format you use, make sure that it reminds you to include all areas and levels of situation awareness and provides an opportunity to compare situation awareness and mental models between teams.

Let us see if we can improve the handover in our scenario between the ED Physician (ED DOC #2) and the ICU Physician (ICU DOC #1). Here is their actual handover:

---

[35] Here, we are addressing what must be included in a handover, but not specifying a format. Formats will be discussed more thoroughly in Section 8.3.

[36] Failure is Level 1 Situation Awareness or what are the indications of a problem. Impact is Level 2 and 3 Situation Awareness on what the problem is and how it will affect the International Space Station. Workaround is the mental model on how the team will resolve the problem.

[37] I, P, A, S, S and B handover all levels of Situation Awareness, and A, T, O and N handover the mental model.

> ED DOC #2: “ Mr. Lopez is a 52-year-old male who presented to the ED for respiratory distress. He reported a 2-day history of shortness of breath and productive cough. When I examined him, Mr. Lopez exhibited dyspnea, as he could not complete a full sentence, along with tachycardia and tachypnea. Mr. Lopez has a history of diabetes and hypertension. We think Mr. Lopez is having a COPD exacerbation and were concerned that he may need intubation. His oxygen saturation, CXR and blood gas were reassuring so we tried non-invasive ventilation which seemed to alleviate his symptoms. Any questions?”
>
> ICU DOC #1: “Do you think he could have a concurrent infection that is the cause for his exacerbation?”
>
> ICU DOC #2: “I thought the same, but don’t think so, since he did not report fever, rhinorrhea, or recent sick contacts. However, we did not send any diagnostic studies.”
>
> ICU DOC #1:“ OK, thanks.”

How well did this handover cover all areas of STEP and all levels of situation awareness? Concerning Status of the Patient, the handover covered Level 1 Situation Awareness (dyspnea, tachycardia and tachypnea), Level 2 Situation Awareness (COPD exacerbation) and Level 3 Situation Awareness (may require intubation). Concerning Status of the Task, the handover covered the status of the ventilation and the lack of diagnosis studies. So, was it a pretty good handover of Status? There was one possibly very significant error.

> ICU DOC #1: “Do you think he could have a concurrent infection that is the cause for his exacerbation?”
>
> ICU DOC #2: “I thought the same, but don’t think so, since he did not report fever, rhinorrhea, or recent sick contacts. However, we did not send any diagnostic studies.”

Who is the “he” to whom the ED physician is referring? The ICU physician probably believes the “he” is the patient: the patient said he had no fever, runny nose, or contact with any sick people. In reality the “he” is the previous shift’s ED physician, who was too busy to ask those questions. The failure to mention all STEP areas in the handover gave the ICU physician an incomplete picture of whether fever, rhinorrhea or sick contacts were possible. Would stating that the ED team was also very busy (Team) with a motor vehicle accident with multiple patients (Environment) at the end of their shift (Progress) have prompted the ICU physician to examine the patient earlier and more completely?

4.3 An Example of Best Practices in Handovers

NASA's Space Shuttle and International Space Station flight controllers have developed a team handover best practice to not only ensure a complete handover of situation awareness and mental models, but also to ensure integration and quality of situation awareness and mental models of the on-coming team. (Park and Kanki 2008) Recall that integration is the final step in Exchanging Information. Do not concentrate on the specifics of a Mission Control Center handover, since their conditions and requirements are different than yours. Just pay attention to their effort to ensure an integrated and quality handover of situation awareness and mental models.

Each on-coming person (officer) gets a handover from the off-going officer (e.g., the on-coming electrical power officer gets a handover of the status of the electrical power system). This would be equivalent to the ED nurses handing over to the ICU nurses. Meanwhile, the on-coming team leader also gets a handover from the off-going team leader, equivalent to the ED physician handing over to the ICU physician.

Fig. 4-1
Off-going Personnel Handover Their Situation Awareness and Mental Models to Their On-coming Counterparts and Any Differences Are Resolved

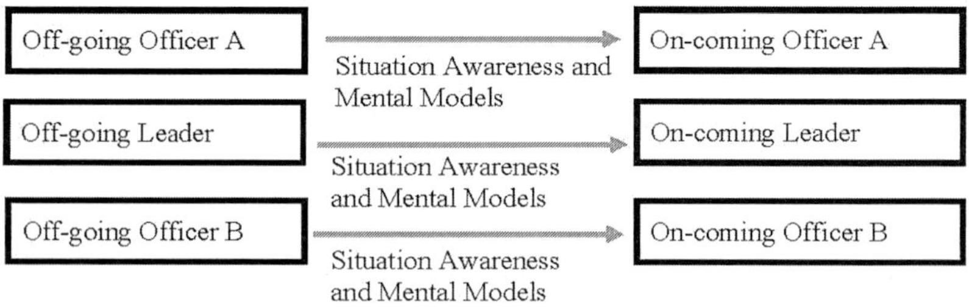

The on-coming officers then have two additional handover responsibilities.

1. Integration of Status and Team Mental Models - all team members should agree on what tasks to undertake during the upcoming shift and why and how each team member interacts with the other team members.

Fig. 4-2
Officers Ensure They Understand How Their Tasks Affect and Are Affected By the Tasks of Others

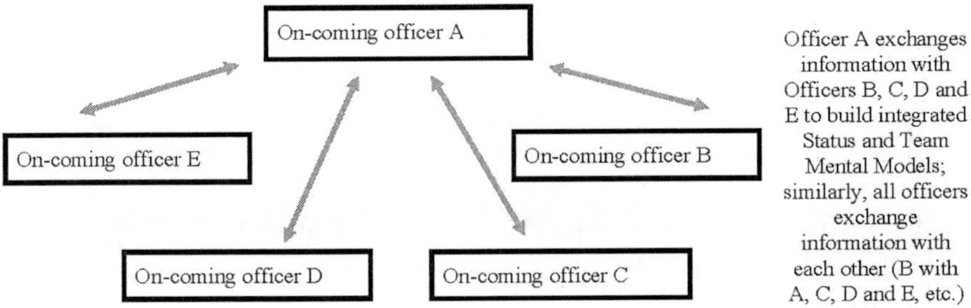

Officer A will tell the other officers that he or she plans to do Task *X*, how that task might affect them, and what help or information is needed. Each officer will tell Officer A what he or she needs to support Task *X*. The other officers will then do the same for their planned tasks. The desired result of these interactions is integration of Task Mental Models—the team members all agree on what should happen and how they need to interact.

2. Integration of the threat and error mental models, or, what in High Reliability Organization theory is called "Preoccupation with Failure" (Christianson, Sutcliffe, Miller, and Iwashyna 2011), or in NASA-speak, "worst case scenario."

As part of the integration of the Task Mental Models, the team discusses what is the worst possible thing that could happen at the worst time, and how they would recognize it. The result of this discussion is the integration of Threat and Error mental models; the team members all agree on what bad things might happen, and what they might look like.

Fig. 4-3
Officers Ensure They Understand How Their Threats and Errors Affect and Are Affected By the Threats and Errors of Others

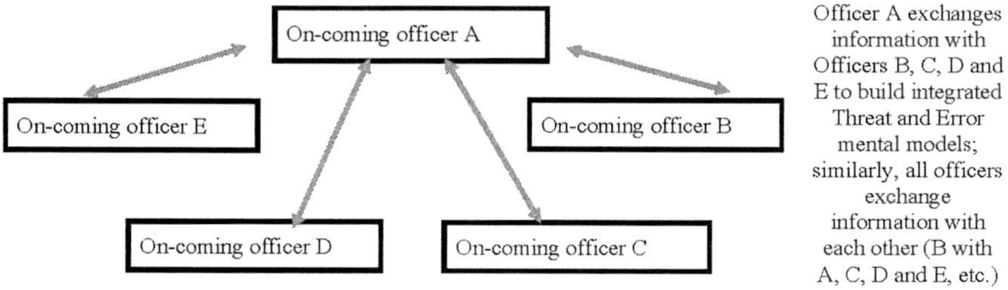

The on-coming officers, then, brief the on-coming team leader on the status of their systems and what they plan to do that shift. Here is the quality check: the on-coming team leader is comparing what the on-coming electrical power officer is saying to what the off-going leader said to expect. If everything matches, then great; if not, time is taken to determine why there is a difference.

Fig. 4-4
On-coming Officers Brief the On-coming Leader Who Compares What He or She Is Hearing to What the Off-going Leader Said to Expect and Any Differences Are Resolved

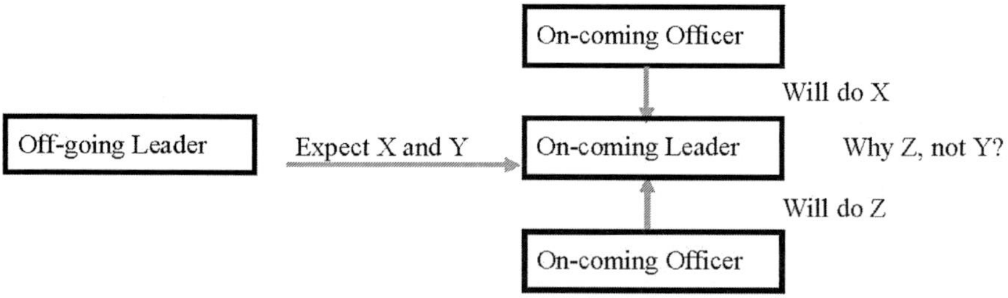

The team leader also checks for integration of mental models by asking each on-coming officer how the tasks they plan to do over the shift affect the tasks of the rest of the team. So, if the electrical power officer plans to shut down a power system, the team leader will ask: "Who might be affected by that shutdown, and have you already coordinated any required actions?" (You do not want to be the officer who says, "I don't know.")

The on-coming team leader then asks: "OK, everyone. If we need to shut down that power system, what is the worst possible failure at the worst possible time that might occur?"

The incoming leader asks questions until he or she is sure that the team knows what tasks the team will do, how team members will interact, what threats and errors might occur, their indications, and the tactics to effectively address them.

By the end of the handover--and it does not take long--the team knows they have good situation awareness and mental models, and should be able to judge if the tasks go well and to identify when problems arise.

Summary Box 4.1
What a Good Handover Does

Does your team ensure that regardless of format, the handover…

- must cover all areas of STEP (i.e., Status-Team-Environment-Progress) and levels (Perception, Comprehension and Projection)?
- allows an opportunity for the on-coming team to resolve differences in situation awareness and mental models?
- allows the on-coming team to ensure the integration and quality of its handover?

If only exchanging information to build situation awareness and mental models were that easy! Unfortunately, you will have to deal with a number of factors, what we call Situation Awareness and Exchanging Information Demons, that greatly complicate the process. These Situation Awareness and Exchanging Information Demons are covered in the next chapter.

Chapter Debriefing

I want to call a quick STAR (Stop-Think-Act-Review): get off your email, stop your side conversations, and turn off the television.[38] Let's see if you can expand upon these statements:

- Handovers are a unique form of Exchanging Information where the who and when are defined. It is the what where many handovers fail.
- The what requires passing all areas (Status, Team, Environment and Progress [STEP]) and all levels of Situation Awareness (Perception, Comprehension and Projection).
- A good handover requires giving the on-coming team member a chance to understand your situation awareness and mental models and ask questions if their situation awareness and mental models do not match yours.

If this was an actual debriefing, we would ask you to expand further on each of these statements. Depending on your response, we would ask open-ended follow-up questions until we were sure you understood the material and had a plan to implement one or more best practices. We might ask, 'What is a specific handover problem that you experience on your job?' We would not be satisfied if you said, "Our handovers aren't as good as we need." Again, we would ask open-ended follow-up questions until you might say, "We see too many errors in the first hour as the team tries to figure out what is happening." We would then ask, "What can you do to fix that problem prior to your next shift?" After a few open-ended questions, you might say, "I need to make sure that for any handover we get, we get all the STEP areas, and we ask questions if the information we are getting does not match our mental models." We might then say, "That will help your team, but what about helping the rest of the teams?" We would then continue to ask open-ended follow-up questions until you might say, "We need to modify our handover guide to discuss all areas of STEP and all levels of situation awareness."

[38] See Chapters 11-15 for information on STAR.

References

Christianson, Marlys K, Kathleen M Sutcliffe, Melissa A Miller, and Theodore J Iwashyna. "Becoming a High Reliability Organization." Critical Care 15, no. 6 (2011): 314. https://doi.org/10.1186/cc10360.

Endsley, Mica R. "Situation Awareness." Handbook of Human Factors and Ergonomics, 2006, 528–42. https://doi.org/10.1002/0470048204.ch20.

Parke, Bonny, and Barbara G. Kanki. "Best Practices in Shift Turnovers: Implications for Reducing Aviation Maintenance Turnover Errors as Revealed in ASRS Reports." The International Journal of Aviation Psychology 18, no. 1 (2008): 72–85. https://doi.org/10.1080/10508410701749464.

CHAPTER 5

RECOGNIZING AND AVOIDING SITUATION AWARENESS AND EXCHANGING INFORMATION DEMONS

Chapter Briefing[39]

I want to call a quick STAR (Stop-Think-Act-Review): get off your email, stop your side conversations, and turn off the television.[40] In this chapter, we will discuss Situation Awareness Demons, or, those factors that make it difficult for a team member to build Total Situation Awareness and STEP Mental Models. We will also discuss Exchanging Information Demons, or, those factors that make it difficult for a team to exchange information in order to integrate Total Situation Awareness and STEP Mental Models. We will be successful if you can list at least 3 Situation Awareness or Exchanging Information Demons in your profession, and possible remedies.

The primary threat that you might experience is the introduction of a large number of concepts and terms, some of which you may have never encountered, and some of which you may think about in a different sense. We will therefore explicitly define and differentiate each term and concept. We also realize how busy you are. We will make sure that the chapter is short enough to be read in approximately thirty minutes. Finally, we provide Summary Boxes. The Summary Boxes serve two functions. First, they emphasize the take-home points in each section, and you can use them to

---

[39] By now, you may feel that repeated use of the chapter briefing format is redundant. However, we believe that it is important to continue to emphasize that a good briefing builds mental models by discussing what is happening, what success looks like, and what threats or errors are possible and how you plan to prevent, avoid or mitigate them. Hence, the repetitive nature is meant to cement this belief with an understanding that you will also immerse yourself in this book on an irregular and/or intermittent basis.

[40] For more information on STAR, see Chapters 11-15.

check your understanding of those take-home points. Second, you can use them to determine if you and your team are implementing those take-home points. If a Summary Box does not make sense to you or you do not understand one or more take-home points, then review the related material before continuing to the next section.

Did I miss anything? Any concerns? Any questions? (Pause) No? Then, let's get started.

List of Abbreviations

CRM	Crew Resource Management
DOC	Physician
FAA	Federal Aviation Administration
ICU	Intensive Care Unit
IM SAFE	Illness-Medication-Stress-Alcohol-Fatigue-Eaten
PA	Physician Assistant
RT	Respiratory Therapist
SBAR	Situation-Background-Assessment-Recommendation
STAR	Stop-Think-Act-Review
STEP	Status-Team-Environment-Progress

A Situation Awareness Demon is anything that prevents you from having good situation awareness. [41] This chapter presents a list of Situation Awareness Demons that Endsley, Bolté, and Jones (2003) developed. We have modified their list to differentiate between Situation Awareness Demons that prevent or hurt Total Situation Awareness (personal Situation Awareness Demons in Section 5.1, and organizational Situation Awareness Demons in Section 5.2), and Exchanging Information Demons that prevent a team from integrating situation awareness (Section 5.3). As you read, keep two questions in the back of your mind. How do these Situation Awareness and Exchanging Information Demons manifest in your team or organization? And, how can you modify your practices and procedures to prevent, avoid or mitigate Situation Awareness and Exchanging Information Demons from affecting your team's next shift?

[41] Even though this book is about team skills (i.e., CRM) and situation awareness is not a team skill, we believe that Situation Awareness Demons are too important a topic to not discuss.

5.1 Personal Situation Awareness Demons that Prevent a Team Member from Developing Total Situation Awareness

What personal factors would prevent a team member from perceiving (Level 1 Situation Awareness) or developing the mental models to comprehend and project (Levels 2 and 3 Situation Awareness)? They are:

- Can Do people: if you are reading this, you are probably a Can Do person. Healthcare professionals are Can Do people. Can Do people, those who are willing to accept any challenge, can achieve remarkable results under very difficult conditions. Unfortunately, they also may have a difficult time admitting when they are wrong, realizing that they should wait for more information, or asking for help. When faced with difficulties, Can Do people may not admit that their situation awareness and mental models are wrong. Instead, they may work harder to force fit the facts into their situation awareness and keep going. If and when they realize that their situation awareness or mental model is wrong, they might be so far along the wrong response pathway that any remedy will be costly in terms of effectiveness, time, finances and other resources. By contrast, people who are willing to envision that their situation awareness or mental model might be inaccurate look for more cues to both confirm and disconfirm their situation awareness or mental model; they more rapidly determine that their situation awareness or mental model requires modification, and they more readily find ways to rebuild them. People who feel safe to admit that they are wrong can be taught to self-reflect, self-discover, and self-correct.

- Performance Shaping Factors: if your team is already fatigued and dealing with a patient with a severe traumatic brain injury, or any other psychological, emotional, or physical stressor that affects performance, they are experiencing Performance Shaping Factors.[42] When a Performance Shaping Factor becomes manifest during a task, make sure that everyone is supporting and backing up one another. Stress is a common Performance Shaping Factor. As a leader, you can reduce stress by staying calm and reminding team members that they have the necessary training to successfully

[42] See Section 19.2 for more information on how to handle Performance Shaping Factors.

manage the situation before them, and have actually handled similar situations in the past, thereby increasing their confidence. You can also use the IM SAFE checklist (FAA 2017) to ensure that no member of your team is:

I	Ill
M	on Medication
S	Stressed
A	on Alcohol or drugs
F	Fatigued
E	hungry or thirsty (has Eaten)

- Lack of experience or training: if you do not have the necessary training or experience, you do not have the necessary mental models. In other words, you cannot have situation awareness if you do not have the training or experience to develop the mental models to turn what you perceive (Level 1 Situation Awareness) into what you comprehend and project (Levels 2 and 3 Situation Awareness). When you and your team show up for work without the necessary mental models, this lack of training or experience is a threat that must be overcome. There are three ways to improve mental models during a shift: the briefing before the task, mentoring or feedback during the task, and the debriefing after the task.[43] Unfortunately, in our scenario, the ICU physician did not brief the team on Mr. Lopez before leaving his bedside, or have a debriefing to improve before the next shift. The physician did some real-time mentoring when she suspected a mainstem intubation by telling the respiratory therapist to pull back on the tube, auscultate, and stop when there are equal breath sounds.

Some organizations may try to compensate for a lack of training or experience with the use of protocols. While protocols may help inexperienced people complete tasks, they may not improve their mental model. As a result, the inexperienced person might not realize that the situation has changed enough to neutralize the protocolized tasks, or, worse, create the potential for harm. Likewise, guidebooks and research articles with decision tables or guiding algorithms often do not include enough information for inexperienced personnel to gauge when a step is inappropriate, or an underlying assumption is not met. Also, too many

---

[43] See Section 7.2 for more information on how to improve mental models during a shift.

procedures do not include the what, who and when required for Exchanging Information: who on what team needs what information from you or can give you, and when can it be given.

- Complexity: by definition, if you are working on a complex system (e.g., the human body), it is impossible to have a complete mental model and therefore absolute Levels 2 and 3 Situation Awareness. For complex systems, you have to rely on the fact that people have different mental models and therefore different holes, so by the "Power of And" process (how might my mental model be right, And your mental model also be right?) team members can come up with better, and more complete, mental models. Even then, you have to constantly remember that your mental model may still have holes and what you anticipate may be wrong. You can rely on shorter range forecasts, hoping the less you project into the future, the less likely any holes will hurt your situation awareness. You can try do-a-little, learn-a-little, plan-a-little with planned STARs where you use your CRM to constantly re-build a new situation awareness and mental model. [44] Finally, you can also try to simplify the situation or use a rule-of-thumb, but be aware that simplifying may hide essential features of the situation and rules-of-thumb do not cover all situations.

- Cognitive biases: if you are normal, you will try to reduce time and effort spent thinking (Kahneman 2011).[45] Thinking is difficult as evident in the large energy requirement of the brain. Humans have found heuristics (i.e., simple, efficient rules used to quickly and easily form judgments and make decisions) to be useful in most circumstances. These mental shortcuts usually involve focusing on one aspect of a complex problem and ignoring others. Most of the time heuristics work fine, but when they do not, they create cognitive biases. For example, you usually look for things that confirm that you are right and things that you expect. As long as you have good situation awareness and mental models and are not too tired, stressed, or busy, there is no problem. But what if your situation awareness and mental models are wrong, and you still only look for information that says you are right and what you expect? Under these circumstances, heuristics create Confirmation

---

[44] See Chapters 11-15 for more information on STAR.

[45] There are researchers who do not believe that cognitive biases exist, especially for experienced people. (Klein 2020)

Bias and Expectation Bias, respectively. Once you consider biases, you realize that your situation awareness or mental models might be wrong, which mitigates the Confirmation Bias, and you will look for disconfirming cues which mitigates the Expectation Bias. Another example of a bias is the Availability Bias. The Availability Bias affects decision making by only using what information comes to mind most readily, and you are more likely to do this when you are tired, stressed, or busy. Yet another example is the "Everyone Knows" Bias (Tannenbaum and Salas 2021), where you believe that if you know something, everyone knows it. There are two problems with that. First, what you know may be unique knowledge: you are the only one who actually possesses it. Second, what you know should be common (i.e., everyone should know it), but due to any number of reasons, someone does not know it. In either case, some team member does not have the information he or she needs. The literature defines dozens of cognitive biases, and it is very difficult for someone to recognize his or her own biases. Teams can limit cognitive bias as members cross-check each other's expectations against their own. So, diversity of mental models, "fresh eyes," and a good briefing that proactively discusses possible biases and their indications are needed to mitigate cognitive biases (e.g., how will we know that we might be giving in to availability, confirmation, or expectation bias?).

The ICU physician was very unusual to be able to overcome Confirmation Bias, especially since the confirmation came from another physician saying, "it looks like symmetrical chest rise…", but recognize disconfirming information (i.e., seeing asymmetrical chest rise).

NOTE: Unfortunately, it can be difficult even for team members to spot someone else's Situation Awareness Demon because those Situation Awareness Demons are just part of their everyday life. Everyday team members are stressed, perform complex tasks with multiple teams across shifts, and so forth, and it typically works out well. This is a form of a cognitive bias known as the Gambler's Fallacy. So, if a team cannot see if a Situation Awareness Demon is materializing in real time, they have to consider it during the planning phase. They can do that by assigning someone specifically to monitor situation awareness or schedule a review by people outside the core team (i.e., "fresh eyes") or Pre-Mortems (Klein 2008) to prove their situation awareness and mental models are correct.[46]

5.2 Organizational Situation Awareness Demons that Prevent a Team Member from Developing Total Situation Awareness

What organizational factors would prevent a team member from perceiving (Level 1 Situation Awareness) or developing the mental models to comprehend and project (Levels 2 and 3 Situation Awareness)? They are:

- Workload: if people have too many tasks to perform, they do not have the time and cognitive resources to adequately perceive, comprehend, project or exchange information. You mitigate that by reducing, moving, or cancelling non-essential tasks; preparing as much as possible before periods of high workload; delegating tasks; and asking for or offering to help. In our scenario, the ICU team prepped the room and equipment to reduce future workload. In the briefing, future cognitive load is reduced by discussing what to perceive and where to look, then designating who is perceiving what, when and how. The briefing should also include what certain perceptions mean in terms of present and future significance. Finally, the briefing must include who needs what portion of the information and when.

- Distractions or Interruptions: if activities not pertinent to the goal keep popping up, these distractions and interruptions use up a team member's working memory. Distractions and interruptions can be eliminated by prohibiting or at least limiting extraneous phone calls, conversations and e-mails. For example, when someone tries to distract you, you can say:

  Team member: "Did you see the game last night!?"
  You: "Let's talk about that later. Meanwhile, we need to discuss …"

[46] We are not specifying use of a Pre-Mortem. We are saying you need to use something to validate your situation awareness. Pre-mortems are discussed in Section 6.1.

You can also request/demand that non-essential personnel leave the area. In commercial aviation, the "sterilized cockpit" concept is used at 10,000 feet and below in preparation for landing (i.e., no distractions are allowed).[47]

If you cannot avoid a distraction or delay, you can project what your situation awareness should look like in the future. Then, after the distraction or delay, compare what you see with the projection. If they are close, then you probably have good situation awareness; if not, you must do something to regain situation awareness. For example: a 55-year-old female came to the ED with a temperature of 102.5 degrees Fahrenheit, heart rate of 130 bpm and a blood pressure of 85/50 (Level 1 Situation Awareness). The ED Physician Assistant (PA) became concerned for septic shock with the presence of fever, tachycardia, and hypotension (Level 2/3 Situation Awareness). The PA immediately placed this patient in a resuscitation room, ordered an anti-pyretic, a bolus of IV fluids and antibiotics, and then notified the physician. Based on the information exchanged between the physician and PA, the physician knew what to expect upon arrival. When, however, the physician arrived at the resuscitation room, the patient's vital signs were worse. Because of the difference between projected values and actual values, the physician knew that that the initial situation awareness and mental model were wrong. New information revealed that rales were heard upon chest auscultation and the history from a caregiver indicated that the patient has cardiac disease (new Level 1 Situation Awareness). Concern for cardiogenic shock (new Level 2/3 Situation Awareness) led to administration of a diuretic, initiation of an epinephrine infusion and a cardiology consultation (new mental model).

- Multitasking - If you are attempting to do two or more tasks simultaneously, you are setting yourself up for errors. Despite the fact that multitasking is believed to be a requirement in today's world and despite your thoughts that you are good at it, no one can handle two cognitively demanding tasks simultaneously. When many people talk about multitasking, they are considering tasks that are so habitual that they have passed into automaticity, and therefore pose little or no cognitive workload (e.g., walking and talking at the same time). However, as cognitive workload

[47] "ECFR :: 14 CFR 121.542 -- Flight Crewmember Duties." Accessed October 28, 2021. https://www.ecfr.gov/current/title-14/chapter-I/subchapter-G/part-121/subpart-T/section-121.542.

increases, even automaticity can be compromised. What happens to our walking pace if the discussion gets deep and heated? Do we slow down? What if I shock you with a statement? Do we stop? If we cannot walk and talk at the same time, how are we going to handle a situation where both tasks require cognitive workload (i.e., neither has passed into automaticity, so we need to think about them)? When people multitask, what they are really doing is either rapid switching (i.e., jumping back and forth between tasks), or interval switching (e.g., doing Task A for 15 minutes, then remembering to go to Task B). The working memory in human brains (the equivalent of a computer's RAM) is a serial processor. This means that switching actually requires you to remember where you were in each task (e.g., you were on Step 4 in Task A, and Step 2 in Task B). In that situation, it is easy to forget what step you were on and then either re-do a step or forget a step. That is called a placekeeping error. Cognitive aids --such as a big red arrow meaning "Resume Here"--can be tremendously helpful in reducing placekeeping errors. Remembering to do a task in the future (e.g., in 15 minutes) is called prospective memory and forgetting to do that future task is called a prospective memory error. A way to avoid prospective memory error is to set a deliberate, salient and associative reminder (Loukopoulos, Dismukes, and Barshi 2009). Another way is to remove the need to multitask. Historically, commercial pilots have had major problems with placekeeping and prospective memory errors during ground operations prior to take off. In response to this, procedures and timelines have been redesigned to reduce multitasking. In our scenario, the ICU team reduced future multitasking by tending to their other patients and tasks in order to free themselves up for when Mr. Lopez arrived.

5.3 Organizational Exchanging Information Demons that Prevent the Team from Integrating Situation Awareness

What organizational factors would prevent a team from exchanging information to integrate situation awareness? They are:

- Simultaneous operations by multiple teams: in today's world, you are frequently working in an environment where your team is working in a coordinated manner with other teams. While your team is carrying out its tasks, other teams are simultaneously undertaking their tasks. Simultaneous operations by multiple teams requires bigger, deeper and more refined Task and Team Mental Model to understand how your actions affect the other teams (and vice versa), and therefore the what, who and when of Exchanging Information. In many situations, there may be no mechanism to achieve this mutual understanding. Often, if such a mechanism exists (e.g., a morning briefing), it is at Level 1 Situation Awareness, a simple statement that another team is doing a task, without sufficient information to support Level 2 or 3 Situation Awareness as to how that task affects your team. You must talk to those other team leaders and ask questions to determine what other teams are working on and how their actions may affect your team and vice versa. An example is the treatment of a patient with a history of deep venous thrombosis, treated with an anticoagulant, who now requires surgery. Communication and coordination among the medical and surgical teams must happen to ensure that the anticoagulant is discontinued in a timely manner prior to surgery in order to reduce the risk of excessive bleeding during and after surgery, but also restarted at some point in order to prevent recurrent thrombosis. Another example is during time-pressured situations such as cardiopulmonary resuscitation, when multiple actions by multiple healthcare professionals take place simultaneously. This makes it challenging for any one individual to be aware of all of the actions that have already occurred, at the same time they need to plan for actions that may need to take place in the future. In locations where resuscitation occurs frequently, such as the ED, ICU, and delivery room, resuscitation algorithms are often posted as cognitive aids to improve Exchanging Information.

In any organization where simultaneous operations are possible, you must assume that there will always be a threat that some team that you did not know about will do a task that you did not expect, and you will be forced to use your CRM to respond. Despite that threat, multiple teams also present opportunities. Different teams have different mental models, each of which has different gaps. Because different teams have different goals, philosophies, policies, procedures, practices, situation awareness and mental models, conflicts may arise. Those diverse situation awareness and mental models, combined with the "Power of And" (how might my mental model be right, And your mental model also be right?) should result in more complete mental models, although it might take time and lots of conflict management.[48]

- Misplaced or different priorities or goals: situation awareness and mental models drive possible priorities and goals (what you can do), and conversely desired priorities and goals (what you want to do) drive mental models (how to accomplish those goals).[49] If you have different priorities or goals than your team or other teams, you will have different situation awareness and mental models. Any difference should be viewed as a threat that must be resolved by the team using CRM.

- Bad reports or handovers: if your reports or handovers only present facts like temperature, blood pressure, heart rate, etc., (Level 1 Situation Awareness), they do little to support comprehension (what the facts mean now) or projection (what the facts will mean in the future). Mnemonics devices, such as SBAR, SOAP, FIW, or I PASS the BATON remind you of the breadth and depth of information required to aid comprehension and projection when passing situation awareness and mental models.

---

[48] See Section 17.2 for more information on Managing Conflict.

[49] An example: you perceive the smoke alarm, comprehend fire, and project that it will spread to where your son is listening to music with his headphones, which drives a goal of warning him and getting him to safety. That goal drives you to consider mental models about escape routes, but also that your son will not hear the fire alarm. Your son does not hear the smoke alarm, and therefore, he does not invoke any Fire Mental Models. His goal is to listen to his favorite songs. That goal drives his mental models on how best to accomplish that.

Table 5.1
Remedies for Situation Awareness and Exchanging Information Demons

Situation Awareness Demon	Why it is a problem	What to do about it
Personal Situation Awareness Demons That Prevent a Team Member from Developing Total Situation Awareness		
Can Do People, Performance-Shaping Factors, Lack of Experience/Training, Complexity, Cognitive Biases	Each of these factors makes it hard for a team member to realize that his or her situation awareness or mental models is wrong.	Realize that in today's complex world, no one can perceive, comprehend, and project all. Team members must ask for/accept back-up behaviors. Also use briefing, feedback, and debriefing to build better situation awareness and mental models.
Organizational Situation Awareness Demons That Prevent a Team Member from Developing Total Situation Awareness		
Workload, Distractions, Interruptions, Multitasking	You do not have the time or cognitive resources to perceive, comprehend, project, and exchange.	Reduce or redistribute workload, eliminate distractions and interruptions, and reschedule tasks that are not required.
Organizational Exchanging Information Demons That Prevent the Team from Integrating Situation Awareness		
Simultaneous Operations/Multiple Teams, Misplaced/Multiple Priorities/Goals	You need to keep track of too many teams performing too many tasks with different situation awareness, mental models, and goals, so you do not know what to pass to whom, and when.	You must consider people and tasks outside your immediate team as you build your situation awareness and mental models.
Bad Reports/Handovers	Bad reports and handovers do not give the information to feed into or build situation awareness and mental models.	Fill out/read reports and perform handovers with the goal of passing on/building all of your situation awareness and mental models.

Before you proceed to the next section, again take some time to note how these Situation Awareness and Exchanging Information Demons manifest themselves in your team or organization. How can you prevent, avoid, or mitigate a demon from affecting your team during your next shift?

Besides these specific fixes for Situation Awareness and Exchanging Information Demons, there are best practices that the best teams use every day to make sure they have and exchange situation awareness and mental models. How many of these best practices does your team do? Let's check in the next chapter.

Chapter Debriefing

I want to call a quick STAR (Stop-Think-Act-Review): get off your email, stop your side conversations, and turn off the television.[50] Let's see if you can expand upon these statements:

To defeat Situation Awareness and Exchanging Information Demons, you must

- use a good briefing to mitigate lack of training or experience.
- use your team members' different situation awareness and mental models to find gaps in your own situation awareness and mental models.
- control workload and distractions to give your team time and the mental resources to perceive, comprehend, project, and exchange.
- realize that in today's world, you must consider a much bigger team than just your core team when determining who gives/needs information to/from you.

If this was an actual debriefing, we would ask you to expand further on each of these statements. Depending on your response, we would ask open-ended follow-up questions until we were sure you understood the material and had a plan to implement one or more best practices. We might ask, 'What is a specific Situation Awareness or Exchanging Information Demon that you experience on your job? 'We would not be satisfied if you said, "Our situation awareness isn't as good as we need." Again, we would ask open-ended follow-up questions until you might say, "We have a problem with new team members not having the mental models they need." We

[50] See Chapters 11-15 for information on STAR.

would then ask, "What can you do to fix that problem prior to your next shift?" After a few open-ended questions, you might say, "I can use the briefing to discuss what will happen, what success will look like, what threats are possible and how we might recognize those threats. During the shift, I can control workload and distractions. Of course, we would debrief any mental model gaps, including mine." We would then say, "That helps your team, but what about other teams?" We would then continue to ask open-ended follow-up questions until you might say, "We need to modify our briefing guide to discuss possible gaps or errors in mental models."

References

"ECFR :: 14 CFR 121.542 -- Flight Crewmember Duties." Accessed October 28, 2021. https://www.ecfr.gov/current/title-14/chapter-I/subchapter-G/part-121/subpart-T/section-121.542.

Endsley, Mica, Betty Bolté, and Debra Jones. "SA Demons." Designing for Situation Awareness, 2003, 31–42. https://doi.org/10.1201/9780203485088.ch3.

Aeronautical Information Manual - aim. Accessed October 30, 2021. https://www.faa.gov/air_traffic/publications/atpubs/aim_html/index.html.

Kahneman, Daniel. Thinking, Fast and Slow. New York: Farrar, Straus and Giroux, 2013.

Le Roy, Grégory. "Critical Decisions - Redeciding Cognitive Biases - Gary Klein (Sources of Power)." HEC Stories, February 5, 2021. https://hecstories.fr/en/redeciding-cognitive-biases-gary-klein-sources-of-power.

Klein, Gary. "Performing a Project Premortem." IEEE Engineering Management Review 36, no. 2 (2008): 103–4. https://doi.org/10.1109/emr.2008.4534313.

Barshi, Immanuel. Multitasking Myth - Handling Complexity in Real-World Operations. Ashgate Publishing Group, 2009.

Tannenbaum, Scott I., and Eduardo Salas. Teams That Work: The Seven Drivers of Team Effectiveness. New York, NY: Oxford University Press, 2021.

CHAPTER 6

IMPLEMENTING SITUATION AWARENESS AND EXCHANGING INFORMATION BEST PRACTICES

Chapter Briefing[51]

I want to call a quick STAR (Stop-Think-Act-Review): get off your email, stop your side conversations, and turn off the television.[52] In this chapter, we will discuss best practices to develop, maintain, and exchange situation awareness and mental models. We will be successful if you can:

- describe best practices to develop, maintain and exchange situation awareness and mental models before a task (Section 6.1); and
- describe best practices to develop, maintain and exchange situation awareness and mental models during a task (Section 6.2).

The primary threat that you might experience is the introduction of a large number of concepts and terms, some of which you may have never encountered, and some of which you may think about in a different sense. We will therefore explicitly define and differentiate each term and concept. We also realize how busy you are. We will make sure that the chapter is short enough to be read in approximately thirty minutes. Finally, we provide Summary Boxes. The Summary Boxes serve two functions. First, they emphasize the take-home points in each section, and you can use them to

---

[51] By now, you may feel that repeated use of the chapter briefing format is redundant. However, we believe that it is important to continue to emphasize that a good briefing builds mental models by discussing what is happening, what success looks like, and what threats or errors are possible and how you plan to prevent, avoid, or mitigate them. Hence, the repetitive nature is meant to cement this belief with an understanding that you will also immerse yourself in this book on an irregular and/or intermittent basis.

[52] For more information on STAR, see Chapters 11-15.

check your understanding of those take-home points. Second, you can use them to determine if you and your team are implementing those take-home points. If a Summary Box does not make sense to you or you do not understand one or more take-home points, then review the related material before continuing to the next section.

Did I miss anything? Any concerns? Any questions? (Pause) No? Then, let's get started.

List of Abbreviations

COPD	Chronic Obstructive Pulmonary Disease
CRM	Crew Resource Management
DOC	Physician
ED	Emergency Department
ICU	Intensive Care Unit
NUR	Nurse
PEEP	Positive End-Expiratory Pressure
PIP	Peak Inspiratory Pressure
STAR	Stop-Think-Act-Review
STEP	Status-Team-Environment-Progress

As you read in Chapter 5, developing situation awareness and mental models, and exchanging information to integrate them is rife with obstacles (i.e., Demons). In this chapter, you will learn best practices from research, but they are also found in teams and organizations that have found ways to consistently build and maintain situation awareness and mental models. You will learn best practices you can do before starting the task (Section 6.1), and then best practices you can do during the task (Section 6.2). As you read the chapter, consider what best practice you can do in your organization or team.

6.1 Best Practices on What to Do Before Starting the Task

A quote often attributed to Albert Einstein goes:

> "If I had an hour to solve a problem, I'd spend 55 minutes thinking about the problem and 5 minutes thinking about solutions."[53]

The upshot of the quote is that too many people and teams spend too little time thinking about the problem (i.e., assessing the situation or developing situation awareness), and then too much time trying to find a solution to a poorly defined situation. Your goal here is to follow Einstein's advice: to develop a clear picture of what is happening, where the problems are, and what, where and when to look for critical information. You also want to determine who needs what critical information and when. To do all that, you need to spend more time:

1. Perceiving. You need to attend to more cues and seek more information within a predetermined timeframe.[54] Your mental model should tell you what information is crucial to your success, and what information might tell you something is wrong. Each additional cue may provide you more information and more differentiation of what the situation really is and what it is not.

Be careful of making assumptions. This check is especially difficult for an individual due to cognitive biases such as Expectation and Confirmation Biases. One way to minimize cognitive bias is to define a specific set of data to look for, and record and plot, as do many healthcare professionals with lab results. If combined with expected values and tight limits, you can more rapidly see unexpected values. By plotting the values, you can see long term

---

[53] Quoteresearch, Author. "I Would Spend 55 Minutes Defining the Problem and Then Five Minutes Solving It." Quote Investigator, November 22, 2018. https://quoteinvestigator.com/2014/05/22/solve/.

[54] One very important point: you need to make a conscious and deliberate effort to determine how much time you can spend doing situation assessment. Whether you have 5 minutes, or 5 hours, or 5 days before something must be done or before something bad happens, you might decide to spend 1/4 of the time in situation assessment. That will leave you with 3/4 of the remaining time to decide on a plan, develop the plan, execute the plan, and then have the actions take effect, with a time margin. The 1/4 might be 1/3 or even 1/2. The important point is to pick a time and monitor it, at least until your situation assessment says you can change it. Once you determine that time, whether 75 seconds, 75 minutes, or 30 hours, assign someone to keep track of that time.

trends. Arguably, the best way to overcome cognitive biases is to ask your team members what they perceive. Because they have different situation awareness and mental models, they might perceive different factors than you do.

2. Comprehending. You start comprehension by trying to understand how you found yourself in the situation. If you are not sure of the background or context, you will not know what string of events brought you to the situation. You want to make sure that you know the possible ways that the situation might have unfolded. The classic example of failure to do this is the USS Vincennes (Cohen, Freeman, and Thompson 1998). On July 3, 1988, the USS Vincennes shot down an Iranian airliner thinking it was under attack from an Iranian military aircraft. Although there were other complicating factors, failure to consider alternate stories (i.e., it was a commercial airliner) contributed to this tragic error. In your world, you see a patient who is complaining about fever, muscle aches, nausea, headaches, and fatigue. It is also the height of flu season. There may be a likely story or explanation (e.g., flu), but there are other possible diseases or stories that would also explain the patient's symptoms (e.g., meningitis). You ask about stiff neck, light sensitivity, and seizures to determine if meningitis is a valid story. Again, encourage the members of your team to offer their mental models and actively listen to their alternative viewpoints. What in his or her mental model suggests that it is possible? What in your mental model says it is not possible? Actively listen to his or her rationale to understand the underlying mental model and decide if your mental model has a hole or error. Or, maybe both are right, and this is a case where the both of you have a piece of the complete mental model. Different stories may represent different situations. Here is one example: A patient presents to the ED with tachycardia (abnormally high heart rate) and the ED immediately implements the Septic Shock Protocol. What goes unnoticed is the fact that the patient has no fever or any other sign of infection or shock. Additionally, the heart rate is fast but is in the range of where one should consider an alternative diagnosis. Despite these findings, the ED team hands off the patient to the ICU with this diagnosis. The ICU team recognizes that the diagnosis may be wrong and considers an alternative story (i.e., diagnosis)—supraventricular tachycardia. This is an example of perception, plugged into an incorrect mental model, activated by the wrong story, leads to incorrect comprehension, while someone who is willing to consider alternate stories may come up with another mental

model and another comprehension. You need to consider all possible stories until additional information rules them out.

Once you understand how you might have arrived at your situation and gathered as much information as time permits, you need to understand what all that information is telling you. Comprehension must be in all areas of situation awareness (i.e., STEP or Status: the Patient and Task; Team: Teamwork and the Team Members; Environment, the physical and organizational context; and finally, Progress, the schedule, time-to-effect, and margin). As part of your Task Mental Model, you need to determine how your task affects and is affected by other tasks. As part of your Team Members' Mental Model, you need to determine who needs information from you and who has information you need. Finally, as part of your Progress Mental Model, you need to determine when to exchange the information. But as in the example of the elephant and the six blindfolded people, your individual mental models may not allow you to come up with the right answer. In a team, we can always go back to actively listening to the inputs of your team members and using the "Power of And".

3. Projecting. In many instances, even more important than realizing what is happening now is realizing what might happen in the future. You and your team must talk about the future: this is what we think will happen, what it will look like if we are right or wrong, and what it will mean in terms of the patient, the team, and so on. A clinical example is a child with asthma who is admitted to the hospital with respiratory distress. With timely and appropriate treatment, the patient can be discharged within 24-48 hrs. If not, then some other problem, such as viral or bacterial pneumonia, exists. When you know what to expect, you can treat any deviation from your expectations as a possible sign that your situation awareness or mental models might be wrong.

If you anticipate a possible threat or error materializing (e.g., viral or bacterial pneumonia) and know what the indications of that threat or error are, you will know what information to look for and therefore will be more likely to detect that threat or error earlier. One set of threats that is sometimes missed is the threats the team themselves pose. Too many teams rate their situation awareness above average, at least until an accident proves they were wrong. While 80% of drivers rate their driving skill as above average (McCormick, Walkey, and Green 1986), it is more likely that 30-50% of drivers may have a poor mental model on their skills and abilities. Good teams realize that they need to look out for team threats. These threats involve poor mental models, inadequate skills to handle the problems that are being faced, and inability to accurately gauge the length of time that a task will require. Good teams accurately estimate the time required to complete a task. One way they do that is by utilizing historical data. If all previous teams took eight hours to accomplish this task, effective teams will not assume that they somehow will finish in less time unless they have compelling information (e.g., the availability of a larger number of appropriately trained personnel) to support that assumption. What about your Status, Team, Environment and Progress situation awareness and mental models tell you that your team is better than every other team?

Now that you have Perceived, Comprehended and Projected, before your team can decide that they have the right situation awareness and mental models, you must check the validity of your situation assessment, preferably with someone with a fresh set of eyes and maybe a different mental model. You could also do a Pre-Mortem (Klein, Snowden, and Pin 2011).[55] A Pre-Mortem assumes that you are now in the future and your task failed. Your team asks itself what caused it to fail. You will get responses like "It could have been *A*" or "Maybe we forgot to do *B*". Your team then spends some time making sure that *A* does not happen, and you do not forget *B*.

There are only two things left to do before you start the task. Firstly, determine who needs to know what (content), when (timing) and how (format). When done formally, this is sometimes called a Communication Plan. It is all about making sure your team can develop situation awareness and mental models by determining ahead of time all information exchanges. Secondly, prepare a briefing for your team (e.g., a pre-procedure timeout [Meginniss, Damian, and Falvo 2012]) that discusses everything that you have learned and ensures that you have complementary situation awareness and mental models.[56] The ICU physician might have done a better job of briefing the ICU team before leaving Mr. Lopez's bedside, especially since they were not sure about possible concurrent infection causing exacerbation of COPD. If the ICU physician had done this, the ICU nurse might have noticed the increased heart rate and lower oxygen levels before talking to Mr. Lopez's wife.

---

[55] We are not specifying use of a Pre-Mortem. We are saying you need to use something to validate your situation assessment.

[56] See Section 14.2 for more information on how to prepare that briefing. See Section 7.2 for more information on mental models.

Summary Box 6.1
Situation Awareness and Exchanging Information Best Practices Before Getting Started

Does your team…
- deliberately determine how much time you can spend doing situation assessment and then monitor time to ensure that you do not exceed it?
- determine what information is crucial to tell you if things are progressing as planned or not?
- remember that perception, comprehension, and projection must include a full STEP (Status-Team-Environment-Progress)?
- find a way to evaluate your situation awareness and mental models?
- brief your team on what to look for if things are going well and if they are going badly, what it means right then and, in the future, and who to tell what and when they should be told?

6.2 What To Do During the Task

During the task, the team should be checking for four things: critical data, deviations, your team, and Situation Awareness and Exchanging Information Demons.

Before the task, you predicted what you should look for (i.e., critical data: oxygen saturation in the scenario) to determine if a threat or error is materializing. If, during the task, that critical data exceeds the value that you consider out of limits (i.e., reaches a trigger: oxygen saturation at 80% or the patient is unresponsive), you should execute your transition to your planned contingency plan (i.e., intubation).[57] There can be no wishful thinking where you hope the data will return to normal soon. Once you execute your contingency plan, you should perform a quick STAR to make sure you know how to Think, Act and Review in the new situation (i.e., a quick STAR post-intubation to ensure that the team is ready to handle any threat or error).

During the task, you might perceive deviations, other indications that do not appear normal, but you did not think that they are crucial to your task or goal, or even indications that you did not expect at all. No matter how small a deviance, even those that are better than expected, do not ignore

[57] When a critical data parameter reaches a trigger, your present margin is zero. See Section 12.3 for more information on margin.

them, or explain them away. They may be signs that your situation awareness or mental model is wrong. Again, perform a quick STAR, just for a minute or two, to make sure that these indications are not an unexpected threat or error.

Besides having situation awareness on possible threats and error, you must have situation awareness on your team members. Watching them gives you a chance to "see into" their heads; their actions reflect their situation awareness and mental models. Compare their actions to what your situation awareness and mental models say they should be doing. If there is a mismatch, then someone's situation awareness or mental models may be wrong. They may be perceiving something you did not expect, or comprehending or projecting it differently. Remember to give them a chance to also "see into" your head. Do that by explaining your actions and decisions (e.g., increasing PIP and PEEP in response to an oxygen saturation level remaining low after intubation). This gives your team a chance to compare their situation awareness and mental models with yours and see if they agree or not (e.g., agree or disagree with increasing PIP and PEEP). If they do not agree, they should assert their situation awareness and mental model and seek to identify, understand, and resolve any differences. You may also notice subtle cues, such as your team is making mistakes, getting behind schedule, or their communication is suggesting that they are unsure of what is happening (e.g., when the ICU Physician says "I think so…"), or are constantly pulling (asking for) information. All these are possible indications of situation awareness and mental model problems. You must find ways to give your team enough time and cognitive resources to rebuild their situation awareness and mental models. Do this through STARs, Timeouts, Stop Works, holding patterns (in aviation), or using any schedule margin to delay tasks. Finally, request and accept help from outside your team—your management and other teams—paying especial attention to any information that conflicts with your situation awareness or mental models. Those outside sources may find and fix holes in your situation awareness and mental models.

Finally, you may notice unplanned Situation Awareness or Exchanging Information Demons, such as higher workloads, frequent multitasking, or more distractions than expected. You compensate by making real-time changes to your plan by moving or cancelling tasks, reducing distracting activities or conversations, or providing more back-up support.

Summary Box 6.2
Best Practices During Task Execution

Do your team members…
- pay attention to critical data, and execute their contingency plan immediately if the data exceeds a trigger?
- pay attention to any indications "not normal" or not expected?
- pay attention to the actions of others to "see into" their heads?
- explain their own actions and decisions to let others "see into" their head?
- treat errors, being behind schedule, or poor communication as indicators of possible bad situation awareness or mental model?
- prevent, avoid and mitigate any Situation Awareness or Exchanging Information Demons?

All the above is considered a High Reliability Organization's Preoccupation with Failure (Weick, Sutcliffe, and Obstfeld 1999), meaning, until you can prove that an abnormal indication is not a threat or error, you should treat it as one.

6.3 What to Do After the Task

The best teams are always learning, so they debrief what they did right and wrong in building, maintaining, and rebuilding their situation awareness and mental models, and exchanging information. They then incorporate what they learned into their practices before their next shift and validate their effectiveness. In our scenario, the Intensive Care Unit (ICU) team failed to do a debriefing, meaning that they may make similar mistakes during the next shift. See Chapter 18 for more information on Debriefing.

Before you go to the next section, how can you modify these best practices to improve situation awareness and mental models for your team during the next shift?

Chapter Debriefing

I want to call a quick STAR (Stop-Think-Act-Review): get off your email, stop your side conversations, and turn off the television.[58] Let's see if you can expand upon these statements:

- Determine how long you can spend on your situation assessment (and then monitor that time).
- Determine what STEP (Status-Team-Environment-Progress) information is crucial to determine if your plan is going well or not.
- Use your briefing to make sure your team knows what to look for and what it means, and who to tell what and when.
- During the task, monitor critical data and the actions of others, and let them know what you are thinking.
- If during the task, if anything happens that you did not expect, treat that difference as a possible situation awareness or mental model problem and do a STAR.
- Debrief!

If this was an actual debriefing, we would ask you to expand further on each of these statements. Depending on your response, we would ask open-ended follow-up questions until we were sure you understood the material and had a plan to implement one or more best practices. We might ask, "What is a specific Situation Awareness or Exchanging Information Demon that you experience on your job?" We would not be satisfied if you said, "Our situation awareness isn't as good as we need." Again, we would ask open-ended follow-up questions until you might say, "We have a problem with team members exchanging information inconsistently." We would then ask, "What specific Situation Awareness or Exchanging Information best practice can you modify to fix that problem prior to your next shift?" You might say, "In the briefing, I can discuss specifically who needs what information, when and how. During the shift, I can provide feedback if I see that team members must pull information. During the debriefings, we can discuss any Exchanging Information problems and how to fix them." We might then say, "That helps your team, but how can you help other teams?" We would then continue to ask open-ended follow-up questions until you might say, "We need to modify our debriefing guide to include who needs what information, when and how."

---

[58] See Chapters 11-15 for information on STAR.

References

"Critical Thinking Skills in Tactical Decision Making: A ..." Accessed October 30, 2021. https://www.researchgate.net/profile/Marvin-Cohen-2/publication/236030478_Critical_Thinking_Skills_in_Tactical_Decision_Making_A_Model_and_A_Training_Strategy/links/02e7e515e220e2e87f000000/Critical-Thinking-Skills-in-Tactical-Decision-Making-A-Model-and-A-Training-Strategy.pdf.

Klein, Gary, David Snowden, and Chew Pin. "Anticipatory Thinking." Essay. In Informed by Knowledge: Expert Performance in Complex Situations; Based on Presentations from the 8th International Conference on Naturalistic Decision Making, edited by Ute M. Fischer and Kathleen L. Mosier, 235–44. New York, NY: Psychology Press, 2011.

McCormick, Iain A., Frank H. Walkey, and Dianne E. Green. "Comparative Perceptions of Driver Ability— a Confirmation and Expansion." Accident Analysis & Prevention 18, no. 3 (1986): 205–8. https://doi.org/10.1016/0001-4575(86)90004-7.

Meginniss, Anne, Frances Damian, and Francine Falvo. "Time out for Patient Safety." Journal of Emergency Nursing 38, no. 1 (2012): 51–53. https://doi.org/10.1016/j.jen.2011.04.007.

Weick, Karl, Kathleen Sutcliffe, and David Obstfeld. "Organizing for High Reliability: Processes of Collective Mindfulness." Essay. In Research in Organizational Behavior: An Annual Series of Analytical Essays and Critical Reviews, edited by Robert I. Sutton, Barry M. Staw, and Larry Cummings, 81–122. Greenwich, CT: JAI Press, 1999.

CHAPTER 7

IMPROVING MENTAL MODELS

Chapter Briefing[59]

I want to call a quick STAR (Stop-Think-Act-Review): get off your email, stop your side conversations, and turn off the television.[60] In this chapter, we will discuss mental models further. We will be successful if you can:

- define all the mental models you need (Section 7.1);
- explain how to improve mental models in the briefing (Section 7.2.1);
- explain how to improve mental models during the task or shift (Section 7.2.2); and
- explain how to improve mental models in the debriefing (Section 7.2.3).

The primary threat that you might experience is the introduction of a large number of concepts and terms, some of which you may have never encountered, and some of which you may think about in a different sense. We will therefore explicitly define and differentiate each term and concept. We also realize how busy you are. We will make sure that the chapter is short enough to be read in approximately thirty minutes. Finally, we provide Summary Boxes. The Summary Boxes serve two functions. First, they emphasize the take-home points in each section, and you can use them to check your understanding of those take-home points. Second, you can use

---

[59] By now, you may feel that repeated use of the chapter briefing format is redundant. However, we believe that it is important to continue to emphasize that a good briefing builds mental models by discussing what is happening, what success looks like, and what threats or errors are possible and how you plan to prevent, avoid, or mitigate them. Hence, the repetitive nature is meant to cement this belief with an understanding that you will also immerse yourself in this book on an irregular and/or intermittent basis.

[60] For more information on STAR, see Chapters 11-15.

them to determine if you and your team are implementing those take-home points. If a Summary Box does not make sense to you or you do not understand one or more take-home points, then review the related material before continuing to the next section.

Important Note to the Reader

You will notice that this chapter brings together the concepts from Chapters 2-6, as well as introducing the proper use of the briefing, cross-checking during the task, and debriefing to improve your team's CRM. The result is you may feel like you are drinking from a firehose. Comprehending this chapter is crucial to implementing good CRM. We know this is a tall task, but we also know that you are up to it.

Did I miss anything? Any concerns? Any questions? (Pause) No? Then, let's get started.

List of Abbreviations

COPD	Chronic Obstructive Pulmonary Disease
CRM	Crew Resource Management
DOC	Physician
ICU	Intensive Care Unit
NIV	Non-Invasive Ventilation
NUR	Nurse
PEEP	Positive End-Expiratory Pressure
PIP	Peak Inspiratory Pressure
PPV	Positive Pressure Ventilation
STEP	Status-Team-Environment-Progress

Why is there now a whole chapter on mental models since we have already discussed them in earlier chapters? Mental models, conceptualized as how and why you believe something works (Rouse and Morris 1986), are crucial to CRM. First, CRM is a Teamwork Mental Model, or how and why team members should work together to be safe and effective. This book is all about getting you to believe that CRM is the way your team must operate. Second, without a full suite of mental models (i.e., mental models in Status, Team, Environment and Progress [STEP]), team members cannot have Total Situation Awareness and a team cannot fully integrate their situation awareness. In too many books, authors do not give their readers concrete and achievable methods to improve situation awareness. Part of the reason for that is the authors do not treat situation awareness as the output of mental models. To improve situation awareness, you must improve mental models. A team can improve their situation awareness by:

- ensuring that the proper mental models are activated in the briefing.
- cross-checking the actions of others during the task, to see if there is a possible mismatch of mental models.
- working to improve their mental models prior to their next task or shift by debriefing.

Let us dive deeper into two scenarios to help you understand the connection between situation awareness and mental models:

1) Team members need mental models to turn Perceptions (Level 1 Situation Awareness) into Comprehension and Projection (Level 2 and 3 Situation Awareness). You can see and hear what is going on, but not realize what the consequences are now and in the future. If you cannot tell what is happening and why, you cannot know if what you see is important or not. Another way to say that is "I see much, but know little." Does this remind you of your first day in a new position or job? It is your responsibility to have mental models in all the areas you need situation awareness (i.e., in Status, Team, Environment and Progress [STEP]), so that you can have Total Situation Awareness. This scenario will be covered more in Section 7.1
2) Team members need correct, complete, complementary, and diverse mental models to accomplish team goals.[61] Unfortunately, since there are different mental models for different situations, the STEP mental models must also be the right ones for the situation. Another way to say that is "He is doing the right thing in the wrong situation." Does this remind you of a team's reactions to an unexpected crisis? It is the responsibility of every team member to make sure that all team members activate the right mental models and fix any errant mental models. This scenario will be covered more in Section 7.2.

[61] Correct = no wrong information; complete = covers all of STEP; complementary = covers task intersections and team interactions; and diverse = based on different knowledge, experiences, goals, roles, responsibilities, tasks, etc.

7.1 How to Prevent "I See Much, But Know Little"

A mental model is how and why you believe something works. A mental model allows you to turn what you see, hear, feel, taste, or smell into present and future consequences. Another way of saying that is what you see or hear (Perception or Level 1 Situation Awareness) are inputs to your mental model and the outputs are your comprehension of present consequences (Level 2 Situation Awareness) and projection of future consequences (Level 3 Situation Awareness) (Endsley 2000).

Fig. 7-1
Mental Models Turn Perception Into Comprehension and Projection

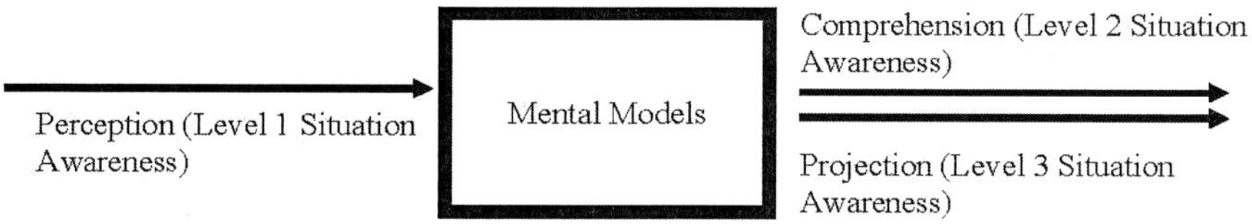

Different mental models are required to cover Status, Team, Environment and Progress (STEP). In healthcare, Status includes the Patient and Tasks; Team includes Teamwork (i.e., CRM) and Team Members; Environment is the physical and organizational context within which the team must work; and Progress includes the schedule, time-to-effect and margin.[62] Some examples are:

Status

- how and why a disease progresses (e.g., how COPD, diabetes, hypertension, or infections would affect breathing).
- how, why, and when (not) to do a task (e.g., when to do an intubation).

Team

- how and why to work as a team (e.g., how your team employs CRM).
- common errors made by teams (e.g., what errors team make when they are tired and overworked).

---

[62] Time-to-effect is how long before something happens. It could be how long before medication takes effect, or how long before major injury occurs. Margin is how much a critical data parameter (temperature, pressure. resource, and so forth) can increase or decrease before you must go to a contingency plan.

Environment

- how your organization's philosophies, policies, procedures, and practices expect you to operate.[63]
- how you manage caring for multiple patients and multiple problems while also preparing for the admission of another patient to the ICU.

Progress

- what tasks must be done before other tasks.
- how long before the good or adverse effects of a task can be detected (e.g., how long you can stay with NIV if the patient's oxygen saturation is 80%).
- how much temperature—or any other critical data parameter—can increase or decrease before you must do something (e.g., if oxygen saturation falls to 80%, an immediate response is required).

This section covers what constitutes a good mental model (7.1.1), why we advocate complementary mental models (7.1.2), the importance of diversity in mental models (7.1.3), and how mental models help build Bottoms-Up and Top-Down Situation Awareness (7.1.4).

7.1.1 What Constitutes Good STEP Mental Models

You may be thinking, "Isn't a mental model just knowledge about conditional relationships?" No. For example, "If A, then B" is an incomplete mental model. A mental model is not just knowing about a relationship between two (real or potential) events but understanding how any such relationship works. "If A, why B" or, more correctly, "How does A turn into B" implies comprehension—and a more complete and accurate mental model—that not only allows you to explain why A causes B, but also why it does not cause C, and, later, why D would happen.

You may also be thinking that you have made a diagnosis (Level 2 Situation Awareness) and prognosis (Level 3 Situation Awareness) without relying on a mental model. An illness script, for example, describes how an experienced clinician can use symptoms alone to determine an illness, as

63 Unfortunately, in some organizations there is a disconnect between how the organization says it wants teams to operate (philosophies, policies, and procedures) and how they actually operate (practices).

well as its prognosis.[64] Illness scripts may be considered to be a class of "Codified Knowledge" about situation awareness (Endsley 2000) where the components of a thorough illness script fall into three main categories: the predisposing conditions (Level 1 Situation Awareness), the pathophysiological insult (Level 2 Situation Awareness), and the clinical consequences (Level 3 Situation Awareness).[65] In the case of this codified situation awareness, the mental model was used to build the illness script and large portions of the mental model (disease's pathophysiology, epidemiology, time course, salient symptoms and signs, and/or diagnostics) are documented.

A clinician uses his or her experience, and the patient's symptoms, to make a diagnosis and determine a prognosis. An experienced clinician has seen the illness and its associated symptoms numerous times, under varying circumstances. Even then, a clinician will use a tacit mental model to critique and correct the diagnosis, checking for indications that the experienced-based diagnosis might be wrong, and correcting it based on this disconfirming information.

Based on your comprehension and projection of what is happening, your mental model will tell you what changes to inputs and outputs to look for. For example, based on the illness script or your experience, your Status Mental Model says that you should be looking for an increasing heat rate in a patient with fever. It will also tell you how much of an increase in heart rate you should see. If the heart rate deviates too much from your mental model, it is possible that your mental model is wrong. Your mental model will also tell you that you should not see decreasing blood pressure. If you do see decreasing blood pressure then, again, it is possible that your mental model is wrong, and the patient might have septic shock. Your mental models for Team, Environment, and Progress provide similar information on what changes to expect, how much, and what not to expect.

Also, based on your comprehension and projection, your STEP Mental Models will also tell you the most likely or the worst possible threat or error. Your mental models will tell you that your patient might react badly to a treatment, a team member might be tired, weather might preclude an air transport, or that the situation has caused fixation, and loss of situation awareness regarding time. Since your mental models tell you what threats

---

[64] An illness script is an organized summary of a provider's mental model of a disease.

[65] For more information on illness scripts, go to https://www.sgim.org/web-only/clinical-reasoning-exercises/illness-scripts-overview.

and errors to look for, you will detect them earlier and react to them more forcefully and correctly.

Summary Box 7.1
What Status-Team-Environment-Progress (STEP) Mental Models Must Do

Does every member on your team possess mental models that…
- fully cover Status, Team, Environment, and Progress (STEP)?
- include:
  - the whys and hows of turning inputs into outputs?
  - what those inputs and outputs should look like?
  - which inputs and outputs would not be valid for your mental model?
  - possible threats and errors and what they would look like?

If your inputs or outputs do not match your mental model, then your mental model may be wrong.

7.1.2 Shared Versus Complementary Mental Models

Much of the research on teamwork and CRM emphasizes the need for shared mental models in which everyone has the same mental model. Some of this research was conducted on airline cockpit crews, where either crew member can do the flying, so both crew members must have the same mental model. But do a physician, nurse and respiratory therapist need to have the same mental model (i.e., perceive, comprehend, and project the exact same things), since they are not required to do the exact same tasks? Our answer is an unequivocal no. Since a mental model is based on your role, knowledge, experience, goals, etc., some researchers believe that it is impossible for any two people to have the exact same mental model. They, however, do need to know how their mental models are related to the mental models of their team members to ensure that patient care is both safe and effective. Those researchers (and the authors of this book) emphasize the need for complementary mental models (DeChurch and Mesmer-Magnus 2010). What is meant by complementary mental models? Mental models are complementary when the mental models of team members have the same task intersections and the same team interactions. Task intersections are how my tasks affect you, and how your tasks affect me. Team interactions are what I need to do, or say, for you to do your job and what you need to do, or say, for me to do my job effectively. In our scenario, the ICU team had complementary mental models on the intubation. As the physician started the intubation, the three nurses checked blood pressure and femoral pulses. They knew how their tasks affected each other (task intersections), and the physician knew what to do and say to the nurses, and vice versa (team interactions).

Let us look at the ICU team again. The patient's oxygen saturation and heart rate were decreasing. Everyone needs to know that fact, but that is just something that everyone needs to hear (i.e., it is a shared Level 1 Situation Awareness requirement, not a shared mental model). The physician will use that information for different tasks than the nurses, and will therefore use different mental models. Even the respiratory therapists will have different mental models, since one is monitoring the PIP and PEEP, and the other is checking on the breath sounds. They all have different mental models based on their role, but the mental models must complement each other if they are to work together as an effective team. If any of the team members has a bad mental model or a mental model that is not complementary with the others, then the patient's care is at risk.

Rather than striving for shared mental models, a team would be better served by ensuring complementary mental models. A notional test of complementary mental models would require that the physician states what she needs from the nurse, what she needs to do for the nurse, and her understanding of how that information should be communicated. The nurse would do the same. The two lists can then be compared. The lists must be mirror images of each other (i.e., what the physician expects from the nurse matches what the nurse expects to provide to the physician, and vice versa). Since such a test of complementary mental models is impractical, then the leader must find other ways to ensure complementary mental models. One way is for the team to use the briefing to ensure that the team's mental models are complementary (See Section 7.2).

Summary Box 7.2
A Team Needs Complementary Mental Models

Rather than worry about everyone having the same mental models, a team is better served if the team has complementary mental models. That means that we agree on what each team member needs…

- to do for all other team members, and how.
- from all other team members, and how.

7.1.3 The Role of Diversity in Mental Models

The bad news is that no matter how much knowledge and experience an individual may have, when working complex problems within complex systems, gaps and holes in mental models are inevitable. The good news is that in teams, your mental models are not my mental models (and vice versa), and together we can have more complete mental models. This is what we consider diversity: not diversity in nationality, gender, culture, but diversity of mental models. Organizations without a diversity of mental models "drift" into failures over time (Dekker 2016). The only remedy for that drift is to leverage those diverse mental models to eliminate gaps in team members' mental models. Teams can prevent that drift by incorporating different mental models. This means listening to the resident or fellow, the surgical technician, the Director of Safety, the "new person" or anyone else who can offer a different perspective without being influenced by "the way we have always done it here…". You must decide if an outsider's mental model is so bad that it adds no value, or if it is exposing a hole in your mental model. How you decide to handle "That's not how I thought it worked…" or "That doesn't make sense to me…" may determine how complete a mental model you have. Many accidents have been averted when the leader asked what the "rookie" meant by "Is it supposed to do that?".

Summary Box 7.3
A Diversity of Mental Models Is Required to Eliminate Gaps

Do your team members actively listen to the questions and statements of others to determine if their mental models may be wrong (or incomplete)?

7.1.4 Mental Models and Top-Down Versus Bottoms-Up Situation Awareness

In our example, the ICU physician sees rapid heart rate and low oxygen saturation. That is Level 1 Situation Awareness. That Level 1 Situation Awareness determined the physician's mental model which allowed her to comprehend that the patient is in respiratory distress (Level 2 Situation Awareness) and project that he may die without an intervention. This is an example of Bottoms-Up Situation Awareness where what you perceive determines what mental model you select which determines what you comprehend and project.

There is also Top-Down Situation Awareness where your goal determines what mental model you select which determines what you should perceive, comprehend, and project. In the clinical scenario when the ICU charge nurse briefed the ICU physician that Mr. Lopez had COPD, diabetes, and hypertension and presented with respiratory distress, the goal of determining if COPD, diabetes, or hypertension contributed to the respiratory distress told the ICU physician to activate a mental model to determine if any of those conditions or even an infection was causing the distress. In this case, the mental model tells the ICU physician what to perceive to determine what is happening.

Any mental model, whether Top-Down or Bottoms-Up, will have feedback indications. Feedback indications are perceptions that either confirm, or disconfirm, a Level 2 comprehension or Level 3 projection. Back to our example, the ICU physician's mental model would tell her that the tube going through the vocal cords, color change on the end tidal CO2 detector, and mist in the tube indicate a good intubation (Level 2 Situation Awareness), but the presence of a low oxygen saturation would indicate that the Level 2 Situation Awareness might be wrong.

Summary Box 7.4
How Mental Models Affect and Are Affected by Situation Awareness

The relationship between situation awareness and mental models:

- What you perceive (Level 1 Situation Awareness) will tell you what mental model to use.
- Your mental model will tell you what you should and should not perceive.

7.2 How to Prevent "He Is Doing the Right Thing in the Wrong Situation"

Ideally, all team members would show up for their shift or task with correct, complete, and complementary STEP Mental Models covering every situation. In today's world of complexity and constant change, yesterday's mental model may no longer be adequate. Even if everyone had "good" mental models, are they the right ones? Back to our example, the ICU team did not know the status of the patient. What if the ICU physician activated the mental model for a patient with a fever, while one ICU nurse activated the mental model for a patient who was breathing comfortably, while a second ICU nurse activated the mental model for a patient requiring intubation? Each individual's mental models might be correct, complete, and complementary, but they may also be inappropriate for the situation. Every team member has the responsibility to make sure that all team members have the correct, complete, complementary, and valid mental models. A leader has three crucial opportunities to improve the team members' mental models: in the briefing (7.2.1), during the task (7.2.2), and in the debriefing (7.2.3). However, all team members have a responsibility to improve their own mental models, but also the mental models of others (7.2.4).

7.2.1 Role of the Leader in the Briefing[66]

The briefing may be the single most important tool to ensure that every team member has the full suite of mental models required for his or her responsibilities. Briefings are especially important for inexperienced team members, or ad hoc teams without strong Standard Operating Procedures. You cannot address every possible mental model, but you can spend a few minutes discussing those mental models that are the most crucial to success, most likely to be new to the team, or be characterized by gaps. You just have to make sure your briefing covers the important whats, whys, and hows to improve mental models.

A leader's goal in the briefing is that the team activates the right mental models and that the mental models are correct, complete, and complementary. The leader can make sure the team activates the right mental models in two ways. The first way is by telling them what mental models to activate (e.g., "We have a 52-year-old male in respiratory distress transitioning from ICU."). That statement tells the team to activate their respiratory distress mental models.[67] The second way is by telling them what to look for (trigger) to determine what mental model to activate (e.g., "Although I assume the patient is stable on ventilation, if we see oxygen saturation of 80%, we have to intubate immediately.").[68] That statement tells the team if

---

[66] Besides the formal leader, we are also considering the informal and situational leaders who must step up when they see a problem with mental models.

[67] It is "respiratory distress mental models," (plural) and not "respiratory distress mental model," (singular) because every member of the team has a different mental model based on each team member's role, knowledge, and experience.

[68] This is a perfect example why you must ensure the team activates the right mental model. That trigger (% oxygen saturation) is relative to the scenario itself. What type

they see 80%, they must change their mental models from monitoring ventilation to doing an intubation.

Checking that each team member has correct and complete mental models is more difficult because even for the same task, each team member has different mental models based on different goals, roles, responsibilities, and experiences. Even if a leader cannot check the mental models directly, a leader can check the outputs of the mental models. If the team perceive the same thing (same Level 1 Situation Awareness), do they comprehend (Level 2 Situation Awareness) and project (Level 3 Situation Awareness) the same thing? Modifying the scenario, what if the ICU physician had heard the fact that the Emergency Department (ED) team did not ask the patient about fever, rhinorrhea, or sick contacts, did not send any diagnostic studies, and the ED physician had not seen the patient in over an hour:

> ICU DOC: "The ED team has been very busy and did not have a lot of time with this patient. There are no diagnostic studies, so we don't have a good grasp on what is causing the respiratory distress and how it might progress, so my plan is…"

By stating a lack of Level 1 Situation Awareness (no diagnostic studies) and what it means now (Level 2 Situation Awareness: undetermined diagnosis), and in the future (Level 3 Situation Awareness: undetermined prognosis), if any team member thought that the plan did not adequately address that uncertainty, then someone's mental model may be wrong. The team must take time to figure out the right mental model.

Finally, a leader must check for complementary mental models by stating "What I expect from you…" and "What I expect to do for you…". If that does not match what the team member expects to do or receive, again, someone's mental model may be wrong. The team must take time to ensure complementary mental models.

---

of patient is experiencing the desaturation (e.g., normal cardiac/pulmonary anatomy/physiology versus cyanotic heart disease or COPD), whether the problem causing the desaturation is acute or chronic, whether the desaturation is precipitous or gradual, how much O2 the patient is receiving at the time, whether the patient is mechanically ventilated or not, what the patient's underlying disease state is, and so forth. If the leader had not briefed the specific percentage, team members with different mental models would have different percentages in their minds.

For ad hoc teams, especially when you know you have inexperienced team members (a very common event in academic medical centers), you may have to ask open-ended questions to check mental models. For example, you could check the first ICU nurse's Task Mental Model by asking "What will you be doing if we need to intubate?" You could check the respiratory therapist's Team Member Mental Model by asking "How can you back up the rest of the team during the intubation?" As a leader, you then need to actively listen to their answers, checking for hesitations and watching their body language, to ensure that they do have valid mental models.[69]

One comment we often hear is, "I don't have time to brief all that!". However, as the saying goes, "An ounce of prevention is worth a pound of cure." The time spent in a briefing to ensure that the task goes well by activating the correct, complete, complementary, and valid mental models will save time, and potentially lives, by preventing any threats or errors that would have occurred.

Summary Box 7.5
A Leader's Goals for Mental Models in the Briefing

Do you ensure that the team…

1. activates valid mental models, including
   - what mental models to use.
   - when to change mental models.
2. has correct and complete mental models, including
   - what to expect and let them compare their Level 2 and 3 Situation Awareness to yours.
3. has complementary mental models, including
   - what you need from them, and how, and what they will get from you, and how.

Make sure that any differences are resolved.

Let us now address the specific mental models in STEP that may need to be covered in the briefing.

[69] A necessary precondition for all this is psychological safety. Ad hoc and inexperienced team members have to feel safe to give an incomplete or even wrong answer without ridicule or reprimand. You have to stress that the purpose of your questions is to find mental models that need improvement.

7.2.1.1 Building Status Mental Models in the Briefing

The Status Mental Models relate to the Patient and the Task. You probably already do an excellent job building mental models on the patient. In our example, this can be done with a statement, such as: "Our patient is a 52-year-old male with respiratory distress on non-invasive ventilation. When he arrives, I want to check oxygen saturation to make sure the ventilation is adequate. I am most concerned about possible exacerbation caused by COPD, diabetes, hypertension or even infections. We must be prepared to intubate.".

The second Status Mental Model is Task, which includes both the procedure and equipment. You probably already do a good job explaining the procedure, but there may be areas for improvement. If your team has done that procedure before, especially recently and well, you might think discussing a procedure is not necessary. Before dismissing a discussion on a procedure, however, you need to recognize that the situation might be subtly different. Is this exactly the same situation or are there other circumstances that might be different and therefore influence whether the team is successful (or fails)? If previously successful, was the team successful because they performed at a high level, or were they just lucky? The discussion could be as simple as "Last time we were in this situation we had a mainstem intubation. So, this time we are going to …." Once the team knows the right way to do the task, they need to know what success looks like (i.e., how they can tell if things are going well). An example of this would be" "If we intubate, we should see increasing oxygen saturation within *X* seconds.". If oxygen saturation is increasing, the team knows they should continue. If things are not going as planned, they know that something might be wrong and that they need to tell you.

The second part of the Task Mental Model involves equipment, supplies, hardware, and software. Different models of hardware with different software, displays, alerts, and modes of failure can lead to confusion and are very common threats. You can discuss threats with your team with as little as "Seeing the tube go through the cords, color change on the detector, mist in the tube, and even apparent symmetric chest rise do not 100% tell us the intubation is successful". You also know the most likely errors that your team might make. An example might be: "The biggest error is trusting these confirming cues too heavily, and not treating any diminished breath sounds found during auscultation as a sign of a bad intubation."

By the end of the Task discussion, all the team members know what you want done, and how, how to tell whether the task is going as planned or not, and what to do if it is not.

7.2.1.2 Building Team Mental Models in the Briefing

The Team Mental Model includes both Team Members and Teamwork. The Team Member Mental Model is about knowing the strengths and weaknesses of your team, the stressors under which they operate, and how to prevent, avoid, or mitigate those stressors. Because you are also a member of the team, you need to know your own strengths, weaknesses, and stressors. Unless you work with the same people every day on the same tasks, or your organization has very strong Standard Operating Procedures, you will also have to discuss everyone's roles and responsibilities (who does what, when, and how). This means that team members must understand the necessary task intersections (how does what I do affect you, and vice versa) and team interactions (what do I know that you need to know, and vice versa). This is vital if you have ad hoc teams, or you want things done your way. In the scenario, if the two ICU physicians have never worked together before, ICU DOC #1 may not know how comfortable ICU DOC #2 is with intubations. ICU DOC #1, if actively listening, will later get an indication of ICU DOC #2's comfort level when she sounds unsure (i.e., saying "I think so…") when asked if the tube is in.

The Teamwork Mental Model is how individuals operate as a team. We believe that involves using CRM. The Teamwork Mental Model may be the most difficult mental model to build, unless your organization and team already have a strong CRM philosophy, policies, training, and practices. Unless you have those strong organizational underpinnings, you need to mention your CRM expectations, standards, techniques, errors and best practices in your briefing.[70]

7.2.1.3 Building Environment Mental Models in the Briefing

The Environment Mental Model includes everything outside of your team and the patient. It could be the fact that this is the last hour of a long shift that included motor vehicle accidents and traumatic brain injuries, or that the family has made a past decision on instituting aggressive care, or the hospital's policies that might affect how your team performs a task.

---

[70] See Section 9.2.7 for an example.

Regardless, if there is anything outside your team and the patient that adversely affects your team's ability to perform effectively, you have to highlight those threats, what they might look like, how they might affect your team, and how to prevent, avoid, or mitigate any problems that they cause.

7.2.1.4 Building Progress Mental Models in the Briefing

The Progress Mental Model includes schedules, any time-to-effect, and margin. Schedules include both individual and team schedules. If your team has tasks that must be done by a specific time, or tasks that are dependent on other tasks, then make sure your team knows them. Time-to-effect is how long before something (bad) happens. In our example, the physician should have briefed the team that if attempts at intubation cannot be completed within 30 seconds, they need to be aborted, and the patient ventilated with an ambu bag before the next attempt is made. How much time has passed? Margin is how much a critical data parameter can increase or decrease before you reach a trigger. In our example, the team might decide that if oxygen saturation falls below 80%, regardless of time, they would need to go to Plan B. How close is the oxygen saturation to 80%? The ICU physician should have also briefed her team on who was going to monitor the time, and margin.

As you discuss the various mental models, actively listen for any questions, and watch for any signs that your team members may have different mental models.

Summary Box 7.6
Your Briefing Builds the Right Mental Models

Does your briefing…

- cover all types of mental models: Status, Team, Environment and Progress (STEP)?
- provide more detail for any mental models that are crucial, error-prone, or new?
- cover CRM expectations, standards, and best practices?
- include open-ended questions to the team to ensure that their mental models are correct?

7.2.1.5 Codifying Mental Models to Reduce Cognitive Load

Mental models can be codified into artifacts, or aids such as whiteboards, overhead displays, or procedures. The goal of codifying is to free up working memory, and to prevent errors when under stress. For example, some Neonatal ICUs use a Neonatal Resuscitation Program algorithm. While not mentioned specifically in our scenario, another example would be illness scripts, where the Level 1, 2 and 3 Situation Awareness items can be documented. What artifacts do you have, or can you make, to codify your mental models?

7.2.2 Role of the Leader During the Task

A leader ensures good mental models by monitoring the actions of the team during the task and looking for signs that someone's mental model may be wrong. Here are some indications of wrong mental models and how to correct them:

1) If you notice an action incongruous to your mental model, ask why the team member did that action. Knowing why is important, because their answer gives you insight into the team member's mental model and where any possible gaps or errors might be. If the team member's mental model is indeed wrong, take time to explain the what, the how, and the why to build a better, more complete mental model for the team member.

2) If the team member looks or sounds confused, treat that as sign of a possibly wrong or incomplete mental model. You should ask a few open-ended, non-confrontational questions to see if there is a mental model problem, and then spend a few seconds improving it.

Table 7.1
List of Possible Open-Ended Questions to Check Mental Models

How do you see this happening?
What do you expect the results to be?
How do you interpret …?
What challenges or obstacles do you anticipate?
What other information do you think is important?
Who else do you think we need to involve?
What could make this no longer a priority?
What are your thoughts?
How do you go about…?
Why is this happening?

3) If a team member has the courage to expose him or herself to possible ridicule by "asking a stupid question", you should respect that courage not only by answering the immediate question, but also by using that question to indicate potential gaps in a mental model, and then spending a few seconds to improve the mental model.

4) If a team member asks you questions about your decisions and actions, you must provide the rationale for your decisions and actions. By doing that, you let them see into your mental models, which they can then compare to theirs. You will not know if there is a difference in mental models, however, unless you explicitly ask them if their mental models or assumptions differ from yours. Team members' willingness to talk about their mental models depends on you creating psychological safety for it and by praising individuals who do talk about their mental models.

5) If you fear that your organization's culture may make team members reluctant to question you, you might tell your team to not let you make a mistake that will hurt a patient. The most important approach to prevent and mitigate an error in mental models may be by admitting you might make an

error. How do you respond when your team member thinks you are making an error? You could rely on rank, title, or seniority to show that you could not possibly be wrong. Or you could ask those open-ended questions and use active listening to find out why the team member thought you were wrong, determine which mental model was wrong, and fix that mental model. You could also proactively invite others to support you. An excellent but short CRM briefing could go, "My mental models are very good, but still have some gaps in them. Hopefully, your mental models can cover those gaps, and my mental models can also cover gaps in yours." By the way, if you will not consider that you might be wrong, then you might as well forget CRM. If you believe you are immune to errors, you will not develop the psychological safety for your team members to question you, or to admit their own errors.

Summary Box 7.7
The Role of the Leader During the Task

Do you…

- monitor for errors, and "strange" questions and actions.
- treat every error, sign of confusion and inquiry as an opportunity to improve a mental model.
- explain your rationale so that the team can see your mental model.
- admit your mental model is incomplete and might be wrong.

7.2.3 The Role of a Leader in the Debriefing

The third tool to ensure good mental models is the debriefing. Without debriefing, experience alone can be inefficient and even counterproductive. Unless trained in self-discovery and self-correction, everyone will need help via debriefing to see how each experience is slightly different and how each difference may require a slightly different response. What is different about treating a 52-year-old male with COPD, diabetes, and hypertension versus a 34-year-old pregnant female with hypertension? Without debriefing, a physician might fail to appreciate the important differences and manage the interventions in the same manner. Worse yet, the physician might make mistakes but still be successful, thus reinforcing an inaccurate mental model that might eventually result in patient harm. In our scenario, the team failed to do a debriefing, so none of that learning occurred.

After the task, the team must take a few minutes to discuss where their mental models were wrong or incomplete. Why did they miss that indication? Why did they not comprehend or project correctly? Why did they not anticipate a threat or error? The team should look at what went well and poorly in all STEP Mental Models. For example, did

- multiple team members miss indications that should have told them that the patient was in trouble? (Status/ Patient Mental Model)
- your team not know why they were doing a procedure, and then became distracted by lower priority tasks? (Status/Task Mental Model)
- they not recognize that a team member was stressed, and then not provide back-up support before that person made an error? (Team/Team Member Mental Model)
- a team member fails to inquire when he or she did not understand why the leader was doing a task? (Team/ Teamwork Mental Model [i.e., CRM])
- the team fail to appreciate the impact of being at the end of a long shift marked by multiple emergencies? (Environment Mental Model)
- a team member fails to notify the team that a task was complete? (Progress/Schedule Mental Model)
- the team fail to monitor the time or margin before something bad happened? (Progress/Time-to-Effect or Margin Mental Model)

A common, but major, debriefing error is to only find a very specific fix to a very specific error. Modifying the scenario, let us assume that the ED physician tried to multitask by doing a handover while performing Positive Pressure Ventilation (PPV). This multitasking resulted in slower than required ventilation rates, a very specific error. A very specific fix would be to increase ventilation rates to 40 breaths per minute. The bigger problem, however, was in the physician's Team Member Mental Model, specifically, his mental model of how his memory and attention work. The physician thought that he could deliver the PPV and the handover simultaneously (i.e., multitask). Luckily for the physician, a nurse's Team Member Mental Model told her that people who attempt multitasking make errors and, therefore, she provided back-up support by monitoring the ventilation rate. In the debriefing, besides commending the nurse for her back-up support, the physician should discuss common errors that occur while multitasking, and what can be done to reduce errors, such as giving some tasks away or asking for back-up support. The physician could extend the debriefing to include high workload, distractions, or interruptions. The physician could also ask other team members what techniques they use to both recognize those situations and how they handle them.

Another example might be seen in a transport situation. The team has to decide between various transport methods. An error in that situation is to not set a definite time for the patient to be at the next facility. The very specific fix would be to say that the patient has to arrive by midnight. The bigger problem might have been a Teamwork (CRM) Mental Model problem if a nurse wondered how they would know if they could afford to wait another hour, but, simultaneously, did not know how best to ask this question. What about the physician's leadership style or the nurse's followership prevented the nurse from asking? The team could also talk about how their communication protocols facilitate, or discourage, inquiry and assertiveness and then discuss alternative strategies for making their communication more effective. By the end of the debriefing, the team should have a better Teamwork Mental Model.

The goal of a CRM portion of a debriefing is not to assess blame, but to fix CRM behaviors or mental model gaps before the next task or shift.

Summary Box 7.8
The Role of Debriefing in Building Mental Models

Does the team…
- address possible problems in all Status-Team-Environment-Progress (STEP) Mental Models?
- extend their debrief beyond specific fixes for specific problems to address gaps in mental models?
- leverage the ideas of the entire team to find techniques and ways to improve?

7.2.4 The Role of Team Members

So far, in Section 7.2, we have only discussed the role of a leader. Every member of the team has a responsibility to ensure correct, complete, complementary, and valid mental models. You have an obligation to inquire when something does not make sense, and then advocate and, if required, assert until any differences are resolved. You must inquire, advocate, and assert if:

- during the briefing, the leader says something that does not match your mental models (e.g., wrong task to do, different projected

outcomes, or you do not understand who, what, when, or how to communicate).
- during the task, any team member (including the leader) is doing something that you did not expect.
- during the debriefing, any team member (including the leader) says something that you do not understand.

While inquiring, advocating, and asserting, you must actively listen and have an open mind in case it is your mental model that is wrong. You may find it useful to ask for help from your leader, mentor, or expert during your time off to improve your mental models.

Chapter Debriefing

I want to call a quick STAR (Stop-Think-Act-Review): get off your email, stop your side conversations, and turn off the television.[71] Let's see if you can expand upon these statements:

- Use the briefing to ensure the correct, complete, complementary, and valid mental models are activated covering all of Status-Team-Environment-Progress (STEP).
- During the task, check for signs that team members may have different situation awareness or mental models.
- During the debriefing, go beyond specific fixes to specific problems to address underlying problems for all STEP Mental Models.
- Every team member has the responsibility to inquire, advocate and assert if there is a possible mismatch of mental models.

If this was an actual debriefing, we would ask you to expand further on each of these statements. Depending on your response, we would ask open-ended follow-up questions until we were sure you understood the material and had a plan to implement one or more best practices. We might ask, 'What is a specific mental model problem that you experience on your job?' We would not be satisfied if you said, "Our mental models aren't as good as we need." Again, we would ask open-ended follow-up questions until you might say, "We have a problem with new team members not having valid mental models." We would then ask, "What can you do to fix that problem prior to your next shift?" You might say, "I will use the briefing to

[71] See Chapters 11-15 for information on STAR.

discuss what mental models we need, but also what might tell us to change mental models. During the shift, if team members are making errors, then I need to call a quick STAR to correct any mental model problems. During the debriefing, we need to find out how our mental models diverged." We might then ask, "That helps your team. How can you help other teams?" We would then continue to ask open-ended follow-up questions until you might say, "We need to modify our briefing guide to discuss how and why what we are doing supports our goals, and possible threats to those goals."

Now that everyone on your team has the situation awareness and mental models to do their tasks, you need to know the best way to communicate that knowledge to your team. Communicating is the next chapter.

References

Cohen, Marvin S., Jared T. Freeman, and Steve Wolf. "Metarecognition in Time-Stressed Decision Making: Recognizing, Critiquing, and Correcting." Human Factors: The Journal of the Human Factors and Ergonomics Society 38, no. 2 (1996): 206–19. https://doi.org/10.1518/001872096779048020.

DeChurch, Leslie A., and Jessica R. Mesmer-Magnus. "The Cognitive Underpinnings of Effective Teamwork: A Meta-Analysis." Journal of Applied Psychology 95, no. 1 (2010): 32–53. https://doi.org/10.1037/a0017328.

Dekker, Sidney. Drift into Failure from Hunting Broken Components to Understanding Complex Systems. London: CRC Press, 2016.

Endsley, Mica R., and Daniel J. Garland. Situation Awareness: Analysis and Measurement. Boca Raton: CRC Press, 2008.

Klein, Gary A., Roberta Calderwood, and Anne Clinton-Cirocco. "Rapid Decision Making on the Fire Ground." Proceedings of the Human Factors Society Annual Meeting 30, no. 6 (1986): 576–80. https://doi.org/10.1177/154193128603000616.

Rouse, William B., and Nancy M. Morris. "On Looking into the Black Box: Prospects and Limits in the Search for Mental Models." Psychological Bulletin 100, no. 3 (1986): 349–63. https://doi.org/10.1037/0033-2909.100.3.349.

PART 1B.

COMMUNICATING, LEADING AND FOLLOWING, AND MUTUALLY SUPPORTING

Briefing[72]

I want to call a quick STAR (Stop-Think-Act-Review): get off your email, stop your side conversations, and turn off the television.[73] Here is what we will do in the next three chapters. We will discuss how team members communicate, what leaders and followers do to enable CRM, and, finally, how team members support each other to prevent errors. We will be successful if you can describe:

- communicating in terms of Delivery, Protocols and Confirmation (Chapter 8);
- the responsibilities of a leader and follower to enable CRM (Chapter 9); and
- how team members in healthcare can overcome organizational and cultural issues to better support each other (Chapter 10).

The primary threat that you might experience is the introduction of a large number of concepts and terms, some of which you may have never encountered, and some of which you may think about in a different sense. We will therefore explicitly define and differentiate each term and concept. We also realize how busy you are. We will make sure that the chapter is

---

[72] We will use the chapter briefing format throughout the book. You may feel the repeated use is redundant. However, we believe that it is important to continue to emphasize that a good briefing builds mental models by discussing what is happening, what success looks like, and what threats or errors are possible and how you plan to prevent, avoid, or mitigate them. Hence, the repetitive nature is meant to cement this belief with an understanding that you will also immerse yourself in this book on an irregular and/or intermittent basis. For more information on briefings and how this briefing embeds into CRM concepts, see Section 14.2.

[73] For more information on STAR, see Chapters 11-15.

short enough to be read in approximately thirty minutes. Finally, we provide Summary Boxes. The Summary Boxes serve two functions. First, they emphasize the take-home points in each section, and you can use them to check your understanding of those take-home points. Second, you can use them to determine if you and your team are implementing those take-home points. If a Summary Box does not make sense to you or you do not understand one or more take-home points, then review the related material before continuing to the next section.

Did I miss anything? Any concerns? Any questions? (Pause) No? Then, let's get started.

List of Abbreviations

BP	Blood Pressure
DOC	Attending Physician
HR	Heart Rate
MET	Medical Emergency Team
NUR	Nurse
ONC	Oncology
RES	Resident
RT	Respiratory Therapist

Personnel Involved in Scenario
Oncology Team - ONC DOC, ONC NUR, ONC RES
Medical Emergency Team – MET DOC, MET NUR, MET RT

Let us start with a scenario that will illustrate good and bad examples of Communicating, Leading and Following, and Mutually Supporting. We will use this scenario as we discuss these CRM skills further in Chapters 8-10.

This is the fifth night shift in a row for the Oncology resident. The team recently completed night rounds, and the Oncology resident was just about to settle in for a brief nap.

[Beep, Beep, Beep! The Oncology resident looks at the pager, then picks up the phone, and dials.]

ONC RES: "Hi, this is the Oncology Resident returning a page."

ONC NUR: "Hi doctor, this is the nurse for Mrs. Jackson. I was calling because she has had abnormal blood pressure readings. I repeated it several times but get the same abnormal results. Can you come and assess her?"

ONC RES: "Yes, I'll come right over."

The Oncology resident heads to the Oncology ward and encounters the Oncology nurse as he arrives at the bedside.

ONC NUR: "Hi doctor, thanks for coming so quickly. Mrs. Jackson's blood pressures (BP) are low. I have checked them 3 times, about 15 minutes apart. I also tried different extremities and even changed out the BP cuff. But the result is consistently 90-95 over 50-55. She is otherwise responsive, follows commands and is warm and well perfused."

ONC RES: "Okay, let me perform a manual measurement to verify."

The Oncology resident gets the manual sphygmomanometer, performs a manual BP measurement on Mrs. Jackson, and gets a result of 89 over 49. The Oncology resident then goes to review Mrs. Jackson's electronic medical record.

ONC RES: "After hearing your concerns, examining Mrs. Jackson and reviewing her chart, I am very concerned. I noticed her heart rate (HR) has been steadily rising and BP declining over the past 24 hours. I also noticed that her sats were relatively lower at the start of your shift and she was started on oxygen via nasal cannula."[74]

ONC NUR: "Yes, I was assigned to Mrs. Jackson last night, and her sats are relatively lower. She dipped into the upper 80s, so I had the respiratory therapist (RT) place her on oxygen. It happened while she was sleeping so I didn't think much of it."

ONC RES: "I wouldn't have either, but now add low BPs and an elevated HR in a patient with cancer receiving chemotherapy through a

---

[74] Oxygen saturation percentage.

central line. I am very concerned that Mrs. Jackson may be developing septic shock. I think we should call the medical emergency response team (MET) but let me speak to the Oncology attending first."

The Oncology resident calls the Oncology attending, ONC DOC.

ONC RES [speaking in a rushed manner, and with a nervous tone]: "Sorry to disturb you but the bedside nurse called me about soft BPs on Mrs. Jackson she tried several retakes and did some troubleshooting but kept getting the same reading so I did a manual BP and verified that her reading was accurate her exam is fine but when I looked at the trend of her vitals there has been a significant change…"

ONC DOC: "Sorry to interrupt you, you seem concerned, but I am not quite understanding what exactly you are concerned about. Take a moment to collect yourself and take a deep breath. I know residents do several nights in a row in our ward, which is challenging."

The Oncology resident takes an audible deep breath.

ONC DOC: "Good job…now, on the Oncology ward we like to use the SBAR format to communicate concerns about acute issues. Are you familiar with the SBAR format?"

ONC RES: "Yes, I do recall that was mentioned in our orientation. Sorry, let me try again."

ONC DOC: "Sure, go ahead."

ONC RES: "Okay so the situation is that I was called about soft BPs on Mrs. Jackson…"

ONC DOC: "Okay, what do you mean by soft"?

ONC RES: "I got a manual reading of 89 over 49 which is lower than what she usually is…"

ONC DOC: "Correct. Okay, so she is relatively hypotensive as she actually has hypertension at baseline. Go on…"

ONC RES: “Her background is that she was recently diagnosed with cancer on this admission, and is receiving her first cycle of chemotherapy. She also has a history of hypertension, as you mentioned. My assessment is that I am very concerned about septic shock in a patient with cancer receiving chemotherapy through a central line who then develops hypotension, an elevated HR, and a need for oxygen. My recommendation would be to call the MET.”

ONC DOC: “Well done. So based on the patient’s background and current vital signs, you think she has developed shock from an infection of which her central line is the most likely source. “

ONC RES: “Yes.”

ONC DOC: “I agree with your recommendation, and you should draw cultures from her central line and start antibiotics. You should also consider cardiogenic shock as an alternative diagnosis, as Mrs. Jackson is at risk for cardiotoxicity from her chemotherapy. Did she have a gallop rhythm on your cardiac exam?”

ONC RES: “I don’t think so, but I’ve only read about it and have never heard it, so I could have missed that.”

ONC DOC: “Okay, well, call the MET and be sure to mention that nuance. I am leaving my house to drive into the hospital now.”

ONC RES: “Okay, will do. Thank you.” [to the ONC NUR] “Can you initiate the call to the MET?”

ONC NUR: “ Yes.″

While the Oncology resident was updating Mrs. Jackson’s wife on the phone, the MET arrives at Mrs. Jackson’s bedside. The Oncology nurse communicates a similar SBAR to the MET, who then go into the room to evaluate Mrs. Jackson. The Oncology nurse and resident also go into the room, trailing behind the MET. The Oncology resident finds the corner of the room and stands there observing the team around Mrs. Jackson’s bedside.

MET DOC: "Hi Mrs. Jackson, I am MET DOC and my team was called because there is concern about your blood pressure. How are you feeling?"

Mrs. Jackson: "Okay, but in the past hour or so, I have been feeling a bit more weak, tired, and short of breath than usual."

Each member of the MET performs their individual assessments.

MET DOC [to MET NUR]: "Her extremities feel cold, and pulses are weak. What are her vitals?"

MET NUR [to MET DOC]: "She is afebrile, her HR is 110 beats per minute, her BP is 80 over 50, and her respiratory rate is 21 breaths per minute."

MET DOC [to MET NUR]: "And her respiratory support?"

MET RT [to MET DOC]: "She is on 4 liters via nasal cannula. Should I put her on a non-rebreather?"

MET DOC [to MET RT]: "Yes."
[to MET NUR and MET RT]: "Okay, I am going to repeat what we discussed on the way over, as we have new personnel that are helping us." [MET NUR and MET RT both nod to MET DOC]

MET DOC [while making eye contact and looking at each team member in the room]: "My name is MET DOC and I will be leading this resuscitation. Mrs. Jackson has a rapid HR, hypotension, cold extremities, and weak pulses. This is concerning for septic shock in the context of her cancer diagnosis and chemotherapy via a central line."
[to MET NUR] "Let's give a 1-liter normal saline bolus."
[returns to addressing each team member in the room] "It is impossible for me to hear, see, and know everything so, as we go, I expect anyone and everyone to communicate any information or observations and what it might mean, to actively listen to our dialogue, and to work together to accomplish our plan while looking out for each other."
[makes eye contact with the ONC RES, who nervously withdraws further into the corner] " And you are?"

ONC RES [nervously responds]: "The Oncology Resident."

MET DOC [to ONC RES]: “Oh, great. Do you know this patient well?”

ONC RES [shakingly]: “Uh…well…yes, I have taken care of her for the past 4 nights.”

MET NUR [to MET DOC]: “1-liter normal saline bolus completed.”

MET DOC [to MET NUR]: “1 liter NS bolus in, got it. Assess her response to the bolus.″

MET NUR re-examines Mrs. Jackson.
[to ONC RES]: “Oh, really? Well do you have any insight or anything further to contribute that will help us care for Mrs. Jackson?”

ONC RES [hesitantly]: “Um…”

MET DOC [to ONC RES]: “Listen, if you are not sure that what you’re thinking is helpful, or not, I would rather hear it than not hear it, as it could influence how I care for Mrs. Jackson.”

ONC RES [to MET DOC]: “Okay, well, I spoke to the Oncology attending and it was mentioned that we should also consider cardiogenic shock as an alternative diagnosis, as Mrs. Jackson is at risk for cardiotoxicity from her chemotherapy.”

MET NUR [to MET DOC]: “I do hear crackles on her lung exam and a gallop rhythm on her cardiac exam.”

MET DOC [to ONC RES]: “That is very helpful information.”

MET DOC [to the team members in the room]: “OK everyone, we were just informed that Mrs. Jackson is at risk for cardiotoxicity because of her chemotherapy regimen. So, Mrs. Jackson’s shock has a cardiogenic component but may or may not have an infectious etiology. This changes our management strategy. We must be judicious with fluid boluses and give only 250-500 milliliters at a time and re-examine her for clinical worsening. We should also start a norepinephrine infusion.”
[to ONC RES]: “Order a norepinephrine infusion at 2 micrograms per minute.”

ONC RES: “Okay.”

MET DOC [to MET NUR]: “Call the cardiac intensive care unit and tell them we need a bed ASAP for Mrs. Jackson.”

MET NUR [to MET DOC]: “Calling now.”

CHAPTER 8

COMMUNICATING

Chapter Briefing[75]

I want to call a quick STAR (Stop-Think-Act-Review): get off your email, stop your side conversations, and turn off the television.[76] Here is what we will do in this chapter. We will discuss the CRM skill Communicating—how team members pass information to one another. We will be successful if you can explain:

- how proper delivery and protocols improve encoding (Sections 8.2 and 8.3);
- how 3-Way Communication and Active Listening improve decoding (Section 8.4); and
- the best practices to ensure good communication (Section 8.6).

The primary threat that you might experience is the introduction of a large number of concepts and terms, some of which you may have never encountered, and some of which you may think about in a different sense. We will therefore explicitly define and differentiate each term and concept. We also realize how busy you are. We will make sure that the chapter is short enough to be read in approximately thirty minutes. Finally, we provide Summary Boxes. The Summary Boxes serve two functions. First, they emphasize the take-home points in each section, and you can use them to check your understanding of those take-home points. Second, you can use

---

[75]By now, you may feel that repeated use of the chapter briefing format is redundant. However, we believe that it is important to continue to emphasize that a good briefing builds mental models by discussing what is happening, what success looks like, and what threats or errors are possible and how you plan to prevent, avoid, or mitigate them. Hence, the repetitive nature is meant to cement this belief with an understanding that you will also immerse yourself in this book on an irregular and/or intermittent basis.

[76] For more information on STAR, see Chapters 11-15.

them to determine if you and your team are implementing those take-home points. If a Summary Box does not make sense to you or you do not understand one or more take-home points, then review the related material before continuing to the next section.

Did I miss anything? Any concerns? Any questions? (Pause) No? Then, let's get started.

List of Abbreviations

CRM	Crew Resource Management
CUS	Concerned-Uncomfortable-Safety
DESC	Describe-Express-Suggest-Consequences
DOC	Doctor (physician)
ED	Emergency Department
MET	Medical Emergency Team
NASA	National Aeronautics and Space Administration
NUR	Nurse
SBAR	Situation-Background-Assessment-Recommendation
STAR	Stop-Think-Act-Review
STEP	Status-Team-Environment-Progress

Communication is the act or process of using words, sounds, signs, or behaviors to express or exchange information or to express your ideas, thoughts, feelings, etc., to someone else.[77] It can be verbal (conversation via face-to-face interaction, phone, video conference), written (an email, letter, form), visual (facial expressions, body language, hand signal), or even physical (a hand on the shoulder, pat on the back). We will concentrate on verbal communication because most teams operating in most environments rely on verbal communication to exchange information and it is a big part of how healthcare is provided. In this chapter, you will learn what is and is not a Communicating error (Section 8.1), how communication is delivered (Section 8.2), under what protocols (Section 8.3), and how understanding is confirmed (Section 8.4). You will also learn about Communication Demons (Section 8.5) and best practices to defeat them (Section 8.6).

[77] Merriam Webster dictionary citation.

8.1 When a Communicating Error Is Not a Communicating Error

We communicate every day, yet poor communication is an oft-cited team deficiency. We will consider Communicating errors solely in terms of Delivery, Protocols, and Confirmation errors, therefore many of the instances classified as "poor communication" are not Communicating errors at all. Instead, they are really errors in Exchanging Information, Leading and Following, or Mutually Supporting that are only noticed when someone articulates them while communicating. Here are examples where an error in other CRM skills may be characterized incorrectly as a Communicating error:

a. Exchanging Information
   - Not communicating the right information in all levels (Perception, Comprehension and Projection) and in all areas (Status, Team, Environment and Progress [STEP]).[78] The real error may be the Exchanging Information error of not knowing what to communicate.
   - Not communicating the information to the right team member. The real error may be the Exchanging Information error of not knowing with whom to communicate.

b. Leading
   - Not communicating using the proper protocols. The real error may be the leader's failure to brief, model, or provide feedback on Communicating expectations and standards.
   - Not communicating when a team member has a question or is unsure of an instruction. The real error may be the leader's failure to establish and maintain a climate of psychological safety to inquire.

c. Following
   - Not communicating another course of action in a convincing but respectful manner. The real error may be a follower not advocating and asserting properly.

d. Mutually Supporting
   - Not communicating when a team member makes an error. The real error may be team members did not know when or how to support each other.

---

[78] See Section 2.4 for more information on STEP.

Failure to differentiate true Communicating errors from errors in other CRM skills results in poor mitigation efforts. Even experienced instructors sometimes fail to differentiate. Let us see if you can differentiate a true Communicating error from an error in another CRM skill articulated in this example: a nurse and physician agree that should a patient's potassium level become greater than 7 meq/L (milliequivalents per liter), the nurse will call the physician to inform her of the result. Here are three different scenarios:

1. The nurse calls the physician to inform her that the potassium level is 4.2 meq/L.
2. The nurse texts the physician that the potassium level is 7.5 meq/L.
3. The nurse calls the physician and states "You wanted me to call you if the potassium level was greater than 7 meq/L. What do you want to do?"

We consider Communicating errors occurred in the second example (wrong protocol: text versus phone call) and third example (poor delivery: the nurse did not mention actual potassium level) but not in the first example (wrong information: the nurse called but the potassium level was less than 7 meq/L). The first example (wrong information) is a knowledge issue: the nurse did not remember what the right potassium level was, and no amount of Communicating training can help that. Communicating training can help in the second and third examples. In our CRM model, Communicating is not about content, or about what information you exchange. Instead, Communicating is about how information in your head gets passed to your team member's head, or how it is encoded and decoded. Why is this distinction important? If you cannot differentiate content errors from Communicating errors, you may implement the wrong solution (e.g., more format training for a content problem, or more situation awareness training for a delivery problem).

Summary
Box: 8.1
Differentiating a Communicating Error from other CRM Errors

Does your team treat a problem in…
• content or what is communicated as a problem in Exchanging Information, Leading and Following, or Mutually Supporting?
• how information is communicated as a problem in how to encode or decode?

"The single biggest problem in communication is the illusion that it has taken place."[79] Let us consider the Communicating process to find where problems may occur. The sender encodes the message and transmits it, and the receiver receives it and decodes it. We will disregard environmental factors such as high ambient noise levels or poor acoustics as threats that the team must address in their planning and execution. We will concentrate on how CRM helps reduce encoding and decoding errors. In CRM, Communicating can be broken down to A) Delivery, B) Protocols, and C) Confirmation. Delivery and Protocols help with better encoding. Confirmation helps with better decoding.

8.2 Delivery

Delivery is all about "the adjectives and adverbs". Delivery that is timely, accurate, clear, concise, confident, consistent, professional, proactive, objective, tailored, and targeted will better encode the message. Let us cover each one of these in some detail.

Timely is about passing the information at the right time; not so early that it is forgotten and not so late that it is no longer needed. In our scenario, the Oncology nurse's communication with the Oncology resident was timely. The Oncology resident's communication to the MET physician was not, which then required the MET physician to change the management strategy.

Accurate implies that the details are correct. The Oncology nurse stated that the blood pressure results were "90 to 95 over 50 to 55."

Clear is about using terms that are not confusing, ambiguous or have different meanings to different individuals or organizations. Words such as "soft" are not clear. What blood pressure constitutes "soft"? The Oncology attending had to ask for clarification. Terms that are not well defined and well accepted across organizations can be very confusing. For example, those in the military joke about the differences in the meaning of the command "Secure the building". The Navy would turn out the lights and lock the doors. The Army would surround the building with defensive fortifications. The Marines would assault the building. The Air Force would take out a three-year lease.

---

[79] A quote usually attributed to George Bernard Shaw.

Concise is not about reducing the length of your message. It is about removing all words that provide no value. Let us critique a possible medic's call to Dispatch:

> "We are en route to your facility with a 28-year-old Caucasian woman in active labor at 34 weeks. Arrival time is 10 to 15 minutes. We'll be coming in through the ED, so please let the ED attending physician know and call me back if they want to talk."

We could remove non-value-added wording without losing any informational content:

> "Enroute direct to ED with 28-year-old Caucasian female, active labor at 34 weeks. Arrival time 10 to 15 minutes. Alert ED. Call back if required."

Note that 24 words were deleted without losing important information. Conciseness can be confused with reducing redundancy. Redundancy can be superfluous such as non-value-added repeating, but it can also help ensure that the message would be understood. Going back to the call "Female" and "Alert ED" could be considered redundant since only females can be in active labor and the medic already stated they were enroute to the ED; but the medic considered them important to ensure that the hospital knew who the patient was, and the necessary actions were taken in the ED.

Confident refers to expressing an appropriate level of certainty in your voice: not too little when you are sure of your information or position, and not too much when you are unsure.[80] Lack of confidence in your delivery of a recommendation will reduce the chances that it will be accepted. In our scenario, the Oncology resident did not sound confident to the MET physician. Luckily, the MET physician actively listened and caught that hesitancy and provided some psychological safety: "... if you are not sure that what you're thinking is helpful or not, I would rather hear it than not hear it…"

Consistent indicates that your words, tone, and body language are aligned. If your words say one thing but your tone or body language say another, do not be surprised if you get a lot of questions about what you mean.

---

[80] An aspect of Confidence will be covered in Assertiveness in Section 9.3.2.

Professional signifies that the content and style of your communication are appropriate for the standards, practices, and culture of your profession, organization, and team. In healthcare, where multiple professions and specialties work together on one team, challenges exist in deciding the most inclusive professional content and style. Depending on tone, phrases by the MET physician such as “Oh, great” or “Oh, really” could be perceived as dismissive or sarcastic. If so, it would diminish any psychological safety that a leader was trying to build.

Proactive implies that information is “pushed” rather than “pulled”. Ideally, you provide or push the information just before it is needed without being asked (having the information pulled). You might push it at the right time (one hour into the shift), in the right place in the timeline (right after Step 4 is done), or at the right trigger (if the heart rate does not increase). In our scenario, the MET physician had to ask for information from the Oncology resident. If a team member has to ask you for information, it is being pulled. Pushing allows people to have information before it is needed; pulling requires the person to stop and ask, possibly delaying an action.

Objective denotes that facts are being presented, not personal opinions disguised as facts. Professional opinions are required, but make sure that it is obvious that it is your assessment based on your situation awareness and mental model. In our scenario, the Oncology attending said, “…you should consider cardiogenic shock…”, expressing a professional opinion based on experience.

Tailored conveys that you are modifying your message based on to whom you are speaking: you use different wording when speaking to a new person with whom you have never worked (e.g., ad hoc teams), compared with the language you use when speaking to someone with whom you have worked for years (e.g., formed teams). Replacing medical terminology with lay terms when speaking with the patient and family is another example.

Targeted means that you are addressing questions and requests to specific individuals rather than making “overhead” statements or delivering “thin air” commands. In our scenario, the MET physician made an effort to make eye contact with anyone to whom she was talking.

Summary Box 8.2
Requirements for Communicating Delivery

Does your team deliver facts as facts and opinions as opinions (Objective) while communicating…
…to specific individuals (Targeted)?
…in a respectful manner (Professional)?
…before being asked (Proactive)?
…just before being needed (Timely)?
…exact details (Accurate)?
…using unambiguous wording (Clear)?
…with no superfluous terms (Concise)?
…with wording, tone, and body language aligned (Consistent)?
…commensurate with your certainty (Confident)?

8.3 Protocols

Communicating protocols are methods for passing on information that are agreed to by the organization, profession, or team to which one belongs. Protocols involve formats, terminology, and standard callouts. Formats refer to presenting all of the required information in a manner and sequence that the receiver expects to hear it. Note: format should be receiver-oriented, not sender-oriented. It is not about how you, as the sender, like to send information, but rather about how the receiver expects to receive it. The approved format enables better encoding because the sender knows what information must be included, and in what order. The approved format also enables better and faster decoding because the receiver is prepared to hear the expected information in an expected sequence. A commonly used format in healthcare to pass information about a patient is SBAR: Situation-Background-Assessment-Recommendation. In our scenario, the Oncology attending required the resident to use SBAR to help the resident determine what information to pass, and in what order. DESC (TeamSTEPPS Pocket Guide 2020, TK) is another format used in healthcare. Its specific purpose is to resolve a conflict.

Summary Box 8.3
DESC format

D: Describe the specific situation or behavior; provide concrete data. E: Express how the situation makes you feel/what are your concerns. S: Suggest other alternatives and seek agreement. C: Consequences should be stated in terms of impact on established team goals. Strive for consensus.

Format could also include conventions such as using the phonetic alphabet (Alpha for A, Bravo for B, etc.) and terminology such as CUS (TeamSTEPPS Pocket Guide 2020) to voice a concern:

I am Concerned!
I am Uncomfortable!
This is a Safety Issue!

Although teams may need to use different formats for different purposes, tasks, or activities, consistently using the same format for the same purpose, task or activity helps to ensure that your team communicates effectively.

Terminology refers to the correct use of words or terms while communicating. The same term should not apply to different objects or actions, or different terms should not apply to the same objects or actions, lest you receive something that is different than what you request. Terminology mismatches commonly occur when team members from different organizations, professions or cultures interact unless they have prior experience working with each other. Lexicons, or dictionaries, help teams develop common terminology.

A standard callout consists of specific information in a specific format given at a specific time (or position), generating a specific response. This is an example of a standard callout from the world of commercial aviation:

Co-pilot: "Passing 18,000 feet."
Captain: "Passing 18,000 feet, set altimeter 29.92."
Co-pilot: "Altimeter checked, 29.92."

Standard callouts build situation awareness. When the Co-pilot called, "Passing 18,000 feet" announcing that they were climbing through 18,000 feet in altitude, the Captain might not have realized that, so the callout fixed his or her situation awareness. Also, if the Co-pilot called "Passing 18,000 feet" and received either no response or a non-standard response (e.g., "Copy"), the Co-pilot would be cued to the possibility that the Captain may be overwhelmed or may not have understood the callout. There are also safety implications to standard callouts. Consider another example of an airline captain preparing to depart the gate and taxi out:

> Captain: "Ready for pushback."
> Ramp Leader: "Clear for pushback."[81]
> Captain: "Pushback now."

The Captain built the Ramp Leader's situation awareness that the Captain was ready to be towed away from the gate. That cued the Ramp Leader to check the position of all of the ramp personnel to make sure they were in safe positions. If either the Captain or the Ramp Leader did not hear the right words in the right format, he or she needed to ask questions in order to elicit clarifications.

An example of a standard call-out in healthcare is illustrated by the following communication between a physician who has just intubated a patient and a respiratory therapist who is confirming endotracheal tube placement:

Physician: "Tube through the cords."

Respiratory Therapist: "Breath sounds normal right, diminished left. Likely right mainstem intubation."

Physician: "Agree, likely right mainstem intubation. Will pull tube back 1 centimeter."

Respiratory Therapist: "Breath sounds normal left, normal right."

Physician: "Breath sounds now equal. Secure the tube in place."

Summary Box 8.4
Communicating Protocols

Does your team use…
• standard formats to help the sender know what information to hand over, and how, and help the receiver to know what information to expect, and how? • the same terms for the same thing, to prevent confusion? • standard callouts to build situation awareness?

---

[81] The Ramp Leader is the leader of the ground support team.

The ultimate protocol is sometimes called a Communication Plan, which is essentially a Communicating Standard Operating Procedure. A Communication Plan can be a formal document built by the organization days, weeks, or even years earlier that discusses all planned communications, including planned sender and receiver, content, format, and timing. A leader can then use the briefing to discuss any changes to the Communication Plan based on any unique circumstances. If the organization does not have a formal Communication Plan, the team could build their own during the briefing. Here is another airline example of a simplified Communication Plan/Standard Operating Procedure for the Pre-flight Briefing.

Summary Box 8.5
Simplified Example of Communication Plan for the Pre-Flight Briefing

	To: Captain	To: Co-pilot	To: Flight Attendants
From: Captain	X	Information on the flight using the Briefing Guide.	Information on the flight using the Briefing Guide.
From: Co-pilot	Expected status of various aircraft systems (e.g., fuel, weight, etc.), and any known non-standard situations. Provide recommendations to mitigate problems using DESC.	X	How any known non-standard situation might affect the cabin (e.g., high ambient temperature and lack of ground cooling will result in hot cabin temperatures until after engine start).
From: Flight Attendants	Expected status of various cabin systems and any non-standard situations. Provide recommendations to mitigate problems using DESC.	Provide recommendations to change system operations to mitigate problems using DESC.	X

We will cover other formats when we discuss Assertiveness in the Leading and Following chapter.

8.4 Confirmation

Whereas proper Delivery and Protocols help the sender to encode properly, Confirmation is about helping the receiver determine if he or she decoded properly. Confirmation is about making sure that the receiver heard properly and more importantly, actually understood the communication. Confirmation is the responsibility of both the sender, the one initiating the flow of information, and the receiver, the one receiving the information. Confirmation consists of 3-Way Communication and Active Listening.

3-Way Communication (in some professions and industries called 2-Way Communication, Closed Loop Communication, or Readback) proceeds as follows: the sender says something, the receiver repeats what he or she heard using his or her own words, and the sender then agrees or disagrees with the receiver's statement. This process confirms that the receiver actually heard and understood the sender's message. For example:

MET DOC: "Let's give a 1-liter saline bolus."
MET NUR: "1-liter normal saline bolus."
MET DOC: "Correct."

3-Way Communication only ensures that the receiver heard the sender, not that the receiver necessarily agrees with the sender. The sender must question whether 3-way communication is working when a receiver does, or says, any of the following:

- exhibits body language consistent with confusion or discomfort.
- repeats back what the sender said verbatim but cannot repeat it back in his or her own words.[82]
- uses verbal caveats ("I think you said…", "I believe you mean…", "If I get you correctly…").
- asks questions that indicate a lack of understanding.
- responds with "Okay," "Yes," "Copy," "Roger," "Wilco," or "Understood."

---

[82] There are times when verbatim repeat back is required, such as when exact numbers are required. Example: You say, "The code is 5-9-1"; I have to repeat verbatim "5-9-1".

The second part of Confirmation is Active Listening. Have you ever received a comment from a team member that seemed totally inappropriate for the situation? Did you just ignore it? Did you try to explain to the sender what he or she did not seem to comprehend? Or did you try to understand the why behind the sender's comment? If you made that effort to understand the why, you were actively listening. Active Listening involves attempting to discover what is going on in the sender's head and understand how that statement makes sense to him or her. When you are actively listening, you are considering the possibility that your team member might have seen or heard something that you did not (different situation awareness), or that your team member's knowledge or previous experience might explain his or her response (different mental model). Active Listening is much different than defensive listening (getting ready to argue), passive listening (failing to process), dismissive listening (immediately rejecting), not listening (completely ignoring), or takeover listening (listening for an opportunity to take over the conversation). Active Listening requires processing and keeping an open mind to the outsider's perspective. Active Listening also involves carefully observing body language and listening for changes in tone of voice, as well as questions and caveats that indicate whether or not your team members understand what you are saying.

Active Listening also lets the sender compare and check the receiver's situation awareness and mental models. Let us modify the earlier scenario and assume the Oncology nurse had mentioned to the MET nurse (but the MET physician did not hear) about the possibility of cardiogenic shock during their handover:

MET DOC: "Let's give a 1-liter normal saline bolus."
MET NUR: "1-liter normal saline bolus?"
MET DOC: "Yes. Why do you ask?"

By actively listening, the MET physician noticed that the response was a question, not a statement. The MET nurse's response showed that she was unsure of the amount or the need for the bolus. The physician asked an open-ended why question to understand the nurse's question. If the conversation had continued, the physician would have learned that the nurse questioned the bolus due to about the possibility of cardiogenic shock.
A slightly different communication follows:

MET DOC: "Let's give a 1-liter normal saline bolus."
MET NUR: "Roger."
MET DOC: "Confirm 1-liter normal saline bolus."

The physician gave an order, and the nurse stated “Roger”. The physician could have left it at that, but because she was actively listening, she readily picked up that she could not confirm whether the nurse understood the order. By telling the nurse to confirm the instruction, the physician recognized the possibility of a misunderstanding.

Third party active listening is Active Listening performed by someone outside of the immediate conversation. You do this when you realize that your team members are discussing two different issues, or are simply talking past one other without actually paying attention to what is being discussed by the other team members. Let us modify the scenario again, and presume that the Oncology resident was both third party active listening and, also, more assertive:

MET DOC (to MET NUR): “Let’s give a 1-liter normal saline bolus.”
ONC RES: “1-liter normal saline bolus?”
MET DOC: “Yes. Why do you ask?”

If the conversation had continued, the MET physician would have learned about the possibility of cardiogenic shock before giving a fluid bolus that was actually contraindicated.

In addition to detecting different mental models, Active Listening will help to identify differences in approach, values, experience, organization, culture, personality, and history. Active Listening is hard work. It requires that you not only follow someone else’s thinking but also ascertain why he or she may be right, too. In Chapter 3, we called this the "Power of And" (how might my mental model be right, And their mental model also be right?). If you actively listen and use the “Power of And”, you may develop an integrated mental model and situation awareness that is greater than the sum of the parts.

Summary Box 8.6
3-Way Communication and Active Listening

Does your team…
- use 3-way communication in which the receiver repeats back in his or her own words what he or she heard, followed by confirmation or corrections by the sender?
- use Active Listening to understand the underlying situation awareness and mental models behind a team member’s comment with the goal of improving the situation awareness and mental model?

8.5 Communicating Demons and How to Defeat Them

Here are some of the demons that make communicating difficult:

Stress: Probably the hardest time to communicate is when the team is stressed. It affects both the sender and receiver. The sender may fail to use the proper format or terminology. The receiver's working memory is overloaded and, therefore, may be capable of processing only one or two new data points. Because the receiver should not be expected to do much (if any) processing, the sender must simplify the message, reducing it in number of details and complexity, and be extremely specific with what is communicated. Let us modify what the Oncology attending said to reduce detail and complexity, and being more specific:

> ONC DOC: "Take a moment to collect yourself. Now, give me the information, in the SBAR format, starting with Situation."

Different backgrounds: The encoding and decoding of the sender and receiver can be compromised when senders and receivers use different languages, or, for whom English is a second language; come from a different culture, experience, or environment; have biases based on the race, gender, age, education, nationality, or organization of the listener; or resort to improper humor, slang, sarcasm, or emotion. In these situations, it is important that the sender quickly determine what potential limitations to encoding and decoding exist, and tailor the message as much as possible. Example: tailoring the explanation of your treatment plan when speaking to a family from a culture different from your own.

Different modes: Face-to-face Communicating allows you to see visual cues, such as body language, and auditory cues, such as tone of voice. Visual cues help to confirm understanding or raise awareness of miscommunication. While voice-only conversation is limited to auditory cues, 3-Way Communication can still be used. Both visual and auditory cues are lost with written communication. In addition, the delay between messages greatly hampers or even prevents 3-Way Communication. As more cues are lost, the opportunities to determine whether the sender's message is properly interpreted by the receiver are correspondingly diminished. Under these circumstances senders must make every effort to be clear and precise in their communication but also be aware that conciseness often must be sacrificed in order to provide a sufficient level of redundancy to increase the probability that they will be understood.

8.6 Best Practices to Ensure Good Communicating

During the briefing:

- Set the expectations for Communicating. In the scenario, the MET physician said:

  > "…I expect anyone and everyone to communicate any information or observations and what it might mean, to actively listen to our dialogue…"

- Plan out expected communication in terms of what is said, how and when it is said, and to whom. You can codify the content, format and any procedures in an informal or formal Communication Plan.

- Discuss possible environmental threats to Communicating such as high ambient noise levels or a highly stressful situation, as well as organizational threats such as working with new team members or using different protocols. It is important to note past errors made by your team, and other teams in similar situations. Also review how team members can determine whether a threat or error is materializing, and how to mitigate it before it causes more significant problems. In the scenario, the Oncology attending knew that the resident was probably tired from working five nights in a row.

- Discuss what protocols the team should follow in any error-prone, safety-critical tasks (e.g., SBAR, when fatigued).

When executing the task:

- Require 3-way Communication and model that behavior.
- Actively listen for signs indicating team members are not on the same page (i.e., do not possess the same mental model).
- Use opportunities to mentor or provide peer-to-peer feedback on proper delivery, protocols, and confirmation. In the scenario, the Oncology attending knew the resident was both tired from long hours and stressed to be in a new situation, so the attending used the opportunity to mentor the resident on the best way to hand over information.

During the debriefing, review lapses in delivery, protocols, and confirmation, and correct the immediate skill error, but also the gap in the mental model that caused it. Also address how to adapt that skill to different situations.[83]

Summary Box: 8.7
Communicating Best Practices

Does your team…
• use the briefing to prepare their communications by going over expected threats and errors, as well as the required formats and terminology? • use mentoring or feedback to fix Communicating errors in real time? • use the debriefing to improve each team member's Communicating Mental Model?

Chapter Debriefing

I want to call a quick STAR (Stop-Think-Act-Review): get off your email, stop your side conversations, and turn off the television.[84] Let's see if you can expand upon these statements:

- "Communicating error" too often, and wrongly, covers both errors in content and errors in delivery, protocols, or confirmation.
- Communicating as a CRM skill covers delivery, protocols and confirmation.
- Delivery must be timely, accurate, clear, concise, confident, consistent, professional, proactive, objective, tailored and targeted.
- Protocol refers to the proper use of format, terminology, and standard callouts.
- A Communication Plan is a pre-determined set of protocols (i.e., a Communicating Standard Operating Procedure).
- Confirmation is achieved via 3-Way Communication and Active Listening.
- There are best practices that a team can perform during the briefing, execution and debriefing to improve Communicating.

If this was an actual debriefing, we would ask you to expand further on each of these statements. Depending on your response, we would ask open-

[83] See the scenario in Part 2b, and Section B.5, for examples.

[84] See Chapters 11-15 for information on STAR.

ended follow-up questions until we were sure you understood the material and had a plan to implement one or more best practices. Finally, we might ask, “What is a specific communication problem that you experience on your job?” We would not be satisfied if you said, “We don’t communicate as well as we need.” Again, we would ask open-ended follow-up questions until you might say, “We have a problem with team members using different terms for the same object.” We would then ask, “What can you do on your next shift to make sure your team uses the right term?” We would then continue to ask open-ended follow-up questions until you might say, “I need to use the briefing to cover any new terms or terms that caused confusion in the past. During the shift, I can actively listen if anyone seems confused by a term. In the debriefing, we can go over any confusing terms and figure out what term we will use next shift.” We would then ask, “That helps your team, but what about other teams?” More open-ended questions until you might say, “I need to work with management to develop a lexicon.”

Reference

TeamSTEPPS: Pocket Guide: Strategies & Tools to Enhance Performance and Patient Safety. Bethesda, MD: U.S. Dept. of Health and Human Services, Agency for Healthcare Research and Quality, 2006.

CHAPTER 9

LEADING AND FOLLOWING

Chapter Briefing[85]

I want to call a quick STAR (Stop-Think-Act-Review): get off your email, stop your side conversations, and turn off the television.[86] In this chapter, we will discuss the CRM responsibilities of leaders and followers. We will be successful if you can:

- explain why CRM is important to you as a leader (Section 9.1);
- list actions you must do as a leader to fulfill your six CRM responsibilities (Section 9.2); and
- list actions you must do as a follower to fulfill your three CRM responsibilities (Section 9.3).

The primary threat that you might experience is the introduction of a large number of concepts and terms, some of which you may have never encountered, and some of which you may think about in a different sense. We will therefore explicitly define and differentiate each term and concept. We also realize how busy you are. We will make sure that the chapter is short enough to be read in approximately thirty minutes. Finally, we provide Summary Boxes. The Summary Boxes serve two functions. First, they emphasize the take-home points in each section, and you can use them to check your understanding of those take-home points. Second, you can use them to determine if you and your team are implementing those take-home

[85] By now, you may feel that repeated use of the chapter briefing format is redundant. However, we believe that it is important to continue to emphasize that a good briefing builds mental models by discussing what is happening, what success looks like, and what threats or errors are possible and how you plan to prevent, avoid, or mitigate them. Hence, the repetitive nature is meant to cement this belief with an understanding that you will also immerse yourself in this book on an irregular and/or intermittent basis.

[86] For more information on STAR, see Chapters 11-15.

points. If a Summary Box does not make sense to you or you do not understand one or more take-home points, then review the related material before continuing to the next section.

Did I miss anything? Any concerns? Any questions? (Pause) No? Then, let's get started.

List of Abbreviations

a-i-d	(specific) action - impact - desired behavior
A-I-D	(generalized) action - impact - desired behavior
CRM	Crew Resource Management
CUS	I am Concerned; I am Uncomfortable; It is a Safety issue
DESC	Describe-Express-Specify-Consequences
DOC	Physician
MET	Medical Emergency Team
ONC	Oncology
RES	Resident
RT	Respiratory Therapist
STAR	Stop-Think-Act-Review
STEP	Status-Team-Environment-Progress
TeamSTEPPS	Team Strategies and Tools to Enhance Performance and Patient Safety

Good leaders, good followers, and good CRM are interrelated. Good leaders enable CRM, but good CRM also makes leaders better. Good followers must do CRM, but good CRM also makes followers more effective. In this chapter, you will learn why CRM makes leaders better (Section 9.1), how leaders enable CRM (Section 9.2), and what followers must do to fulfill their CRM responsibilities (Section 9.3).

9.1 What You, as a Leader, Get Out of CRM

Before we do a deep dive into CRM leaders and followers, we want to cover two misconceptions. The first misconception happened when CRM was first introduced to airline flight crews 40 years ago. Some captains considered CRM as simply "charm school", the 1970s equivalent of today's political correctness: make followers feel listened to, empowered, and appreciated. Empowerment is an indirect side benefit of CRM, and follower engagement is a tool used in CRM. However, neither follower empowerment nor engagement is the reason why you as a leader should do and encourage CRM. The second misconception is even more incorrect: that CRM forces you, as a leader, to get follower buy-in to your decisions. CRM does not turn decision making into a democratic or even a consensus process. CRM does not decrease your authority to make the decisions you need to make. Instead, CRM ensures that you have all the information that you need to make informed decisions and allows your team to be both safe and effective. That is what you, as a leader, get out of CRM. In the scenario, the MET physician specifically stated that the Oncology resident's information was needed to make a good decision on treatment.

By the way, if you can see all and know all without input from others, you do not need to do CRM. If you never make mistakes, you do not need to do CRM. If you will never admit to a mistake, you cannot effectively do, or enable, CRM. If, however, you realize that you need information from your team, that they may have good ideas on how to fix problems, and that you may make mistakes, then you need CRM.

As you read the following sections, you will see the word "leader" repeatedly. Even if you are not the formal leader, you may be an informal leader. Further, everyone must be prepared to be a situational leader.

Summary Box 9.1
Why Leaders Need CRM

All leaders need CRM to make sure that they get all the information they need.

9.2 Leading

There are thousands of books on leadership. We will address only one specific aspect of leadership: how a leader enables the team to do good CRM. First, we need to define a leader. A formal leader, or the final decision maker, is a naturally assumed definition. But a leader is also an informal leader, the person to whom people look or go for advice. A leader is also a situational leader, the person who in that second has the most knowledge or expertise in what is going on, and who must advocate and even assert a perspective or recommendation that the rest of the team might not be seeing. The situational leader may not be the person with the most seniority or highest title. The situational leader may be the most junior person—or least educated person—if that person is the one who actually sees or knows what is going on.

If a leader wants a team to work together effectively, there are six CRM Leading responsibilities. Those CRM responsibilities are 1) setting expectations and standards, 2) developing the team climate, 3) activating, quality checking, and re-establishing situation awareness and mental models, 4) deferring to expertise, 5) providing feedback, and 6) removing CRM barriers.

9.2.1 Leading Responsibility #1: Setting Expectations and Standards

A leader must set the CRM expectations. The main expectation is that team members must use their CRM skills if they are to work interdependently to accomplish the goal. The MET physician said: "I expect anyone and everyone to communicate any information or observations and what it might mean, to actively listen to our dialogue, and to work together to accomplish our plan while looking out for each other."

Setting expectations alone is not enough if the team does not know what good and bad CRM looks like (i.e., what the CRM standards are). The leader must define acceptable and unacceptable behaviors[87]. Once the leader defines those behaviors, he or she must then be the role model, meaning, "walk the CRM skills walk". If you do not do good CRM, do not expect that your team will. Next, you need to enforce CRM standards. You can do that by rewarding good CRM (even if the outcome was not as desired) and correcting bad CRM (even though the outcome was as desired). As a leader you will get what you reward. Never reward bad CRM, such as praising the person who never communicates, regardless how successful. In our scenario, the Oncology attending did not let the resident get away with using the term "soft", even though the attending may have known exactly what the resident meant. Instead, the attending made the resident specifically state the blood pressure.

---

[87] Hopefully, your training organization has already developed a Behaviorally Anchored Rating Scales (BARS). See Appendix A for more information on BARS.

Summary Box 9.2
Setting CRM Expectations and Standards

As a leader, are you… • telling your team your CRM expectations? • providing your team examples of good CRM behaviors through briefings and role modeling during clinical events? • rewarding good CRM, and, correcting bad CRM?

9.2.2 Leading Responsibility #2: Developing the Team Climate

A leader must develop the appropriate CRM team climate, one that includes the concept of psychological safety. When team members feel psychologically safe, they believe that it is safe to voice a risky or conflicting opinion, and that it is safe to admit mistakes without worrying about punishment. In our scenario, there might have been two places where the MET physician might have undermined psychological safety. Depending on the exact tone used, the use of terms such as "Oh, great" and "Oh, really" might have seemed dismissive and discouraged further inputs from the Oncology resident. Something as unintended and subtle as tone could destroy the psychological safety you tried so hard to build. A very short briefing could establish the climate that admitting mistakes is okay, and that the team is there to support each other. Also, by stating that the leader is not perfect, it makes it easier for followers to inquire, advocate, and assert. By inquire, we mean a follower feels safe to ask questions to understand the situation or the leader's intent. By advocate and assert, we mean a follower feels safe to make and defend a recommendation. Although not explicitly saying so in the scenario, by stating "It is impossible for me to … know everything…", the MET physician let the team know they might have to inquire, advocate and even assert to help the physician "know everything". Recognizing that hierarchies exist in healthcare and that no one can possibly know everything that is going on with a patient, one of the authors of this book briefs his team on the importance of speaking up by handing out index cards that encourage every member of the team to speak up and "not let him screw up."[88]

Good leaders praise the right behaviors, not the right outcome. The hallmark of a good team climate is not only one that rewards someone who calls for a work stop or time out when right, but, rather, also thanks the

---

[88] See Appendix C for a copy of the index cards.

person who halts the task when wrong. If a person is instead counseled to have all the data before acting, that person and probably others will never speak up unless they are one-hundred-percent sure that they are right. Unfortunately, by then it might be too late. Without psychological safety, your team will not provide you all the information—especially the bad news—you need to be a safe and effective leader.

Part of developing psychological safety requires you, as a leader, to protect a follower from the organization and other team members. LeSage, Dyar, and Evans (2011) tell a story of a flight paramedic who insisted that a rescue flight abort due to weather conditions well below limits, even though the pilot wanted to continue. The paramedic then picked up a reputation as a coward and was ridiculed on subsequent flights. A leader who wants to develop psychological safety must defend the person to the team, other teams, and management. A leader must explain why an action counter to an organization or profession's culture is required, and the person who makes that action is worthy of respect, not ridicule. A leader who allows a culture, team, or management to punish people who have the courage to inquire, advocate, and assert will not be able to sustain CRM. Developing psychological safety provides the indirect side benefit of CRM: followers who feel empowered to provide their knowledge and insights.

Summary Box 9.3
Developing the Team Climate

As a leader, are you establishing psychological safety by…
- admitting you are not perfect?
- praising team members who inquire, advocate, and assert, even if wrong?
- protecting your team members from ridicule?

9.2.3 Leading Responsibility #3: Activating, Quality Checking, and Re-Establishing Situation Awareness and Mental Models

A leader is responsible for ensuring that everyone has the situation awareness and mental models required to fulfil their responsibilities. First, the leader ensures the team members activate the proper mental models in the briefing. In the scenario briefing, the MET physician said "Mrs. Jackson has a rapid heart rate, hypotension, cold extremities, and weak pulses. This is concerning for septic shock in the context of her cancer diagnosis and chemotherapy via a central line…" ensuring that everyone activated the septic shock mental model. Later in the scenario, the physician made sure that the team knew to change their mental models to include possible cardiotoxicity.

Second, as a leader, you can then help the team check the quality of their situation awareness and mental model by explaining your decisions and actions so that the team can "see into" your head to evaluate whether their situation awareness and mental model matches yours. In the scenario, the MET physician did this twice. By mentioning Mrs. Jackson's rapid heart rate, hypotension, cold extremities, and weak pulses, the team could match their situation awareness and mental models for symptoms of septic shock. Later, the physician mentioned that fluid boluses must be restricted to 250-500 milliliters due to possible cardiotoxicity, which allowed the team to determine if their situation awareness and mental models agreed that was the proper amount.

Finally, during the task, the leader can provide real-time corrections to a team member's situation awareness and mental model. If during the task, the MET respiratory therapist is not doing something that the MET physician expects, then their situation awareness and mental model may be different. For example, the physician sees that the respiratory therapist is not preparing for an intubation, something the physician expects. The physician can then ask questions to understand if the respiratory therapist is seeing something different or knows something different (i.e., has a different situation awareness or mental model).

Unfortunately, the one constant in today's world is change. No matter how good your situation awareness and mental models are at the beginning of a task, something in the status, team, environment, or progress will not be as expected. Therefore, one's situation awareness, mental model, goal, or plan will have to change. The leader is required to re-establish everyone's situation awareness and mental model. Re-establishing means after a period of heavy workload, distractions, or change, or, just before a complex task, the leader is responsible to make sure every follower knows what is happening (Situation Awareness Level 1) and what it means now, as well as in the future (mental models feeding Situation Awareness Levels 2 and 3). With an updated situation awareness and mental models, each follower understands the new situation, goal, or plan and their part in it. An example of re-establishing might be: "Team, we now hear crackles on her lung exam and a gallop rhythm on her exam (new Situation Awareness Level 1). We have to worry about cardiotoxicity (Situation Awareness Levels 2 and 3).

We must be judicious with fluid boluses and give only 250-500 milliliters at a time and re-examine her. We should also start a norepinephrine infusion. Anyone see any problems with that plan?" Finally, the leader needs to monitor the team to make sure that they have correct, complete, complementary, and valid situation awareness and mental models. If the team is making too many errors or does things that do not match the leader's situation awareness and mental models, the leader should call a STAR to re-establish everyone's situation awareness and mental models.[89]

Summary Box 9.4
Activating, Quality Checking and Re-Establishing the Situation Awareness and Mental Models

As a leader, are you... • ensuring that each team member is using the correct mental models? • providing opportunities for each team member to check his or her mental models? • updating everyone's situation awareness and mental models before or after periods of change or stress?

9.2.4 Leading Responsibility #4: Deferring to Expertise

The fourth responsibility of a leader is to defer to expertise. Deferring to expertise is also the mark of a High Reliability Organization (Weick, Sutcliffe, and Obstfeld 1999). By definition, no one on a team has all the knowledge and skills to accomplish the task. If someone did, there would be no reason to have a team. Each member has unique knowledge, skills and experiences. A leader must realize that depending on the circumstances, any follower might be the "smartest person in the room" (i.e., the one who best knows what is happening and what should be done). That person may be the newest member on the team. Let us change up the scenario a little:

> ONC RES (to MET DOC): "Could it also be cardiotoxicity?"
> MET DOC (to MET NUR): "Do you hear any crackles on her lung exam, or a gallop rhythm on her cardiac exam?"
> MET NUR (to MET DOC): "Not sure."

[89] See Chapters 11-15 for more information on STAR.

Without knowing that the Oncology attending was the one suggesting possible cardiotoxicity, would the MET physician have treated the suggestion seriously from the resident (who already seemed hesitant)?

Simply getting recommendations from the followers is not enough. The team leader who actively seeks recommendations must set up ways for team members to provide those recommendations.[90] The MET physician actively sought the inputs from the resident, to the point of assuring the resident that the physician wanted to hear any inputs regardless of whether the resident was sure if the information was helpful or not. The team leader must then actively listen to those recommendations—and use the "Power of And"—to improve the situation awareness and mental models. That does not mean the team leader abdicates decision making or authority to the follower. The final decision always rests with the team leader. The team leader must seek recommendations, and actively listen to them, but is not required to accept the recommendations of the team. It also means that the team leader will not automatically take the recommendation of the most senior person or the one with the most impressive title, but instead listen to the person who has the most intimate knowledge of what is happening, regardless of rank.

Summary Box 9.5
Deferring to Expertise

As a leader, do you…

- listen to the person with the most first-hand knowledge, and not the person with the highest rank or most seniority?
- seek out recommendations, including developing ways to get those recommendations?
- actively listen to those recommendations to build or confirm situation awareness and mental models?

9.2.5 Leading Responsibility #5: Providing Feedback

A leader must provide feedback on a team member's CRM. Where a debriefing is about providing feedback to the team, this responsibility deals with helping an individual follower with his or her own CRM. We advocate

[90] One of the Space Shuttle Columbia Accident Investigation Board findings was that management never set up ways to receive information on the impact of tile damage. (CAIB, 2003)

for facilitation.[91] Effective facilitation requires the leader to ask open-ended questions to the maximum extent possible in order to help a follower self-discover and self-correct. One format to help with those open-ended questions is a-i-d/A-I-D, or action-impact-desired behavior/Action-Impact-Desired Behavior. The a-i-d addresses the specific CRM erroneous action, the impact of that error, and the desired behavior (i.e., the specific skill error and fix). The capitalized A-I-D addresses the generalized erroneous action, the impact of that class of errors, and generalized desired behavior (i.e., fixing the general mental model hole). Let us expand the scenario to possible feedback by the Oncology attending (ONC DOC) to the Oncology resident (ONC RES):

> ONC DOC: "How was your communication?"
>
> ONC RES: "I thought it was pretty good."[92]
>
> ONC DOC: "I was thinking specifically of your phone call to me."
>
> ONC RES: "Well, at first I was rushed, and a little nervous. Then I didn't use the right format. Finally, I used the word "soft", which wasn't clear or accurate. On second thought, my communication was awful."
>
> ONC DOC: "Don't beat yourself up. Everyone's communication can use improvement. What would you have done differently?"
>
> ONC RES: "Well, I will use SBAR next time (specific action). That way I will give you the information in the manner you expect (specific impact). I will address situation first, then background, then assessment, and finally recommendation (specific desired behavior)."
>
> ONC DOC: "That covers this specific situation. Can you generalize?"
>
> ONC RES: "We need to use protocols that we all agree to (Generalized Action) to make sure there is no missed information (Generalized

[91] See Appendix B for more information on Facilitated Debriefings.

[92] This is a very common response. Until they learn about CRM behaviors and standards, the follower does not know what he or she does not know, and so, wrongly, thinks that his or her CRM was "pretty good". A facilitated debriefing may be required to help the follower to self-discover any CRM problems and then think of ways to improve (self-correct).

Impact). Next time, I will take a few seconds to make sure that I have all the information in the right format (Generalized Desired Behavior)."

Summary Box 9.6
Providing Feedback

As a leader, are you…
• providing feedback to each team member on his or her CRM?
• providing feedback on both the specific and general behaviors?

9.2.6 Leading Responsibility #6: Removing CRM Barriers

A leader removes barriers for the team doing CRM. Barriers could be CRM Demons, or that it is two in the morning, cold, and the twentieth straight day of work, or an organization or culture that does not fully support CRM.[93] Whatever the barriers the leader—formal, informal, or situational—is responsible for preventing, avoiding, or mitigating any barrier from affecting your team's safety or effectiveness.

Summary Box 9.7
Removing CRM Barriers

As a leader, are you removing barriers that make it difficult for your team to do CRM?

9.2.7 A CRM Briefing Showing a Leader Covering All the Responsibilities

Below is an example of a shift or pre-task CRM briefing.[94] It contains many more items than you would want to mention in a single briefing, but you could spread out some of the items over several briefings.

By the way: this briefing contains CRM concepts not yet covered (e.g., STAR). When you are done reading the entire book, come back to this section and see if everything makes sense. Also, compare this with what you do at your organization.

---

[93] See Chapter 5 for more information on Situation Awareness and Exchanging Information Demons.
[94] A real briefing would also include the technical tasks, and how CRM is embedded in the technical aspects. See Section 14.2 for more information on briefings.

"I know we haven't had a single problem, but that doesn't guarantee today will go as expected. I expect you to have your head up, and to be seeing and hearing what is going on around you. I expect you to figure out what anything you see or hear means now, and in the future, especially for any upcoming crucial events. You need situation awareness not just about your silo, but also about how you are affecting other team members, and vice versa. You need to know the schedule, today's goal, what will happen during the next shift, and tomorrow's shifts. Further, you need to know about what threats and errors are possible, and what we can do to first spot them, and then prevent or mitigate them.

You must also pass on your situation awareness so that we can integrate it with everyone else's, and be smarter as a team than as individuals. If you see or hear something that does not match your situation awareness, speak up.

You must provide the right information to the right person in the right format at the right time, preferably just before needed. Use 3-way Communication, and actively listen. Use tone, body language and questions to check for understanding.[95]

We will use STAR if we run across anything unexpected.[96] To do this, we will:

Stop to focus, eliminate workload and distractions, get control of our fight-or-flight response and to make a first guess on how much time we have.

Think, so we can do a good problem definition before looking at courses of action, determine critical factors, and check for applicable policies or experiences. If required, we will evaluate courses of action against critical factors, benefits, costs, threats and errors, and contingencies.

Act, in order to embed CRM into our procedures. Before execution, we will make sure we are ready. During execution we will support and back each other up. Ask if you have questions and stop if unsure.

Review at the end of the Problem Definition, Course of Action Selection, and Planning Phases, and after each step of execution. If we aren't getting exactly what we expect, we go back to STAR. When we are done, we will do a debriefing, including both technical and CRM issues, and work with management to incorporate and verify those changes we can't make ourselves.

---

[95] 3-way communication is addressed in Section 8.4.

[96] STAR is addressed in Chapters 11-15.

> Finally, if you don't understand something, have a question, or a concern, speak up. If you think I am not listening, use CUS to get my attention."

NOTE: No matter how strong you think CRM is embedded in your organization, never brief CRM as "per Standard Operating Procedures". Always spend at least a minute or two on some specific aspect of CRM that is most important to the coming task.

9.3 Following

A related topic to Leading is Following. A leader needs effective followers. Being a follower is more than blind obedience to the leader's direction. If a follower is to effectively support the leader, there are three CRM Following responsibilities: 1) a follower must inquire when he or she does not understand what the leader says or wants; 2) advocate, and even assert, if he or she believes the leader has made a safety-related decision without all the knowledge available; and 3) use the right format and terminology.

9.3.1 Following Responsibility #1: Inquire

A follower may not understand what the leader wants or is saying. What the follower is experiencing may be an incompatible, or different, situation awareness. What the leader perceives may not match what the follower perceives. Another way of saying that is, "That is not what I am seeing". The leader needs the followers to have the same perception of what is happening, or Level 1 Situation Awareness. The followers may also have a different understanding of what those perceptions mean now, or in the future (Level 2 or 3 Situation Awareness), because they might have different mental models on the hows or whys. Another way to say that is, "That is not why I think it is happening". A follower must inquire when unsure about the what's, why's or how's. Questions could be about:

- Situation: "I don't understand what is happening."
- Goal: "I am unclear where we are going."
- Plan: "I have a question about how."
- Role: "I don't understand what you want me to do."

9.3.2 Following Responsibility #2: Advocate and Assert

In today's complex world, no one person can see or know everything. Therefore, a leader needs followers who feel comfortable providing a recommendation or advocating an alternative course of action. If a follower feels strongly that a decision is being made without the leader having or understanding all the information and that decision might have adverse (safety or goal) impacts, a follower needs to be assertive, to continue to advocate until the follower is sure that the leader understands the risk and is able to make a well-thought-out decision.[97] Another way to look at the leader-follower relationship is the follower is the expert in his or her area. The follower will perceive things that the leader does not and will know his or her tasks and its threats and errors to a depth, breadth, and refinement that the leader cannot. Let us change up the scenario a little to provide an example of a follower advocating and asserting. Let us assume that the MET physician does not draw out the Oncology resident, and therefore does not hear the Oncology attending's thoughts on possible cardiotoxicity. Instead, the dialogue goes like this:

MET DOC: "This is concerning for septic shock in the context of her cancer diagnosis and chemotherapy via a central line. Let's give a 1-liter normal saline bolus."

MET NUR: "I might be hearing crackles on her lung exam and a gallop rhythm on her cardiac exam."

MET DOC: "Did you hear that I want a 1-liter saline bolus?"

MET NUR: "I think we need to consider cardiotoxicity."

MET DOC: "Okay."

MET NUR: "Then should we limit fluid boluses?"

MET DOC: "You are right. Let's …"

There are many reasons why a follower may not be assertive. There could be a problem with a high authority gradient: the difference in authority, experience, or status between the leader and the follower. Depending on the authority gradient, followers mitigate or tone down their

---

[97] Another time that a follower might provide a recommendation is if the follower sees that the leader is overwhelmed. In that instance, a recommendation on what to do, why, and how risks are mitigated will reduce the cognitive load on the leader. Instead of trying to determine what to do, the leader only has to agree if the recommendation matches the leader's assessment of STEP or disagree if it does not.

assertion. There are six levels of mitigation that the MET nurse might have used:

1. Hint and Hope: “I might be hearing crackles on her lung exam and a gallop rhythm on her cardiac exam.” (Hoping this hint will prompt the MET physician to think of cardiotoxicity and therefore limit fluid boluses.)

2. Preference: “I think it would be smart to limit fluid boluses.”

3. Query: “Then should we limit fluid boluses?”

4. Joint suggestion: “I think we should limit fluid boluses.”

5. Joint obligation statement: “I think we need to limit fluid boluses.”

6. Command: “We need to limit fluid boluses!”

Improper mitigation may result in the assertion getting lost by a busy or distracted leader. At times, good followers have to increase the level of assertion, or persist in asserting until they are acknowledged by the leader, to ensure that their concern is not lost in the distractions.

9.3.3 Following Responsibility #3: Use the Right Format and Terminology

Many accidents have happened because the follower hinted and hoped, and the leader did not pick up on the concern. Some healthcare organizations have come up with CUS (TeamSTEPPS 2020), a set of terms that, when heard by the leader, the leader knows that the follower is asserting a safety issue. CUS stands for:

I am Concerned!
I am Uncomfortable!
This is a Safety Issue!

To help the leader understand what the concern is, some organizations have designed specific communication formats. TeamSTEPPS suggests the DESC model for healthcare (TeamSTEPPS 2020):

D — Describe the specific situation or behavior; provide concrete data.
E — Express how the situation makes you feel/what your concerns are.
S — Suggest other alternatives and seek agreement.
C — Consequences should be stated in terms of impact on established team goals.

In the alternate scenario in Section 9.3.2, would the MET physician have understood more quickly if the nurse had said:

> "MET DOC, I am concerned. I may be hearing crackles on her lung exam, and a gallop rhythm on her cardiac exam. It might be signs of cardiotoxicity. We might limit fluid boluses for the present time. What do you think?"

Summary Box 9.8
A Follower's CRM Responsibilities

Do your followers…
• inquire when unsure of situation, goal, plan, or role?
• advocate and assert at the right level when safety is an issue?
• use the right format and terminology?

Chapter Debriefing

I want to call a quick STAR (Stop-Think-Act-Review): get off your email, stop your side conversations, and turn off the television.[98] Let's see if you can expand upon these statements:

- CRM does not diminish the authority of the formal leader.
- CRM ensures that a leader has all the information he or she needs to make fully informed decisions, and to make the team safe and effective.
- You can be a formal leader, an informal leader, or, depending on the circumstances, a situational leader.
- A leader shall:
    - set the CRM expectations and standards, model them, acknowledge those followers doing good CRM and correct those who are not.

[98] See Chapters 11-15 for information on STAR.

    - establish psychological safety by acknowledging that he or she is not perfect, and rewarding followers who inquire, advocate, and assert, even if they are incorrect.
    - defend the follower from false narratives when a follower advocates and asserts a position counter to an organization's culture.
    - ensure that each team member activates the right mental models.
    - provide opportunities for each team member to check his or her mental models.
    - re-establish everyone's situation awareness and mental models after high workload, distractions, or significant changes, as well as before any crucial task.
    - monitor for signs of poor situation awareness and mental models, and call a STAR if required.
    - defer to expertise, not to title or seniority.
    - seek recommendations, actively listen, and use the "Power of And".
    - help followers to self-discover and self-correct.
    - remove CRM Demons.
- Followers shall:
    - inquire when they are unsure of what the leader wants, or if there is a difference between their situation awareness or mental models.
    - advocate and assert if they believe the leader is making a safety-related decision without all the information.
    - use the right format and terminology, so that the leader can more easily understand the concern.

If this was an actual debriefing, we would ask you to expand further on each of these statements. Depending on your response, we would ask open-ended follow-up questions until we were sure you understood the material and had a plan to implement one or more best practices. We might ask, "What is a specific leading or following problem that you experience on your job?" We would not be satisfied if you said, "Our team members aren't as assertive as we need." Again, we would ask open-ended follow-up questions until you might say, "We have a problem with new team members not knowing how to be effectively assertive." We would then ask, "What can you do during your next shift to fix that problem?" We would then continue to ask open-ended follow-up questions until you might say, "In the briefing, I can discuss how to use CUS and DESC. I could also say that I am not perfect and need their help. During the shift, I need to be open if a team member asks a question or provides a recommendation. In the debriefing, we need to discuss why someone did not know how to be assertive in a situation." We would then ask, "That helps your team, but what about other teams?" More open-ended questions until you might say, "I need to work with management to add more training on when and how to be assertive."

References

"Columbia Accident Investigation Board." NASA. NASA. Accessed October 30, 2021. https://history.nasa.gov/columbia/CAIB.html.

Klein, Gary. "Performing a Project Premortem." IEEE Engineering Management Review 36, no. 2 (2008): 103–4. https://doi.org/10.1109/emr.2008.4534313.

LeSage, Paul, Jeff T. Dyar, and Bruce E. Evans. Crew Resource Management Principles and Practice. Sudbury, MA: Jones and Bartlett Publ, 2011.

TeamSTEPPS: Pocket Guide: Strategies & Tools to Enhance Performance and Patient Safety. Bethesda, MD: U.S. Dept. of Health and Human Services, Agency for Healthcare Research and Quality, 2006.

Weick, Karl, Kathleen Sutcliffe, and David Obstfeld. "Organizing for High Reliability: Processes of Collective Mindfulness." Essay. In Research in Organizational Behavior: An Annual Series of Analytical Essays and Critical Reviews, edited by Robert I. Sutton, Barry M. Staw, and Larry Cummings, 81–122. Greenwich, CT: JAI Press, 1999.

CHAPTER 10

MUTUALLY SUPPORTING

Chapter Briefing[99]

I want to call a quick STAR (Stop-Think-Act-Review): get off your email, stop your side conversations, and turn off the television.[100] Here is what we will do in this chapter. We will discuss the CRM skill of Mutually Supporting, or how team members support each other. We will be successful if you can explain:

- the three aspects of Mutually Supporting (Section 10.1);
- why it is difficult to provide Mutually Supporting in healthcare (Section 10.2);
- best practices to overcome system threats to Mutually Supporting (Section 10.3.1); and
- best practices to overcome human threats to Mutually Supporting (Section 10.3.2).

The primary threat that you might experience is the introduction of a large number of concepts and terms, some of which you may have never encountered, and some of which you may think about in a different sense. We will therefore explicitly define and differentiate each term and concept. We also realize how busy you are. We will make sure that the chapter is short enough to be read in approximately thirty minutes. Finally, we provide Summary Boxes. The Summary Boxes serve two functions. First, they

---

[99] By now, you may feel that repeated use of the chapter briefing format is redundant. However, we believe that it is important to continue to emphasize that a good briefing builds mental models by discussing what is happening, what success looks like, and what threats or errors are possible and how you plan to prevent, avoid, or mitigate them. Hence, the repetitive nature is meant to cement this belief with an understanding that you will also immerse yourself in this book on an irregular and/or intermittent basis.

[100] For more information on STAR, see Chapters 11-15.

emphasize the take-home points in each section, and you can use them to check your understanding of those take-home points. Second, you can use them to determine if you and your team are implementing those take-home points. If a Summary Box does not make sense to you or you do not understand one or more take-home points, then review the related material before continuing to the next section.

Did I miss anything? Any concerns? Any questions? (Pause) No? Then, let's get started.

List of Abbreviations

CRM	Crew Resource Management
DOC	Physician
ED	Emergency Department
IM SAFE	Illness, Medication, Stress, Alcohol, Fatigue, Eaten
NUR	Nurse
PED	Pediatrics
PPV	Positive Pressure Ventilation

Most people would agree that team members should support each other—what we call Mutually Supporting—but what exactly does Mutually Supporting mean in healthcare? You will learn that in Section 10.1, along with the threats that make Mutually Supporting difficult to do in healthcare (Section 10.2) and best practices that will allow you to do Mutually Supporting (Section 10.3).

10.1 Definition of Mutually Supporting

We have modified the definition used by the American Psychological Association (2015) for Mutually Supporting behaviors as follows: Mutually Supporting refers to offering and accepting:

- Task Assistance, or Back-up Support: help doing a task to ensure safe and effective execution.
- Social Support: help combating any Performance Shaping Factor.
- Feedback: advice provided in real-time to improve performance or prevent errors.

We will modify and expand upon each of these concepts and apply them to healthcare.

10.2 Threats That Make Mutually Supporting Difficult to Do in Healthcare

10.2.1 System Threats

Unfortunately, Mutually Supporting may be the most difficult set of CRM behaviors to instill in your team. The airlines are the most frequently mentioned benchmark for CRM, but for the specific topic of Mutually Supporting, the airlines may actually provide a poor example for healthcare. Here is why:

Table 10-1
Differences That Make Aviation a Bad Example for Mutually Supporting in Healthcare

	Airline cockpit crew	Interdisciplinary healthcare team	Impact
Team size	2	2 to many	The bigger the team, the harder to develop complementary mental models of Mutually Supporting.
Authority Gradient (actual or perceived difference in experience, expertise, or authority)	Was very steep, now can be relatively flat	Can be very steep (e.g., between doctors, nurses, and families)	The steeper the authority gradient, the more difficult it is for a follower to tell the leader that he or she may have made an error.
Role, Responsibilities, and Knowledge Differences	Practically identical, since either can be the pilot doing the flying or the pilot mutually supporting	Very distinct and differentiated (e.g., between doctors, nurses, and ancillary staff from different specialties, etc.)	The more distinct and differentiated, the more difficult for a team member to know if another team member is making an error.
Organizational/ Professional Membership	Same organization/ profession	Different organizations and professions	Different organizations and professions have different cultures, processes, and practices, which make it more difficult for a team member to differentiate between cultural differences and errors.

Standardized Operating Procedures	Yes	Few	Without Standard Operating Procedures, everyone does a procedure his or her own way, which makes it more difficult for a team member to differentiate between technique differences and errors.
Safety Culture	Evolving to a culture which stresses fixing the systemic source of errors	Can still be a culture of blame	A culture that is concerned with assessing blame will not have the psychological safety needed for team members to admit errors and accept assistance.

Of all the threats above, the most direct systems threat for a team about to start a task or shift may be the differences in roles, responsibilities, and knowledge. Since both pilots are equally trained to fly the airplane, either pilot can easily tell when the other pilot has made or is about to make an error. In healthcare, that is almost never the case, even if both individuals are physicians. For example, since a surgeon and anesthesiologist have different roles, responsibilities and knowledge, how would an anesthesiologist recognize that a surgeon might be making an error (see Section 10.3.1 for some ideas)?

10.2.2 Human Threats

To become a healthcare professional, you and your team members completed years of training, during which you likely excelled in most, if not all, aspects. You probably have a reputation, and also a self-image, of an over-achieving perfectionist who can overcome any obstacle to deliver quality patient care. You deserve to have that opinion. The problem comes when one's ego runs into the reality of complex, ambiguous, and stressful situations. If ego prevents any team member from either admitting that he or she might make an error, or, asking for or accepting assistance, then Mutually Supporting is impossible. Commercial aviation had the same problem, early on. There was an anecdote of a Captain who, when his piloting was questioned by his First Officer, told the First Officer to "shut up and look out the window". Whether the story is true is not as important as the fact that it was widely accepted as indicative of the state of culture in commercial aviation fifty years ago. Similarly, physicians are often overly trained to be self-sufficient, to the point of rugged and persistent individualism. While individualism is not itself a bad thing, over-reliance on an individualist mindset crowds out the cooperative thinking necessary to support superior team performance. A group of highly talented individuals may be outperformed by a team of moderately talented professionals who cooperate and coordinate well together. Through training and retirement of those who refused to do CRM, the frequency of those types of individualistic behaviors have greatly diminished in the cockpits of the major US airlines, but isolated incidents still occur. If the airline profession can overcome ego, then healthcare professionals can do the same.

The above discussion is not meant to scare you from attempting to engage in Mutually Supporting. Instead, it is meant to list the threats that you face, so that you can identify ways to mitigate those threats. We want to illustrate that healthcare has threats that do not exist in commercial aviation, and therefore the model employed by the airlines cannot simply be dropped into a healthcare organization and be expected to work. All levels of healthcare—profession, organization, team, individual—will need to develop its own unique set of Mutually Supporting behaviors. What we will next address is how you as a formal, informal, or situational leader or team member can help your team develop Mutually Supporting behaviors, despite the potential threats.

10.3 Best Practices

10.3.1 Best Practices Against System Threats

System threats exist in healthcare because team members have different roles, responsibilities, and knowledge; they are from different organizations; and they may not consistently apply standardized procedures. In these situations, team members have no complementary mental models on how to assist each other in their assigned tasks. The best remedy for this is to use the briefing to build those mental models and, thus, provide the basis for Mutually Supporting. First, each team member must tell the team what he or she will be doing, what it will look like if things are going well, how long it will take, what threats are possible (including what they might look like), and what support is expected from each of them. Building a de facto mini-Standard Operating Procedure for your team makes up for tasks that lack formal Standard Operating Procedures. Second, each team member with a safety-critical, error-prone task must use the briefing to tell the team his or her CRM expectations and standards, so they know what behaviors are expected. This partially remedies differences in organizational cultures. With improved mental models, they can ask questions when encountering unexpected events, or when seeing signs indicating that the plan is not working. Third, when each team member also talks through decisions and actions (i.e., thinking out loud), the team members can constantly compare their mental models. Let us look at a possible scenario:

> Anesthesiologist: "You said that if the surgery took longer than expected the patient might become hypotensive from blood loss and require a blood transfusion."
>
> Surgeon: "When I saw oozing from the surgical site, I decided to change my suturing technique. This change is successful if cessation of oozing occurs, but unsuccessful if the oozing continues. Back me up by monitoring his vital signs, in particular, his blood pressure."

If the surgeon had talked through that decision when it was made, the anesthesiologist would not have needed to voice a concern.

When members of your team do ask questions, you must actively listen to their concerns, and answer with the goal of improving their situation awareness and mental models.

Summary Box 10.1
Mutually Supporting Best Practices

To combat system threats to Mutually Supporting, for every safety-critical, error-prone task for which no Standard Operating Procedure exists, does your team…

- prior to the task, brief each other on:
  - what the planned task is, how it will look, what threats are possible (and what they might look like), how long it will take, and what support is expected?
  - CRM expectations and standards?
- during the task's execution:
  - explain decisions and actions?
  - actively listen to team member's questions with the goal of building their situation awareness and mental models?

10.3.2. Best Practices Against Human Threats

The human threats to Mutually Supporting are steep authority gradients; differences in roles, responsibilities, and knowledge among team members; and differences in culture. As we discussed in the Leading and Following chapter, the formal, informal, and situational leaders have a responsibility to both establish psychological safety and to set the expectation and standards for CRM. Without those, Mutually Supporting is impossible. Mutually Supporting, however, goes beyond what a leader does to establish psychological safety.

Besides Task Assistance, it requires two other behaviors among team members. The first additional behavior is offering and accepting social support. Social support is a realization that people work in situations not conducive to safe and effective performance. We expect our healthcare professionals to perform flawlessly while performing complex, time- and safety-critical tasks under adverse environmental conditions, while they themselves are stressed or fatigued. Social support is providing the assistance necessary to resolve or work-around any Performance Shaping Factor or being "IM SAFE" – ensuring that no team member is ill, adversely affected by medication, stressed, under the influence of alcohol or drugs, fatigued, or has not eaten (i.e., not "hangry" or dehydrated). Social support means making team members feel professionally cared for, that you all have assistance available from other team members when needed to ensure quality patient care, and most popularly, that each team member is part of a supportive social entity (i.e., a team). As a team member, you have a responsibility to recognize when colleagues need physical, psychological, or emotional support, and provide that as necessary with your actions or referrals to other professionals, as long as it does not detract from the care that you need to deliver to the patient. In our scenario, the Oncology attending knew that the resident was stressed and fatigued: "Take a moment to collect yourself and take a deep breath. I know residents do several nights in a row in our ward, which is challenging." If your position is, however, "They have to suck it up, just like I do", and they are unable to manage the situation, then errors will occur, and patients will be harmed. Also are you sure that you can really "suck it up" and also perform properly? Similarly, if you wait to provide support until you feel supported, or a team member offers you support, then your team's performance will suffer at some point. As we discussed in the last section, physical support in the form of task assistance may be the most difficult to accomplish, given that team members often have different skills and perform different tasks. For example, a nurse cannot take over for a task-overloaded physician, and vice versa. Instead, physical support may have to rely on techniques that buy your teammates more time to do a task, such as offering to locate equipment, double-checking a reading, or taking on one of your team member's other tasks for which you are well-positioned. Often, Mutually Supporting in healthcare may be more emotional and psychological. It can be as little as "You can do this!", "Take a deep breath…", "Would you like to talk through the pros and cons out loud?" or, "The situation set you up for an error.".

The second additional behavior required by Mutually Supporting is offering and accepting feedback. Feedback, while less formal than a debriefing, is more immediate, and more team member-to-team member. Although feedback usually refers to advice after the action, it can also be proactive. For example: you look over someone's shoulder and see that he or she is about to make an error, you could say, "Before you do that, you need to check …." or "Before you do that, a safer thing is to …" The goal of feedback is to improve the actions of a team member in real-time. In our scenario, the Oncology attending offered, and the resident accepted, feedback on the resident's communication behavior.

Now that you know the four CRM skills, the next section of the book will present tools that are enabled by and enable CRM.

Chapter Debriefing

I want to call a quick STAR (Stop-Think-Act-Review): get off your email, stop your side conversations, and turn off the television.[101]. Let's see if you can expand upon these statements:

- Mutually Supporting consists of team members offering and accepting 1) task assistance, 2) social support and 3) feedback.
- The main system threats to Mutually Supporting in healthcare are:
    - distinct and differentiated roles, responsibilities and knowledge;
    - different organizations, professions, disciplines and cultures; and
    - lack or inconsistent use of Standard Operating Procedures.
- The main human threat to Mutually Supporting in healthcare is fear of retribution.
- A good briefing enables Mutually Supporting by:
    - building psychological safety between you as a leader and the team members, but also among team members (e.g., "This is

[101] See Chapters 11-15 for information on STAR

a complex procedure that sets us up to make errors. Luckily, we will back each other up.");

- setting explanations and standards (e.g., "If it looks like a team member is overwhelmed, stressed, or about to make a mistake, jump in and help."); and
- building mental models to help ad hoc team members who may be from different backgrounds, have different roles and do not have or use Standard Operating Procedures to better support each other.

- Because there are so many Performance Shaping Factors (e.g., stress, fatigue), it is important for team members to support one another's physical, psychological, and emotional needs either directly or by referral.
- Provide feedback, before, during, or after a task, to improve a team member's proficiency or mental models.

If this was an actual debriefing, we would ask you to expand further on each of these statements. Depending on your response, we would ask open-ended follow-up questions until we were sure you understood the material and had a plan to implement one or more best practices. We might then ask, "What is a specific Mutually Supporting problem that you experience on your job?" We would not be satisfied if you said, "We can't do Mutually Supporting as well as we need." Again, we would ask open-ended follow-up questions until you might say, "We have a problem with team members not Mutually Supporting because our responsibilities are so different." We would then ask, "What can you do on your next shift to fix that problem?" We would then continue to ask open-ended follow-up questions until you might say, "I need to modify my briefing so that each team member discusses what they are doing and how they want the team to support them. During the shift, I need to check if team members seem stressed or fatigued, and provide support. In the debriefing, we need to discuss why we did or did not mutually support each other and how to improve next shift." We might then ask, "That helps your team, but what about other teams?" More open-ended questions until you might say, "I need to work with management to change the briefing guide to include mutually supporting."

Reference

"Teach Teamwork." American Psychological Association. American Psychological Association. Accessed October 30, 2021. https://www.apa.org/education/k12/teach-teamwork.

Part 2:

CRM Tools

PART 2A.

STAR (STOP-THINK-ACT-REVIEW)

Briefing[102]

I want to call a quick STAR (Stop-Think-Act-Review): get off your email, stop your side conversations, and turn off the television. Here is what we will do in the next 5 chapters.[103] We will discuss STAR, which stands for Stop-Think-Act-Review. When faced with a situation during planning or execution in which the team is not sure what is going on or what to do, they call for a STAR. Using STARs, which both enables and is enabled by CRM, will help make your team be safe and effective. We will be successful if you can describe what constitutes a good:

- Stop (Chapter 11);
- Think - Define the Problem (Chapter 12);
- Think - Determine a Course of Action (Chapter 13);
- Act - Develop the Plan (Chapter 14);
- Act - Execute the Plan (Chapter 14); and
- Review (Chapter 15).

The primary threat that you might experience is the introduction of a large number of concepts and terms, some of which you may have never encountered, and some of which you may think about in a different sense. We will therefore explicitly define and differentiate each term and concept. We also realize how busy you are. We will make sure that the chapter is short enough to be read in approximately thirty minutes. Finally, we provide

[102] By now, you may feel that repeated use of the chapter briefing format is redundant. However, we believe that it is important to continue to emphasize that a good briefing builds mental models by discussing what is happening, what success looks like, and what threats or errors are possible and how you plan to prevent, avoid, or mitigate them. Hence, the repetitive nature is meant to cement this belief with an understanding that you will also immerse yourself in this book on an irregular and/or intermittent basis.

[103] Chapter 16 provides more information on Decision Making methods.

Summary Boxes. The Summary Boxes serve two functions. First, they emphasize the take-home points in each section, and you can use them to check your understanding of those take-home points. Second, you can use them to determine if you and your team are implementing those take-home points. If a Summary Box does not make sense to you or you do not understand one or more take-home points, then review the related material before continuing to the next section.

Did I miss anything? Any concerns? Any questions? (Pause) No? Then, let's get started.

List of Abbreviations

CPAP	Continuous Positive Airway Pressure
DOC	Physician
ED	Emergency Department
EMS	Emergency Medical Services
EMT	Emergency Medical Technician
L&D	Labor and Delivery
NRP	Neonatal Resuscitation Program
NUR	Nurse
OB	Obstetrics or Obstetrician
PED	Pediatrics
STAR	Stop-Think-Act-Review

When NASA's Johnson Space Center Mission Operations Directorate was looking for Crew Resource Management training for the International Space Station flight controllers and astronauts, it benchmarked several organizations, including the Callaway Nuclear Power Plant in Missouri. There, the NASA team learned about a program that Callaway uses to help their people be safe and effective. When faced with a situation during execution in which the team is not sure what is going on or what to do, they call for a STAR moment. STAR stands for Stop-Think-Act-Review, or if you see something you did not expect, you:

Stop: to get over the startle effect and manage workload and distractions.
Think: to define the problem and determine a course of action.
Act: to develop, and then execute, a plan.
Review: at the end of every step, but also the end of every task and phase.

If, when you review the outcome of each step, task, or phase, you notice that something is not what you expected, you start another cycle of STAR.

Let us start with a scenario that will show good, and bad, examples of doing a STAR. We will use this scenario as we discuss the separate parts of STAR further in Chapters 11-15.

Personnel Involved in Scenario

Emergency Medical Technician: EMT
Emergency Department Team: ED DOC, ED NUR #1, ED NUR #2
Obstetric Team: OB DOC
Pediatric Team: PED DOC, PED NUR #1, PED NUR #2

ED DOC (to ED NUR #1 and ED NUR #2): "I just got off the phone with Dispatch. EMS responded to a call from a neighbor about a woman in active labor. They told me that we are the closest ED, and they will be here in 10 minutes. Let's take one minute for a briefing. She does not speak English, so we don't know anything about her or her pregnancy except that she is already pushing. She may deliver here in the ED before we can move her up to L&D. I need the two of you to do the following as quickly as possible…"
(to ED NUR #1): Notify the OB on call tonight that we need her to come in ASAP. Also, page our pediatric hospitalist to the ED in case she delivers before we can move her to L&D."
(to ED NUR #2): Open the delivery pack and set up for a vaginal delivery in the trauma bay. Also, move the radiant warmer to that room, plug it in, and turn it on."
(to both ED NUR #1 and NUR #2): "Do you need anything from me? From each other? (both ED NURs shake their heads 'No'.)

PED DOC, PED NUR #1 and PED NUR #2 arrive in the ED within two minutes.

PED DOC (to ED DOC): "I'm the pediatric hospitalist on call tonight, and these are two of our newborn nursery nurses…"

ED DOC (to ED NUR #1, ED NUR #2, PED DOC, PED NUR #1, PED NUR #2): "I'm calling a STAR. Let's get everyone together for one minute to brief this situation. First, stop and catch your breath, because we may be very busy very soon. Here's what I know. EMS will be here in about five minutes with a woman in active labor. She does not speak English, so we do not know anything about her pregnancy, including her due date. (to ED NUR#1): Did you reach the obstetrician on call?"

ED NUR #1 (to ED DOC): "I did, but she is about 15 minutes out."

ED DOC: "Okay, we need to assume that she won't be here when the patient arrives, so let's plan to either transport the patient to L&D if we have time or deliver her here. I am comfortable managing a vaginal delivery with my team."
(to ED NUR #2): "Is the trauma bay set up for delivery?"

ED NUR #2: "Yes, the birthing bed and the delivery tray are set up in the trauma bay."

ED DOC: "When the OB shows up, she can take over, but until then, I will lead the delivery."

PED DOC: "I will lead my team in the care of the neonate. I see that the radiant warmer is already in the room and turned on. We brought our neonatal resuscitation pack with us and will get set up." (to ED DOC): "Do you have any idea about the gestational age?"

ED DOC: "None."

PED DOC: "Understood."
(to PED NUR #1 and PED NUR #2): "We need to anticipate that this could be a full-term newborn with problems—like meconium passage and respiratory distress—or even a preterm neonate with respiratory failure. If resuscitation is needed, we'll follow the Neonatal Resuscitation Program guidelines, so make sure that the laminated algorithm is out of the pack, and in a place where we can see it. We have a few minutes, so let's check our equipment and supplies."

ED DOC (to PED DOC): "Do you or your team need anything else from us?"

PED DOC (after looking at the PED NURs who shake their heads from side to side): "No."

ED DOC: "Are we missing anything?"

ED NUR #1: "The OB may be unfamiliar with the location of the trauma bay. Shall I ask the unit clerk to watch for her and lead her to us when she arrives?"

ED DOC: "Yes, call that person now." (to All) "Anything else?"

All: "No, not that we can think of."

ED DOC: "Okay, let's finish setting up and get ready to do our best for this woman and her baby."

Both of the 3-person teams prepare for the patient's arrival.

A faint siren is heard in the background, growing steadily louder as the ambulance pulls into the ED parking lot.

EMS (to the teams assembled in the ED, as she pushes the patient on the gurney toward them): "She's actively pushing, and I can see the baby's hair."

ED DOC quickly introduces himself to the patient, reassures her that both she and her baby will be well cared for, and begins to manage the delivery.

PED DOC (to PED NUR #1 and PED NUR #2): "Remember, we start with the basics on the algorithm: drying, warming, and stimulating. If the patient appears to be less than 32-week gestation, or, under 1.7 kilograms or so, we should NOT dry the patient, but instead cover him or her with the plastic wrap in our supplies. If the patient is apneic, I will deliver positive pressure ventilation and intubate if necessary." (to PED NUR #1) "Place the SpO2 sensor on the right wrist." (to PED RN #2) "Listen to the heart rate and verbalize it. Any questions?"

PED NUR #1 and PED NUR #2: "No, we are ready."

The fetal head is clearly visible on the perineum, indicating to the ED team that delivery is imminent, and therefore transport to L&D is not possible. A preterm neonate appearing to be approximately 33-34 weeks gestation and weighing approximately 2 kilograms is delivered. The ED DOC hands the newborn off to the PED DOC, then delivers the placenta. At this time the

OB DOC arrives, as well as a translator. While the ED DOC provides a verbal handover to the OB DOC, ED NUR#1 updates the mother via the translator.

The PED team resuscitates the neonate, following the NRP algorithm. The patient's heart rate rises to 150 (normal for a newborn) and she breathes spontaneously but at a rate of 80 breaths per minute (high for a newborn), with the use of accessory muscles (evidenced by retractions and nasal flaring), and audible grunting, all of which are signs of respiratory distress requiring proportional intervention. Her SpO2 was at 87% while on room air. Her respiratory rate came down into the normal range (40-60 breaths per minute) and her respiratory distress improved after starting continuous positive airway pressure (CPAP) with a mask and T-piece resuscitator at a pressure of 7 cm H2O. Similarly, her SpO2 rose to an acceptable range (85-95% by ten minutes of age) with the addition of oxygen (FiO2 = 30%).

PED DOC (to PED NUR #1 and PED NUR #2): "Okay, her heart rate is above 100, so let's stop and think about this for a minute."

PED NUR #2: "That would be helpful—she's not like the term newborns I usually care for."

PED DOC: "Is that because she appears to be preterm?"

PED NUR #2: "Yes, the vast majority of babies that I care for deliver at full-term or very close to their due date."

PED DOC: "Her weight of 1.9 kilograms and her physical exam is consistent with a gestational age of 33-34 weeks, a little more than a month-and-a-half early. She is requiring CPAP and oxygen, likely due to surfactant deficiency, but infection is also a possible etiology. Anything else in terms of problems that we need to treat?"

PED NUR #1: "At that weight she probably won't be able to maintain normal body temperature without exogenous heat, like she's getting now under the radiant warmer."

PED NUR #2: "And she probably won't be able to nipple feed well enough to maintain her serum glucose level in the normal range."

PED DOC: "Okay, let's list her main problems, in the order in which we need to address them. Number one: respiratory distress. Thus far, CPAP is enough support, but the natural history of surfactant deficiency is to worsen over the first 72 hours and then slowly resolve. We need to anticipate that her respiratory distress will worsen, and she will need CPAP, and possibly intubation and mechanical ventilation, for hours to days. If her need for oxygen or pressure increases, she may need to be treated with exogenous surfactant."

PED NUR #1: "We have only a Level I nursery, so she can't stay there, we don't have the equipment nor the personnel to manage a neonate on a ventilator for any length of time."

PED NUR #2: "But she certainly can't stay here in the ED."

PED DOC: "We have more resources to care for a newborn in the nursery, so let's plan to move her there. We will need to arrange to transport her to a Level 3 neonatal intensive care unit. We typically send our patients to University Hospital, so I will call the neonatologist there to arrange transport. But in the meantime, what else do we need to do while she is here with us?"

PED NUR #1: "Problem number two is hypothermia: as a premie, she doesn't have enough body fat to maintain a normal temperature. We'll need to keep her warm. I recommend that we cover her with warm blankets and keep her on the radiant warmer to help reduce her heat loss, until we can place her in an incubator in the nursery."

PED NUR #2: "Problem number three is the risk of hypoglycemia. We need to check a glucose level now, and we should place a peripheral IV, anticipating that her level may be or become low. Later, we can see if she can feed, but she will likely need a continuous infusion of IV glucose, at least initially."

PED DOC: "And given the many unknowns about her mother's pregnancy, such as her Group B Strep status, coupled with her respiratory distress and O2 need, we also need to consider the possibility of infection as an etiology and therefore evaluate and treat her for it. We'll need to draw a blood culture and start broad spectrum IV antibacterial therapy, specifically ampicillin and gentamicin, so placing a peripheral IV will be useful in at least two ways. We'll also need a chest x-ray. Anything else that anyone can think of?"

PED NUR #1 and PED NUR #2: "No, that sounds like a good start."

PED DOC: "Okay, let's quickly review then execute our plan. We'll keep her on CPAP and monitor her breathing and SpO2s closely. If her respiratory distress worsens, I will increase her CPAP and if that doesn't fix the problem, I will intubate her."

PED NUR #1: "I will call the nursery and tell them to set up an incubator and await our arrival. Until then, the radiant warmer should maintain her temperature in the normal range."

PED NUR #2: "I will do a venipuncture for a glucose level and a blood culture. I will also start a peripheral IV." (to PED DOC) "I will inform you when the result is available."

PED DOC (to PED NUR #2): "If that level is less than 40 milligrams per deciliter, you can anticipate that I will order a 4-milliliter bolus of D10W, increase the IV infusion rate and order a repeat glucose level in 15 minutes."

PED DOC (to both PED NURs): "Because we all agree that she can't stay at our hospital, I will call University Hospital and arrange for transport as soon as I've written the orders for CPAP, a blood culture, D10W to infuse at 80 ml/kg/day, antibiotics and a chest x-ray. Okay, let's get to work."

CHAPTER 11

STOP

Chapter Briefing[104]

I want to call a quick STAR (Stop-Think-Act-Review): get off your email, stop your side conversations, and turn off the television. In this chapter, we will discuss the Stop phase of STAR (Stop-Think-Act-Review). We will be successful if you can describe what your team must do to accomplish a Stop.

The primary threat that you might experience is the introduction of a large number of concepts and terms, some of which you may have never encountered, and some of which you may think about in a different sense. We will therefore explicitly define and differentiate each term and concept. We also realize how busy you are. We will make sure that the chapter is short enough to be read in approximately thirty minutes. Finally, we provide Summary Boxes. The Summary Boxes serve two functions. First, they emphasize the take-home points in each section, and you can use them to check your understanding of those take-home points. Second, you can use them to determine if you and your team are implementing those take-home points. If a Summary Box does not make sense to you or you do not understand one or more take-home points, then review the related material before continuing to the next section.

Did I miss anything? Any concerns? Any questions? (Pause) No? Then, let's get started.

---

104 By now, you may feel that repeated use of the chapter briefing format is redundant. However, we believe that it is important to continue to emphasize that a good briefing builds mental models by discussing what is happening, what success looks like, and what threats or errors are possible and how you plan to prevent, avoid, or mitigate them. Hence, the repetitive nature is meant to cement this belief with an understanding that you will also immerse yourself in this book on an irregular and/or intermittent basis.

List of Abbreviations

CRM	Crew Resource Management
STAR	Stop-Think-Act-Review

S stands for Stop

Stop literally means cease what you are doing to the extent possible. Others might call it a Time Out or Stop Work. If you see that something bad or unexpected is happening, do not dig the hole any deeper by continuing what you are doing.

Stop helps people get over the startle effect or from going into the Ready-Fire-Aim mode, where you start acting before you spend time to understand the situation. Stop is about taking a deep breath or two, counting to 10, or taking as much time as possible. Stop can be for one second, one minute, one hour, or one day, depending on the circumstance. How much time you have to Stop may be the first thing you need to consider (you will refine that time estimate later in the Think phase, but do not let a stressful situation force you to needlessly rush a decision). In our scenario, when the ED physician found out there was a woman in active labor inbound, she called a quick Stop ("no more than a minute") to get everyone's attention and get over the startle effect.

Stop also means stopping any multitasking, non-critical activities, interruptions, and distractions. Regardless of how good you think you are at multitasking or even how much your job requires it, research shows that multitasking is rife with potential errors. (Loukopoulos, Dismukes, and Barshi 2009) Stop gives your team the mental resources and time to do CRM and complete a STAR. Stop is not a normal response for can-do, action-oriented people or organizations.

Finally, Stop means stopping at the end of any stressful, time-critical, or safety-critical activity to make sure that you accomplished what you needed to do and to rebuild situation awareness and mental models. In our scenario, the Pediatrics team did call for a quick Stop after the newborn's heart rate was in the normal range. They decided to take a minute to discuss the patient's present and possible future status (i.e., all levels of Situation Awareness), possible threats and how they would handle each, and what they needed to do for each other.

In many organizations, any individual can call a STAR. In other organizations, only the team leader can call for a STAR, but any individual can request one and expect the team leader to honor that request. Regardless, it is all about psychological safety—does an individual feel safe to call for a STAR? Every organization will reward someone who called for a STAR when in hindsight a STAR was the right thing to do to prevent an accident. But what does the organization do when only in hindsight a STAR was not required, and operations were needlessly stopped at some cost and delay? Does the organization discourage calling for a STAR unless there is absolute certainty a problem exists? If so, then the next time, not only will that individual wait until absolutely sure, but every individual in the organization also will. By then, however, it may be too late to prevent a small problem from turning into a major incident. If, instead, the organization thanks the individual and states that it would rather stop an activity when uncertainty exists in order to enhance safety, it has developed psychological safety.

Summary Box 11.1
What Constitutes a Good Stop

Does your team…

- call a STAR (Stop-Think-Act-Review) when something unexpected happens or after a time-critical, safety-critical event to (re)gain situation awareness?
- take a deep breath, or count to 10, to get over the startle effect?
- make an initial guess if this is a 10-second, 10-minute, or 10-hour problem?
- stop all tasks and distractions to get the mental resources and time to do a STAR?
- feel safe to call a STAR and potentially be wrong?

Your brain is again in control, and you are now focused on the problem. What do you do next? You figure out what the problem is, which is the subject of the next chapter.

Reference

Barshi, Immanuel. Multitasking Myth - Handling Complexity in Real-World Operations. Ashgate Publishing Group, 2009.

CHAPTER 12

THINK:
DEFINE THE PROBLEM

Chapter Briefing[105]

I want to call a quick STAR (Stop-Think-Act-Review): get off your email, stop your side conversations, and turn off the television. In this chapter, we will discuss the first part of the Think phase where the team defines the problem or Problem Definition. We will be successful if you can:

- list the six questions that must be answered to do a good Problem Definition (Section 12.1);
- describe the factors that must be considered in determining how much time you have to Think (Section 12.3);
- clarify why you should consider different stories (Section 12.4);
- delineate the reasons for considering critical factors (Section 12.5);
- specify the rationale for considering intermediate goals (Section 12.6); and
- explain how you might find holes in your Problem Definition (Section 12.7).

The primary threat that you might experience is the introduction of a large number of concepts and terms, some of which you may have never encountered, and some of which you may think about in a different sense. We will therefore explicitly define and differentiate each term and concept. We also realize how busy you are. We will make sure that the chapter is

[105] By now, you may feel that repeated use of the chapter briefing format is redundant. However, we believe that it is important to continue to emphasize that a good briefing builds mental models by discussing what is happening, what success looks like, and what threats or errors are possible and how you plan to prevent, avoid, or mitigate them. Hence, the repetitive nature is meant to cement this belief with an understanding that you will also immerse yourself in this book on an irregular and/or intermittent basis.

short enough to be read in approximately thirty minutes. Finally, we provide Summary Boxes. The Summary Boxes serve two functions. First, they emphasize the take-home points in each section, and you can use them to check your understanding of those take-home points. Second, you can use them to determine if you and your team are implementing those take-home points. If a Summary Box does not make sense to you or you do not understand one or more take-home points, then review the related material before continuing to the next section.

Did I miss anything? Any concerns? Any questions? (Pause) No? Then, let's get started.

List of Abbreviations

CRM	Crew Resource Management
ED	Emergency Department
DOC	Physician
IV	Intravenous
NICU	Neonatal Intensive Care Unit
NUR	Nurse
PED	Pediatrics
STAR	Stop-Think-Act-Review
STEP	Status-Team-Environment-Progress

The T in STAR stands for Think. Think is basically CRM-enabled decision making.[106] We break up Think into 2 phases: Problem Definition and Course of Action Selection. In this chapter, you will learn what Problem Definition is (Section 12.1), and the six questions you must answer to demonstrate that you have done Problem Definition properly (Sections 12.2 through 12.7).

12.1 Think to Define the Problem

If you recall, we previously shared a quote attributed to Einstein: "If I had an hour to solve a problem, I'd spend 55 minutes thinking about the problem, and five minutes thinking about solutions." The 55-to-5 ratio may not be right, but too many organizations do the opposite: spend 5 minutes thinking

[106] Decision making is considered a CRM skill in many of the CRM models with 6-8 skills. In our CRM model, decision making is not a skill. Instead, good decision making is a product of good CRM.

about the problem and 55 minutes thinking about solutions. That 5-to-55 ratio may be why your great plan failed to solve your problem. Think back to any incident or failure in your organization. Was it due to a good problem definition followed by a bad plan, or a bad problem definition followed by an inappropriate plan? Research (Klein, Orasanu, Calderwood, and Zsambok 1993) shows that good teams treat decision making as a two-step process. The first step is good Problem Definition, followed by the second step, Course of Action Selection. Take as much time as the situation allows to first understand the problem, and, only after doing that, start looking at possible solutions.

Problem Definition takes your situation awareness and focuses it to determine if you have a problem and how best to define it. Think of Problem Definition as developing situation awareness about the problem. Problem Definition makes sure that you are solving the right problem. A Problem Definition is complete if you can answer these 6 questions:

1. Are there any quick response actions required? (Section 12.2)
2. How much time or margin do you have, or can you have? (Section 12.3)
3. What is the problem? (Section 12.4)
4. What are the critical factors? (Section 12.5)
5. What is your first goal? (Section 12.6)
6. How do you validate your Problem Definition? (Section 12.7)

Do not start Course of Action Selection until after you answer these questions.

Each of these questions is addressed in the following paragraphs.

12.2 Are There Any Quick Response Actions Required?

If you are in an emergency situation, you usually need to take a certain number of immediate actions to achieve a stable or safe condition. In these situations, decisions usually have been codified and actions are proceduralized, trained, and practiced to the point that decision and actions come automatically. If so, perform those actions. In our scenario, the Pediatrics team needed to ensure the newborn was breathing properly, and the decision and actions were codified in the Neonatal Resuscitation Program algorithm (which they had laminated in their pack). Once you are in a safe condition, you have time to answer the next 5 questions.

Summary Box 12.1
Quick Response Action Question

Does your team need to undertake any immediate actions to get into a stable or safe condition?

12.3 How Much Time or Margin Do You Have, or Can You Have?

Now that the situation is stable, you have the time and mental resources needed to start refining your initial estimate from the Stop phase on how much time you can spend in Problem Definition. Once done with the Quick Response Actions, you do not want to make a decision in 5 minutes if you have 5 days, and you do not want to take 5 days if you only have 5 minutes. You also need to make sure that you can make the decision, develop the plan, execute the plan, and have the actions produce the desired effects before anything bad happens, probably with some margin. In our scenario, the physician knew that the baby would need to be transferred to a Level 3 Neonatal Intensive Care Unit (NICU), most likely using the NICU Transport Team. Let us add a complication. What if that transport was delayed? The team would need to decide what to do and make that decision soon enough for the team to decide on the best transport option, develop a plan to do it safely, and allow time for the transport and the team at the NICU to admit the patient, all within a reasonable time with margin. Maybe your estimate of the time available to make a decision is 1/10th, 1/5th or 1/3rd of the total time available, which you may continue to refine later. A conscious assessment of how much time you have to make a decision will prevent you from either deciding too quickly and making the wrong decision, or, from deciding too slowly and being overcome by events. One possible CRM error the team made in our example is that the physician never specifically stated how quickly the patient needed to be admitted to a NICU. Everyone assumed "as soon as possible". Without a specific time, the team would not know what other transport options were acceptable if the NICU Transport Team was delayed.

When variables such as time limits are not specified, it is impossible for the team to know if they are exceeding those limits. In 2005, physicians spent over 21 minutes trying to gain a secure airway while Elaine Bromiley's hemoglobin oxygen saturation was 40% (McClelland 2016). No member of the team specified a length of time which, once exceeded, would require the team to try something else. If a time limit is agreed upon, a team member should be assigned to ensure that the limit is not exceeded. Because no time limit was specified and no team member was monitoring the passage of time, Elaine Bromiley died a preventable death. Monitoring time is an example of planning to Mutually Support.

You should also look for ways to "buy" more time. In the scenario, the team prepped the room and equipment so that when the mother arrived, they could devote their entire attention to her. Be aware that too many teams underestimate how long a procedure might take, or, worse yet, allow wishful thinking or ego to bias their estimation. If you know that most teams take five hours to perform a procedure (i.e., the base rate), why would you think that your team can do it in only two hours?[107] Is your team that much different and extraordinary? Most likely, your team will take much closer to five hours than two hours to perform the same task. Unless you have overwhelming proof that your team is truly exceptional, always use the base rate and then adjust up or down, based on the circumstances.

Closely related to buying time is increasing margin. A team must also find ways to monitor, manage, and even increase margin. There are 2 types of margin: present and in depth. Present margin is how much a critical data parameter (e.g., pressure, temperature, resource, etc.) can increase or decrease before something bad happens, or before you must go to a contingency plan. Present margin is gone when you reach a trigger. In the Bromiley case, the team could have decided that when oxygen saturation reached 80 percent, regardless of time, they would try something different. Margin in depth is how many contingency plans you have. Margin in depth is gone when you run out of contingencies (i.e., you are all in).

Both types of margin are determined in the planning phase, discussed in the briefing, monitored during execution, and debriefed in the end. In the planning phase, the team determines what threats are possible, and, when that threat has used up all margin (reached a trigger, meaning loss of present margin), what contingencies are possible, and how to transition to them (using up margin in depth). By the end of the briefing, the team knows what to look for to determine how much margin they have, can comprehend the significance of margin, and can project when margin will run out. During execution, the team is looking at critical data in all areas of STEP to determine margins and knows when a margin is all used up (hits a trigger)

---

[107] Prior data across multiple teams determines the base rate. In this example, the base rate is 5 hours.

and they therefore need to transition to a contingency plan (loss of present margin). When they transition to a contingency, they must realize how much margin is left in that contingency before they need to go to Plan C. Also, the team is always looking for ways to increase margin. A debriefing is all about fixing STEP Mental Models: why did we not know about that Status threat (what affects margin); why did we not know how that Team threat would grow (how it affects margins); why did we not know when the hospital policies would require a change (when margin runs out); and why did we not notice the change (why did we not monitor the margin).

Many people think of margin only in terms of time-to-effect, or how much time do we have left. But a patient might have margin in how much his fever can increase before it reaches an unacceptable point, equipment exceeds its pressure limits, a team member is exhausted, or when an organizational policy says we must quit. Although many of these may be converted into a time-to-effect, it is temperature, pressure, fatigue, or policy that you must find ways to mitigate to increase margin. All the STEP Mental Models must be considered to realize the full suite of margins and how close a team is operating to one.

Another way to buy more time is to keep as many options open as possible, avoiding eliminating any options before absolutely necessary. In our scenario, if the team had learned that the Level 3 NICU Transport might be delayed, they could have worked to see if they could bring in people to do the transport themselves. That way, if they found out later that the NICU Transport was unavailable, they were ahead of the game in knowing whether they could transport the newborn themselves.

Summary Box 12.2
The Time/Margin Question

Does your team…
- proactively determine how much time you have before something bad happens, or you need to achieve a particular result?
- determine how much time to use for Problem Definition?
- assign someone to monitor time and margin?
- find ways to buy time or increase margin?
- determine how long a task will take by adjusting up or down from the base rate?
- keep as many options open for as long as possible?

12.4 What Is the Problem?

The ship *Titanic* hit an iceberg and was sinking. What was the problem that the crew had to solve? The problem the *Titanic* crew faced was that there were not enough lifeboats for all the passengers and crew. They could not solve that problem. A common error during the Think phase is when people have a problem that they cannot solve, they subconsciously change it to a simpler problem that they can solve. The *Titanic* crew did exactly that. Since the crew could not figure out how to get everyone off the sinking boat, they simplified the problem to deciding who would get on the lifeboats. If they had instead reframed the problem to be "how do we find things that will float and get our people on them", would they have decided to do something different? If they had approached the problem from this perspective, would they have thought about the biggest floating object around—the iceberg that caused the original problem—as a potential solution? Although getting the people on the iceberg might not have been practical or might not have saved any more people, simply reframing the problem might have changed the solutions that they were considering. In our example, the problem was defined as the patient needed to get to a Level 3 NICU as soon as possible. What if they had phrased the problem as, "...we do not have the expertise or equipment to manage the patient...", would they have thought of other options such as consulting with another physician who had experience in caring for sick newborns, or getting the necessary equipment to care for the patient? Even though those actions may not represent viable options, they do illustrate that how a problem is framed increases or decreases possible options.[108] One remedy is to use your team and their diversity of mental models to frame the problem. Ask them what they think the true problem is and then actively listen.

An organization's philosophies, policies, procedures, and practices (i.e., culture) affects how it frames a problem, and later in Course of Action Selection, what possible courses of action it is even willing to consider. Your culture and organization can help or hurt your Problem Definition.

After any Quick Response Actions, your next goal may be to obtain more information. Before you can define the problem, you may need more accurate information to build better situation awareness and mental models. If there is missing, unreliable, ambiguous, or conflicting information, you

---

[108] Another place where framing is important is when determining the acceptability of risk. A risk assessment framed as a gain (e.g., 60% chance of a gain) will generate a different response than when framed as a loss (e.g., 40% chance of a loss).

may need to find a way to get the information, make it higher quality, or resolve conflicts. In the scenario, the Pediatrics hospitalist ordered a blood culture to get more information on a possible infection. You need to be careful to not get caught in the trap of trying to get all the possible information. This sometimes results in "paralysis by analysis". More information does not necessarily guarantee better decisions; too much information can result in poorer decisions (Zheng, Marsh, Nickerson, and Kleinberg 2020). Sometimes the request for more information comes from outside the core team. For example, when a team must triage pediatric transports, ultimately their goal is to stabilize the child to a point where the team can get the child to an appropriate hospital safely. But people outside the core team, not typically triaging transports, may ask for extraneous information or lab tests that delay the transport. It is critical that the core team understand what information is required to achieve their first goal (safe transport) and focus only on that information. Get as much information as you can in the time that is available, and then address any remaining uncertainties. You may have to determine how much time you will devote to gathering information, then assign someone to monitor that time.

When building situation awareness and faced with complexity, incomplete data, ambiguity, and uncertainty, experienced people will develop stories (also known as explanation building) (Weick, Sutcliffe, and Obstfeld 2005). In our discussion on situation awareness, we discussed why it is important to consider other stories that would have arrived at the same situation. With incomplete data (i.e., missing, unreliable, ambiguous, or conflicting data), you might not be able to be sure of the exact event timeline. To compensate, experienced people try to make sense of the situation by building possible stories that explain how they arrived at the current situation. Stories use information from the past and present, along with experience to fill in the blanks, and develop a logical flow of events to get to the current state. In our scenario, the most logical story to explain why the mother was alone, and her husband was unreachable was that they were not expecting labor (i.e., the labor was premature). Even if the team finds a story that seems to fit, a good team will ask, "what else?". What else would get us into this situation? An alternate story on why the mother was alone and her husband was unreachable, might be that the mother received no prenatal care and did not know when to expect birth. Both stories end up with the mother alone and pushing, but one story tells the team to look for a premature birth, while the other tells the team to look for a possible full-term birth, but with the potential for maternal and/or neonatal complications. Stories allow experts to check for inconsistencies, to determine what additional data to look for

(Level 1 Situation Awareness) and provide context to make projections into the future (Level 3 Situation Awareness). If the first story is too full of inconsistencies, or additional information does not confirm it, or future projections are wrong, then another story is likely to be a better fit. In healthcare, stories are hypotheses as to what events or conditions could have led a patient to present in their current state of health (or disease). This is similar to the differential diagnoses that healthcare professionals develop to explain a patient's (objective) clinical signs and (subjective) symptoms. They then select the most likely diagnosis based on those signs and symptoms, initiate a treatment plan, and then monitor the patient to determine whether the symptoms are improving (increasing the likelihood that the initial diagnosis is accurate). If the patient is not improving, either the diagnosis is accurate, but the treatment plan needs to be modified (by invoking one or more contingency plans), or, the diagnosis is inaccurate, and a completely new treatment plan must be developed and implemented. Consider the case of a decompensating patient and a physician sharing her thoughts as to possible etiologies for the event with the team. The team leader states, "this could be a pneumothorax, cardiac failure, or fluid overload…". The respiratory therapist who intubated the patient adds, "…it could also be a mainstem intubation...". The team leader then asks what information would allow the team to determine which etiology was the cause. The respiratory therapist responds that asymmetrical breath sounds and/or chest rise would indicate the presence of a mainstem intubation. If multiple stories might explain the current situation, you need to think of what indications in the future will help you determine the right story. We call this "critical data". Defining and monitoring for critical data will help you define your current situation. Therefore, asymmetrical breath sounds and/or chest rise would be critical data, something the team needed to look for.

Summary Box 12.3
The Problem Question

Does your team…

- properly frame the original problem or switch to an alternate simpler problem?
- take advantage of the diversity of their mental models?
- assign someone to monitor the time?
- get as much data in the time available?
- determine other stories that would explain the current situation?
- define critical data that will let you confirm or refute a possible story?

12.5 What Are the Critical Factors?

Critical factors are anything that defines your success, or limits or enables your choices. If you need to get the newborn to a Level 3 NICU, that is a success critical factor (i.e., any course of action that does not get the newborn to that level is unacceptable). If you have limitations on a specific resource such as time, personnel, experience, or equipment (i.e., a limiting critical factor), do not come up with a plan that needs more of that resource than you have. For example, if you only have six hours before something bad happens, then six hours is a critical factor. Do not come up with a plan that exceeds six hours. The presence of a critical factor may also enable options. For example, the presence of an Emergency Department nurse who previously worked in a Level 3 NICU provides a useful resource when a laboring patient presents to the Emergency Department. You also need to determine if what you consider a critical factor is really critical. By definition, a critical factor is non-negotiable. Therefore, you need to be sure that any factor labeled as critical is really that important. Are time constraints that your team places on a procedure necessary, or can they be relaxed to allow more time to safely and effectively achieve your patient care goals? Maybe a critical factor is just an unreasonable, under-defined or artificial constraint produced by your organization's culture, such as "as soon as possible". You must consciously assess anything labeled as critical. Listing a factor that is not truly critical will over-constrain your plan to meet false constraints. Failing to list a factor that is truly critical, however, may cause you to develop a plan that does not meet your needs. Wishful thinking (e.g., "Maybe I don't really need that...") is not allowed.

WARNING: When executing your plan, if a critical factor upon which you were depending does not materialize (e.g., a team member with a specific skill), then, by definition, your plan is wrong. You must restart the STAR process all over again.

Summary Box 12.4
The Critical Factor Question

Does your team determine what...

- must be achieved to be successful? (Success Criteria)?
- prevents consideration of a particular Course of Action? (Limiting Criteria)?
- would allow a Course of Action to be considered if it appeared? (Enabling Criteria)?
- what factors are really critical (non-negotiable)?

12.6 What Is Your First Goal?

Some problems are too complex to be solved all at once but must be solved in stages. There are several reasons why a problem must be solved incrementally. First, a previous step is required before you can do the next step. In our scenario, the first goal was to ensure the newborn was breathing adequately. That step was required before the team could consider any other actions. Some goals are, by definition, sequential.

The second reason why goals may have to be managed incrementally is that you need to perform some actions to see what future options might be available. This is do-a-little, observe-a-little, STAR-a-little, or multiple cycles where you try a small action, see the result, and then perform a mini-STAR to determine what to do next (Plant and Stanton 2015). In our scenario, the Pediatrics team placed a peripheral IV to address the need for IV fluids to prevent hypoglycemia and the need for broad spectrum antibacterial therapy to treat a presumed infection.

A third reason for setting incremental goals occurs when resources are insufficient or temporarily unavailable to complete a goal. In our scenario, the team had to treat the newborn in their nursery until transport to a Level 3 NICU was possible.

A final reason underlying the need to achieve goals incrementally lies in the concept of a team of teams, where collaborating teams each have their own set of priorities and responsibilities. One team may need to help another team achieve that team's goals before it can rely on their help to accomplish its own goals. By consciously assessing goals, you avoid wasting time trying to achieve goals out of priority order for the larger team of teams.

Summary Box 12.5
The Goal Question

Does your team determine if…

- it can solve this problem in one step, or incrementally?
- it must do-a-little, then see where you are, then STAR (Stop-Think-Act-Review), then repeat?
- a goal may be constrained by current resources?
- it must perform some tasks to meet the needs of other teams?

12.7 How Do You Validate Your Problem Definition?

The best teams find ways to validate their Problem Definition, just like they validate their Situation Awareness. The goal of validation is to find holes and errors in your Problem Definition. One way they can validate their Problem Definition is by bringing in a fresh set of eyes to look at what the team did and ask questions, challenge assumptions, and require the team to prove that they thought of everything. Consider opening the validation to a "Red Team", or people outside the core team who can provide a different perspective (i.e., have a different mental model). In our example, the Pediatric team discussed the situation among themselves. They might have considered bringing in a fresh set of eyes or, preferably, consulting a neonatologist, to see if that person could find holes in their Problem Definition. That different perspective may come from the person on your team who "doesn't know how we operate", or "works for that other department" or "is the new guy".

If the team cannot find a fresh set of eyes, they could try a Pre-Mortem (Klein 2008).[109] In a Pre-Mortem, even before they start the Course of Action phase, they assume their Problem Definition was flawed. They hypothesize all the possible reasons why their Problem Definition was flawed. In our scenario, after the Pediatrics team discussed the four threats and how they were going to handle them, the physician could say, "Okay, it is now 2 hours from now and the newborn's condition is worsening. What did we do wrong? What did we miss?" A nurse might say, "Could the patient have some kind of undiagnosed congenital anomaly?". The team could then develop a plan to look for that possible problem.

Instead of a Pre-Mortem, some teams use a Devil's Advocate. There are problems with using a Devil's Advocate approach, however, especially if the person in the Devil's Advocate role was part of the original Problem Definition. He or she may either be reluctant to criticize the team or may have the same holes in thinking.

[109] We are not specifying use of a Pre-Mortem. We are saying that you need to use something to validate your Problem Definition.

Summary Box 12.6
The Validation Question

Does your team…
• seek a fresh perspective from a new set of eyes? • open the validation to people outside the core team? • find other ways to validate their Problem Definition even if a new set of eyes or people outside the core team are unavailable?

How well did the team in the scenario do in defining the problem? How well did the team state:

- whether any quick action responses were required?
- how much time they (can) had to complete a task?
- what was the actual problem?
- the critical factor(s) inherent in this situation?
- its first goal?
- how to validate its Problem Definition?

The Emergency Department and Pediatrics teams took a series of Quick Response Actions to deliver the newborn and ensure that she had an adequate heart rate and hemoglobin oxygen saturation. Because the pediatrician knew that the patient required a higher level of care, he told his team that transport must be accomplished but failed to be specific in the amount of time that they had to achieve the goal of safe transport to a Level 3 NICU. He did, however, define the problem as a need to manage a newborn with surfactant deficiency or infection. The critical factors included time (but in this case it was unspecified), the expertise of a neonatologist, and equipment and supplies found in a Level 3 NICU. The Pediatric team correctly identified its first goal (resuscitate and stabilize the newborn) before proceeding to address its second goal (safely transport the neonate to a Level 3 NICU). The Pediatric team could have sought additional input to validate its Problem Definition, from colleagues in the Emergency Department, others in their own hospital, or professionals based at other hospitals.

Now that you are sure that you have done a complete Problem Definition, you can start thinking about possible courses of action, which is the subject of the next chapter.

Chapter Debriefing

I want to call a quick STAR (Stop-Think-Act-Review): get off your email, stop your side conversations, and turn off the television. Let's see if you can expand upon these statements. Your team needs to determine and then monitor…

- how much time and margin you have;
- critical data to confirm or refute a possible story;
- critical factors;
- intermediate goals; and
- how it will validate its Problem Definition.

If this was an actual debriefing, we would ask you to expand further on each of these statements. Depending on your response, we would ask open-ended follow-up questions until we were sure you understood the material and had a plan to implement one or more best practices. We might ask, "What is a specific Problem Definition problem that you experience on your job?" We would not be satisfied if you said, "We can't do Problem Definition as well as we need." Again, we would ask open-ended follow-up questions until you might say "We have a problem with teams either taking too little, or too much, time to define the problem." We would then ask, "What can you do prior to your next shift to fix that problem?" We would then continue to ask open-ended follow-up questions until you might say, "Prior to Problem Definition, I need to determine times-to-effect and margins to determine how much time we can spend in Problem Definition. During Problem Definition, I need to assign someone to monitor time. During the debriefing, we need to discuss why we took too little or too much time." We would then ask, "That helps your team. What about other teams?" We would ask more open-ended questions until you say, "I need to work with management to change our training to include more discussion on critical data and factors, and times-to-effect and margin."

References

Klein, Gary. "Performing a Project Premortem." IEEE Engineering Management Review 36, no. 2 (2008): 103–4. https://doi.org/10.1109/emr.2008.4534313.

Klein, Gary A. Decision Making in Action: Models and Methods. Norwood, NJ: Ablex, 1995.

McClelland, G, and MB Smith. "Just a Routine Operation: A Critical Discussion." Journal of Perioperative Practice 26, no. 5 (2016): 114–17. https://doi.org/10.1177/175045891602600504.

Plant, Katherine L., and Neville A. Stanton. "The Process of Processing: Exploring the Validity of Neisser's Perceptual Cycle Model with Accounts from Critical Decision-Making in the Cockpit." Ergonomics 58, no. 6 (2014): 909–23. https://doi.org/10.1080/00140139.2014.991765.

quoteresearch, Author. "I Would Spend 55 Minutes Defining the Problem and Then Five Minutes Solving It." Quote Investigator, November 22, 2018. https://quoteinvestigator.com/2014/05/22/solve/.

Weick, Karl E., Kathleen M. Sutcliffe, and David Obstfeld. "Organizing and the Process of Sensemaking." Organization Science 16, no. 4 (2005): 409–21. https://doi.org/10.1287/orsc.1050.0133.

Zheng, Min, Jessecae K. Marsh, Jeffrey V. Nickerson, and Samantha Kleinberg. "How Causal Information Affects Decisions." Cognitive Research: Principles and Implications. Springer International Publishing, February 13, 2020. https://cognitiveresearchjournal.springeropen.com/articles/10.1186/s41235-020-0206-z.

CHAPTER 13

THINK: DETERMINE A COURSE OF ACTION

Chapter Briefing[110]

I want to call a quick STAR (Stop-Think-Act-Review): get off your email, stop your side conversations, and turn off the television. In this chapter, we will discuss the second part of the Think phase, which is to Determine a Course of Action. We will be successful if you can:

- explain when and when not to use Codified Decision Making (Section 13.1);
- explain when and when not to use Naturalistic Decision Making (Section 13.2);
- explain when and when not to use Deliberate Decision Making (Section 13.3); and[111]
- list what you must consider when validating your course of action selection (13.4)

The primary threat that you might experience is the introduction of a large number of concepts and terms, some of which you may have never encountered, and some of which you may think about in a different sense. We will therefore explicitly define and differentiate each term and concept. We also realize how busy you are. We will make sure that the chapter is short enough to be read in approximately thirty minutes. Finally, we provide

---

[110] By now, you may feel that repeated use of the chapter briefing format is redundant. However, we believe that it is important to continue to emphasize that a good briefing builds mental models by discussing what is happening, what success looks like, and what threats or errors are possible and how you plan to prevent, avoid, or mitigate them. Hence, the repetitive nature is meant to cement this belief with an understanding that you will also immerse yourself in this book on an irregular and/or intermittent basis.

[111] See Chapter 16 for more information on Decision Making.

Summary Boxes. The Summary Boxes serve two functions. First, they emphasize the take-home points in each section, and you can use them to check your understanding of those take-home points. Second, you can use them to determine if you and your team are implementing those take-home points. If a Summary Box does not make sense to you or you do not understand one or more take-home points, then review the related material before continuing to the next section.

Did I miss anything? Any concerns? Any questions? (Pause) No? Then, let's get started.

List of Abbreviations

CRM	Crew Resource Management
DOC	Physician
ED	Emergency Department
NICU	Neonatal Intensive Care Unit
PED	Pediatrics

The T in STAR stands for Think. Think is basically CRM-enabled decision making.[112] We break up Think into 2 phases: Problem Definition and Course of Action Selection. In this chapter, you will learn the various decision-making models you can use to decide on the proper course of action, which is when to and when not to use Codified Decision Making (Section 13.1), Naturalistic Decision Making (Section 13.2) and Deliberate Decision Making (Section 13.3). You will also learn how to validate your course of action selection (Section 13.4).

13.1 Codified (or Rule-Based) Decision Making

Codified Decision Making is decision making based on pre-made rules. A resuscitation algorithm is an example of Codified Decision Making. Codified Decision Making often appears as a pre-made conditional statement: if the team sees *X*, then they shall do *Y*. The rules could be documented in an organization's philosophies, policies, procedures, and practices days, weeks, or even years before the team shows up for their task

[112] Decision Making is considered a CRM skill in many of the CRM models with 6-8 skills. In our CRM model, decision making is not a skill. Instead, good decision making is a product of good CRM.

or shift. The rules could also be decided by the team minutes or hours before the task during the team briefing. In the scenario, the Pediatrics team decided before the ambulance arrived that if the patient appears to be less than 32-week gestation or under 1.7 kilogram, they would cover the patient with the plastic wrap. Or, if the patient was apneic, they would deliver positive pressure ventilation. The main point is that the decision has been made beforehand, and the team just has to decide to use it.

The advantage of Codified Decision Making is that the decisions were made without the stress of being in the actual situation and with the help of all the experts, information, and time. It is also the simplest and quickest form of decision making. It is best for inexperienced decision makers, in situations that require rapid response, where entry conditions can be well defined (e.g., 32-week gestation, 1.7 kilograms, apneic) therefore possible alternate stories are limited, and uniformity of response is required.[113]

The problem with Codified Decision Making is that it is impossible to cover every possible variation of a situation. Since Codified Decision Making is a conditional statement ("if you see Situation *X*, then perform Procedure *Y*"), you must decide if you are in Situation *X*. In many cases, Situation *X* is simplified to meet defined entry criteria while ignoring complexity, uncertainty, and alternate stories. Therefore, the main error in Codified Decision Making is applying a codified decision when the entry criteria are different or more complex, or when alternate stories do exist. You must make sure that this is really the situation that the rule makers envisioned, and not something subtly different (e.g., performing Procedure *Y* was not meant for this set of slightly different conditions). In Chapter 3 on Situation Awareness, you compared what is happening to what your situation awareness and mental model say should happen. Here you are using your CRM to compare what is happening to what the rule-makers' situation awareness and mental model say should happen. You are evaluating their situation awareness and mental model. Did they perceive the right things, and do those perceptions match what is happening in your situation? Are their mental models adequate to comprehend and project the situation you are in? In our example, the team used a codified rule (the Neonatal Resuscitation Program algorithm) to resuscitate the newborn. The assumption of the rule is that the physician's assessment of the gestational age, weight and physiologic status is accurate, and that there are no unique

[113] Entry conditions are factors that got you into this situation.

patient anatomic or physiologic characteristics that would necessitate a deviation from the algorithm.

Summary Box 13.1
Codified Decision Making

Does your team…
• consider that the situation may be more complex, or otherwise different, than what is assumed by the rule? • allow for the possibility that there are alternate stories that might explain this situation? • have a mental model that produces a different outcome than the rule predicts?

If your team answered "yes" to any of these questions, then actively listen to your team to fix any errors in situation awareness or mental models, or, maybe Codified Decision Making is not appropriate in this case, and you must use one of the other decision making methods instead.

13.2 Naturalistic (or Experience-Based) Decision Making

Rather than basing decisions on rules, Naturalistic Decision Making is based on previous experience. Naturalistic Decision Making is the "been there, done that" approach of decision making. Naturalistic Decision Making is how experienced people naturally make decisions. Highly experienced people have a repertoire of past experiences upon which to draw and can rapidly decide what to do. In fact, the root of the word "expert" implies significant experience on which to base predictions. Some people confuse this with the word intuition because experts may not be able to articulate what specifically they noticed or how they knew what to do. Our definition of intuition is merely tacit knowledge. Experts recognize a situation and remember what they did that worked last time (Klein 1998). Experts can do a quick review for missing, unreliable, or conflicting data and then run a mental simulation to make sure the plan works. If Plan A does not work, they will check Plan B.[114] They pick the first plan that works. In the scenario, the Emergency Department physician's experience with her team performing vaginal deliveries allowed her to make the decision to do the delivery.

---

[114] In Naturalistic Decision Making, options are evaluated sequentially with the decision maker taking the first option that works. In Deliberate Decision Making, options are evaluated against each other, and the optimal option selected.

The advantage of Naturalistic Decision Making is it allows an experienced person to decide on an adequate, but not optimal, solution very quickly, even under high stress. The problem is that Naturalistic Decision Making requires a broad, deep, and refined repertoire of diverse experiences. Therefore, the main error in Naturalistic Decision Making is that people who do not have that diverse experience think they recognize the situation. In reality, the situation is just different enough to invalidate their limited experience.

In Codified Decision Making, you were using your CRM to compare what is happening to what the rule-makers' situation awareness and mental model say should happen. In Naturalistic Decision Making, you are using your CRM to compare what is happening to what your experience says should happen. You are essentially evaluating the diversity of your experience.[115] You must make sure that what you are perceiving today is the same as what you experienced in the past. You must also make sure that the results needed today are the same as what resulted in the past. While obviously there may be small variations, do not simply explain them away. Instead, use your situation awareness and mental model to ensure the variations do not invalidate your previous experience.

It may be very difficult for an individual to evaluate his or her experience. An individual without a broad repertoire of experiences by definition does not have the situation awareness or mental model to fully understand the situation. What is an important versus a minor difference? How does that difference affect the situation now and in the future? In our scenario, how does the delivery of a 2 kilogram, 33-34 week estimated gestational age neonate differ from that of a 3.5 kilogram full-term neonate in terms of the preparations carried out by the pediatric team? A team has diverse situation awareness and mental models. A diverse Level 1 Situation Awareness will mean that they perceive things differently than you, and that their diverse mental models will mean that they will have different ideas on how and why it is happening. You must actively listen in order to determine if their diverse situation awareness and mental models are exposing holes in yours.

[115] Hopefully, you have been using your previous experiences to broaden, deepen, and refine your mental models, and update your own mental model to understand why subtle changes in what you saw or heard (changes in Level 1 Situation Awareness) resulted in changes in the outcome (changes in Levels 2 and 3 Situation Awareness).

Summary Box 13.2
Naturalistic Decision Making

Does your team…
• perceive information that is different than your previous experience (different Level 1 Situation Awareness)?
• see results that your experience did not expect (different Level 2 or 3 Situation Awareness)?
• have a different explanation for any of the differences (different mental models)?

If your team answered "yes" to any of these questions, then actively listen to your team to fix any errors in situation awareness or mental models. You must also consider the possibility that Naturalistic Decision Making is not an appropriate method for determining a course of action and that you must use an alternative method.

13.3 Deliberate (or Analytical, or Classical) Decision Making

How do you make decisions if you have no rules or previous experience? You must use Deliberate Decision Making. Deliberate Decision Making requires you to list various possible courses of action, evaluate each course of action against various discriminating factors (determining possible benefits, costs, and risks for each course of action), and pick the course of action that scores the best.

The advantage of Deliberate Decision Making is that it should find the optimal solution. The problem with Deliberate Decision Making is it requires a lot of time and data, and you must score various courses of action against discriminating factors that may not be easily quantifiable. There are three potential problems in employing Deliberate Decision Making. First, you may use Deliberate Decision Making when it is not actually required. Using Deliberate Decision Making when not required is usually caused by an erroneous organizational emphasis to always find the optimal solution. In an effort to always achieve the optimal solution, the organization requires you to always evaluate more than one possible course of action without regard to possible pre-existing rules or experience. When forced to do Deliberate Decision Making, experienced professionals will alter the possible courses of action, factors, and scores to get the result that they want. The second problem employing Deliberate Decision Making is that you may develop a set of courses of action that is unnecessarily restricted because "this is the way we've always done it" (i.e., your organizational culture does not allow you to '"think outside of the box" or even enable you to see that you are in a box). The third problem employing Deliberate Decision Making is that you may pick discriminating factors and scores that only weakly tie to the quality of a course of action. Basing a course of treatment primarily on monetary cost is an example. Is cost one of the best factors in determining the optimal treatment plan? Poorly determined courses of action, discriminating factors, or scoring can result in a flawed course of action selection.

Similar to Naturalistic Decision Making, your best CRM defense against bad Deliberate Decision Making is a diversity of situation awareness and mental models. One method to leverage that diversity of situation awareness and mental models is to ask each team member to think of possible courses of action, emphasizing to your team that you want one or two "out of the box" possibilities. You might also start with the least experienced or lowest ranked person to make sure that a higher ranked person, speaking first, does not hijack the exploration process. The goal is to involve everyone in coming up with a diverse set of possible courses of action. You discuss the resulting list of courses of action until you agree to a set of possible courses of action, hopefully with one or two "out of the box" options. Then do the same for discriminating factors: get ideas from everyone, discuss, then agree to the best discriminating factors. Finally, have each team member score the possible courses of action against the discriminating factors, then discuss any differences, and come up with the final scores. By doing this in a three-step process, you get to examine their mental models on possible courses of action, then on possible discriminating factors, and then on scoring. Of course, you must actively listen to see why their ideas make sense to them, and how that links to possible holes and errors in your situation awareness and mental models.

Summary Box 13.3
Deliberate Decision Making

Does your team have…
• a rule to cover this situation, or have experience in it?
• other possible courses of action?
• other possible discriminating factors?
• different scores for a discriminating factor?

If your team answered "yes" to any of these questions, then actively listen to your team to fix any errors in situation awareness or mental models, or, maybe Deliberate Decision making is not appropriate in this case, and you must use the Codified Decision Making or Naturalistic Decision Making method instead.

13.4 How Will You Validate Your Course of Action Selection?

The first thing you need to check is to make sure that any proposed course of action meets any critical factors.[116] For example, if the newborn is failing care at the hospital of birth and needs to be transported as soon as possible to a Level 3 NICU, any proposed course of action that includes unnecessary delays is unacceptable. Any proposed course of action should provide you access to critical data.[117] For example, if you need to continuously monitor hemoglobin oxygen saturation to determine the health of the newborn, any course of action that does not give you access to that critical data is unacceptable. Also, although not necessarily a deal-breaker, does a course of action have contingency plans? For a course of action where there is no possible contingency plan, you should exert extra effort to validate that course of action as the best decision before proceeding.

Just as in Problem Definition, you will need to find a way to validate your course of action selection, whether through Pre-Mortem or a fresh set of eyes.[118] A fresh set of eyes usually requires the involvement of professionals who are not members of your core team in order to provide an objective, comprehensive review. To determine which additional people to involve, you should ask:

- Who needs to be involved in the determination of possible courses of action?
- Who needs to be involved in the determination of a recommended course of action?
- Who will do the validation?

---

[116] A critical factor is any condition that must be met for a course of action to be successful.

[117] Critical data is any information you need in order to determine if the course of action is being successful.

[118] An exercise where the team assumes the course of action failed, they then list possible factors that caused that failure, and modify the course of action to prevent, avoid or mitigate those factors.

- Who approves the final course of action? Who is the final decision maker?

Let us see how the team in our example thought through their course of action selection.

Summary Box 13.4
Decision Making in the Scenario

- Did the pediatric team follow any rules (Codified Decision Making) when resuscitating the newborn? Yes, the Neonatal Resuscitation Program (NPR) algorithm.
    - Did anything about the situation (maternal history, the neonate's condition, available equipment) change that? No, but the neonate's condition did affect follow-on treatment.
- Did experience (Naturalistic Decision Making) influence the ED physician's plans for delivery of the newborn? Yes, the team had performed other vaginal deliveries.
    - Did anything about the situation (the maternal condition, available personnel) change that? No, despite the fact that the newborn might be premature or have other complications (outside their experience), the absence of the OB team required the ED team to perform the delivery.
- What factors were discussed (Deliberate Decision Making) by the pediatric team in order to determine whether the newborn would be cared for in the birth hospital or be transported to another facility? They did not have the equipment nor the personnel (limiting factors) to manage a neonate on a ventilator for any length of time.
    - Did anything about the situation (availability or timing of a transport team) change that? Unknown, since they had not yet called the Level 3 NICU to find out about bed availability or timing.
- How did the pediatric team validate its Course of Action selection? They discussed the options among their team members.
    - Was that sufficient to ensure a good decision? Unknown, since they did not include anyone outside the team (e.g., a neonatologist from the Level 3 NICU) to provide an outside perspective.

Once you have a course of action, you must develop a plan to make it happen, which is the subject of the next chapter.

Chapter Debriefing

I want to call a quick STAR (Stop-Think-Act-Review): get off your email, stop your side conversations, and turn off the television. Let's see if you can expand upon these statements:

- Use Codified Decision Making if a decision has been documented or briefed earlier, and the actual conditions and expected outcome match what was documented or briefed.
- Use Naturalistic Decision Making if you have extensive and diverse experience on what actions will work.
- Use Deliberate Decision Making if you have no rules or previous experience and have the time and data to compare various courses of action.

If this was an actual debriefing, we would ask you to expand further on each of these statements. Depending on your response, we would ask open-ended follow-up questions until we were sure you understood the material and had a plan to implement one or more best practices. We might ask, "What is a specific course of action selection problem that you experience on your job?" We would not be satisfied if you said, "We don't always select the proper course of action." Again, we would ask open-ended follow-up questions until you might say, "We have a problem with team members applying procedures in the wrong situation." We would then ask, "What can you do to on your next shift to fix that problem?" We would then continue to ask open-ended follow-up questions until you might say, "We need to determine if the procedure is designed for the situation that we are in. If we are unsure, we need to do a quick STAR to consider what we should do next." We would then ask, "That helps your team. What about other teams?" More open-ended questions until you might say, "I need to work with management to document what conditions dictate when to use and not use a procedure."

Reference

Klein, Gary. Sources of Power: How People Make Decisions. Cambridge, MA: MIT Press, 1999.

CHAPTER 14

ACT: DEVELOP AND EXECUTE THE PLAN

Chapter Briefing[119]

I want to call a quick STAR (Stop-Think-Act-Review): get off your email, stop your side conversations, and turn off the television. In this chapter, we will discuss using CRM to develop the plan (Plan to Act), and then execute the plan (Act on the Plan) to accomplish the selected course of action. We will be successful if you can:

- explain the CRM best practices to develop the plan (Section 14.1);
- list the CRM items to include in the briefing (Section 14.2);
- annotate the CRM items shown in the example briefing (Section 14.3); and
- list the CRM best practices to execute the plan (14.4).

The primary threat that you might experience is the introduction of a large number of concepts and terms, some of which you may have never encountered, and some of which you may think about in a different sense. We will therefore explicitly define and differentiate each term and concept. We also realize how busy you are. We will make sure that the chapter is short enough to be read in approximately thirty minutes. Finally, we provide Summary Boxes. The Summary Boxes serve two functions. First, they emphasize the take-home points in each section, and you can use them to check your understanding of those take-home points. Second, you can use

---

[119] By now, you may feel that repeated use of the chapter briefing format is redundant. However, we believe that it is important to continue to emphasize that a good briefing builds mental models by discussing what is happening, what success looks like, and what threats or errors are possible and how you plan to prevent, avoid, or mitigate them. Hence, the repetitive nature is meant to cement this belief with an understanding that you will also immerse yourself in this book on an irregular and/or intermittent basis.

them to determine if you and your team are implementing those take-home points. If a Summary Box does not make sense to you or you do not understand one or more take-home points, then review the related material before continuing to the next section.

Did I miss anything? Any concerns? Any questions? (Pause) No? Then, let's get started.

List of Abbreviations

CRM	Crew Resource Management
DOC	Physician
ED	Emergency Department
L&D	Labor and Delivery
NICU	Neonatal Intensive Care Unit
NUR	Nurse
PED	Pediatrics
RT	Respiratory Therapist
STAR	Stop-Think-Act-Review

The A in STAR stands for Act. Once you decide on a course of action, you must develop a plan that accomplishes that course of action, and then execute that plan. In other words, Plan to Act, then Act on the Plan.

As with leadership, there are thousands of books on planning, so we will address only one specific aspect of planning: how a plan is enabled by, and enables, good CRM. A plan is enabled by CRM when CRM best practices are used to develop the plan (Section 14.1). A plan enables CRM when CRM best practices are embedded into the plan, specifically by mentioning in the briefing when and how CRM will be used (Section 14.2). Finally, CRM must be used to execute the plan (Section 14.4).

14.1 Use CRM Best Practices to Develop the Plan

Your team must first determine, and share their goals and priorities. Well-defined goals will keep the team focused on what is important when faced with distractions, high workload, and multitasking. Once the team identifies the goals and priorities, they can determine clear roles and responsibilities. Most importantly, for CRM, they can then determine where their roles and responsibilities intersect (i.e., how one's actions affects others and vice versa), and what information is required. The team can then determine what information needs to be exchanged with whom, when and how. They can even develop specific formats and guides and embed them into the plan. Once your team understands its goals and priorities, they can look for possible threats and errors. They can anticipate where possible threats or errors might arise and what, where, how, and when to look for information that might tell them that the threat or error is happening. One risk the team must consider is the risk caused by the team itself. Are they inexperienced? Are they tired? Is this an error-prone procedure that other teams have had difficulty performing? Once threats and errors are determined, the team can determine possible contingency plans.

One of the products of this phase is a list of expected outcomes when the team Acts on the Plan. They will know what indications to look for (i.e., critical data) to determine how well the plan is working. Some of the indications may be subtle or weak but a team that knows to look for them will be more vigilant in looking for them, detect them earlier, and react faster and more confidently. They will also be less likely to look for only those things that confirm that they were right (Confirmation Bias), or things that they expected (Expectation Bias) or explain away small variances (Normalization of Deviance). The team can then decide on triggers, or at what point an indication of a possible threat turns into an actual threat. For example, rising body temperature (critical data) is an indication of a possible infection. Action Plan A for a fever is typically an oral antipyretic, such as acetaminophen. A persistently elevated temperature coupled with a stiff neck (trigger), is an indication of a potential meningitis, and prompts a transition to Action Plan B: a spinal tap and intravenous antibacterial therapy. In our example, the team set the trigger of gestation age (32 weeks) or weight (1.7 kilograms) to determine the Pediatric Team's plan to dry the newborn (or not).

The team, however, failed to set several other triggers:

- when to move from transferring the mother to L&D to delivering in the ED;
- when to transition from positive pressure ventilation to intubation; and
- what level of oxygen concentration or inspiratory pressure would necessitate treatment with exogenous surfactant.[120]

[120] You can also think of this as a margin reaching zero: the present pressure reached the pressure that required exogenous surfactant.

Once a trigger has been exceeded, the team must have a transition plan to go from Plan A to Plan B. Planning for critical data, triggers, and transitions is best accomplished when there is no time pressure (or other stressors) and all the necessary expertise and time that are needed are available. Some of the decisions, especially the ones that are time-critical or safety-critical, can be codified, documented in procedures, trained, and practiced, if required. Assessment and planning can then be validated by fresh eyes, a Pre-Mortem, walk-through, and so forth.[121]

When a leader asks what to consider in developing a good plan, he or she is asking the team to consider all the following elements:

Summary Box 14.1
CRM Best Practices for Developing the Plan

Does your team…
- define team goals and priorities?
- identify roles and responsibilities, including all intersections?
- determine who needs to know what, when, and how?
- assess risk, including team risks?
- specify what the plan will look like if it is working or not working?
- develop contingency plans including critical data, triggers, and transition?
- codify time-critical, safety-critical decisions?
- validate the plan?

14.2 Incorporate CRM into the Briefing

The last step in the Plan to Act phase is briefing the team who will perform the task. The briefing may be the most important CRM tool you have. If done properly, the briefing embeds the CRM best practices and can also help less experienced people by helping build their situation awareness and mental models. A briefing brings together the entry conditions, goals, risks, critical data, critical factors, and so forth, from the Problem Definition phase (covered in Chapter 12) with the approved course of action that covers how each will be met (covered in Chapter 13). The briefing also includes each team member's roles, responsibilities, and tasks; coordination and

[121] We are not specifying use of a Pre-Mortem. We are saying that you need to use something to validate your assessment and planning.

communication plan; as well as possible contingencies. Some organizations have briefing guides to ensure the briefing includes all necessary items and to present the information in the most effective and efficient manner. Even if the organization does not have a formal briefing guide, many team leaders have personal informal guides.

Here are the CRM constituents of a good briefing:[122]

1. Call a mini-Stop to prevent the team from multitasking or being distracted during the briefing.
2. Introduce the team.
   a. Develop team cohesion, efficacy, and trust (this is especially critical for ad hoc teams).
   b. Establish situation awareness of the team itself: who do I (not) know, who appears to be (in)experienced, who do I go to when I need something, and so forth.
3. Describe the past and present situation.
   a. Explain how we got to this situation (story building).
   b. Build situation awareness and mental models at all levels.
4. Define goals and priorities.
   a. Clarify success criteria (what meeting a goal looks like).
   b. Delineate critical factors (builds situation awareness on what you cannot forget, otherwise you will violate a constraint).
   c. List critical data (informs team members what must be perceived in order to determine if the team's actions are, or are not, achieving its goals).
5. Specify tasks to be performed.
   a. Who is doing what, when, how, and why.
   b. Start situation awareness on how success will be achieved.
   c. Help team members determine how their individual actions might affect others, and vice versa (intersections).
   d. Specify what action is contingent on what other action, and what coordination is required.
   e. Determine where you can buy time (or any slack or slip) or increase margin.
   f. Facilitate talking/walking through any new, complex, or error-prone procedures (to identify possible threats and errors).

[122] Although this appears to be a lot of points which would take a lot of time to brief, with a briefing guide and a little practice, a team familiar with CRM concepts can move swiftly through the points without missing any elements.

6. Determine the resources required and whether those are available? (Resources include hardware, software, people, training, procedures, and so forth.).
   a. Designate who back ups whom (include people outside of the core team).
   b. Identify available alternative resources.
      NOTE: If a required resource is not available, then, by definition, your plan is unworkable, so you will then need to conduct a STAR.
7. Clarify the communication plan.
   a. Who needs to know what, when, and how.
   b. Who has information that will be needed.
   c. Who outside the core team should be involved.
8. Develop contingency plans.
   a. Ascertain the most likely, or worst possible, threat or error seen in the past.
   b. Describe what it will look like if a threat or error is materializing (critical data), when to switch to Plan B (trigger) and how to transition to the contingency plan.
9. Set expectations for CRM.
   a. What does good CRM look like.
   b. What does bad CRM look like.
   c. How are you going to fix bad CRM in real-time.
10. Incorporate lessons learned and best practices, including CRM.[123]
11. Ask if there are any questions or concerns.[124]

NOTE: This process requires active listening and observations of body language, as well as other nonverbal communication.

---

[123] In a perfect world, review of lessons learned and best practices would not be required because any fixes would already been incorporated and validated in the organization's procedures and practices. Until your organization incorporates and validates fixes, you will have to review lessons learned, and so forth.

[124] Do not ask, "Does everyone understand?" or "Does everyone agree?". The first question may seem like you are asking, "Is anyone too stupid to understand?". The second question may seem like you are asking, "Does anyone want to be ostracized for disagreeing?"

Summary Box 14.2
Incorporating CRM into the Briefing

Did you…
• use a briefing guide, even an informal one?
• call a mini-Stop?
• introduce the team?
• describe past and present situations?
• define goals and priorities?
• specify tasks to be performed?
• determine resources required?
• clarify who needs to know what, when and how?
• develop contingency plans?
• set expectations for CRM?
• ensure that no questions or concerns go unaddressed?

14.3 Example Briefing, with CRM Incorporated

How well does this briefing incorporate the elements of a good CRM briefing? Let us modify the scenario, where the Level 3 NICU Transport Team is unavailable, and the team at the birth hospital decides to transport the patient themselves. This is how the briefing might go, with an ad hoc team:

> PED DOC: "I know you are busy, but I need a few minutes of your time." *(waits for team to stop their tasks and walk over)*
> *(looks down at some notes)* "First, introductions. My name is John Jones. I am a pediatric hospitalist here." *(looks at the other 2 people)*
>
> PED NUR: "I am Diana Smith, a pediatric nurse in the normal newborn nursery."
>
> RT: "I am Mike Scott, your RT."
>
> PED DOC: "Since we have never worked together before, and have not performed a neonatal transport before…"
>
> PED NUR: "Actually, I have done several neonatal transports, working with Doctors without Borders, in Africa."

PED DOC: "Great! Speak up if we are doing anything that doesn't match your experience."

PED DOC: "As you know, we are transporting a 32-week female neonate delivered approximately 2.5 hours ago, who has worsening respiratory failure secondary to surfactant deficiency, infection, or both. We must do the transport because University Hospital's neonatal transport team will not be available for another 4 hours and we need to get her to a Level 3 NICU as soon as possible. Given the patient's rate of decompensation, I hope to leave here in the next 30 minutes by ambulance; the trip should take another 30 minutes."

RT: "Is the patient intubated? What are the ventilator settings?"

PED DOC: "Yes, she is. She is on an FiO2 of 60%, PIP of 26, PEEP of 6, and an inspiratory time of 0.35 seconds."

PED DOC: "Our goal is to keep her hemoglobin oxygen saturation above 92% during the trip. That means we may need to increase her oxygen and/or pressures. During the transport, I will be monitoring her breathing and her saturation as well as communicating with the accepting neonatologist. Diana, I need you to assist me with monitoring those variables. Mike, I need you to let me know if her tidal volumes are decreasing. What do you need from me?"

PED NUR: "I will be monitoring her saturations and breathing."
(to PED DOC) "I need to know if you want me to draw a blood gas."
(to RT) "Mike, let me know if you need any help with the transport ventilator."

RT: "I will be managing the settings on her ventilator and following her tidal volumes closely. I need both of you to let me know if you notice anything that requires a change in the ventilator."

PED DOC: "The two things that I am the most worried about during transport are persistent desaturation and a pneumothorax. Let me know about any saturation less than 93% that persists for more than 3 minutes. If that happens, we can increase the inspired oxygen concentration or increase the ventilator pressures. Also, tell me if you hear diminished breath sounds at any time – that can be an indication of a pneumothorax.

If that occurs, I will auscultate to confirm your impression, and perform a needle thoracostomy, if the patient is decompensating."

PED NUR: "I can watch for desaturation and tell you if it falls below 93% for more than 3 minutes."

RT: "I will auscultate the chest frequently, and let you know if I hear diminished breath sounds."

PED DOC: "What are the two of you most worried about?"

PED NUR: "I am most worried about desaturation, but I also will monitor all vital signs."

RT: (to PED NUR) "If you get busy, I can also help with monitoring vital signs."
(to PED DOC) "I am worried about hearing breath sounds in a moving ambulance – it can be tough to discriminate differential breath sounds with lots of background noise."

PED DOC: "If we are concerned about a pneumothorax, we can always pull over and stop the ambulance to be sure about it before we needle the chest. And remember, we will be in radio contact with the neonatologist at University Hospital, if we need advice."

PED DOC: (to all) "Some quick reminders:

* We're a team - look out for each other.
* If something doesn't look right, call a STAR.
* We will also call a STAR if we see something unexpected.
* If you don't understand, ask.
* Remember, everyone makes mistakes, including me. If you see me doing something that doesn't make sense to you, ask me. If you make any error, tell me. We can't fix what we don't know about.
* What have I missed? Anyone have any additional concerns? Anyone have any questions?" *(In addition to asking questions, PED DOC is also reading body language and other nonverbal communication.)*

NOTE: The stronger your organization's Standard Operating Procedures, the shorter your briefing will be. You will need to mention only the exceptions to Standard Operating Procedures or where Standard Operating Procedures are not available or do not apply. In our example, if your organization has a strong Standard Operating Procedure to use the Resuscitation Algorithm, then that briefing item could be as little as "Resuscitation in accordance with Standard Operating Procedure". If your organization does not have a strong Standard Operating Procedure (i.e., each physician does it differently), then you will be required to brief in detail who is doing what, when, how, and why, and so on.

Summary Box 14.3
CRM in the Scenario Briefing

Did the physician…
- use a briefing guide, even an informal one? (PED DOC had some notes.)
- call a mini-Stop? (PED DOC asked for a few minutes and waited until the team came over.)
- introduce the team? (Physician, nurse, and respiratory therapist introduced themselves.)
- define past and present situation? (Neonate born 2.5 hours ago with surfactant deficiency and/or infection.)
- define goals, priorities? (Keep the neonate stable while transporting to a Level 3 NICU.)
- define tasks to be performed? (Each team member discussed what they planned to do.)
- define resources required? (PED DOC discussed seeking advice from the accepting neonatologist.)
- define who needs to know what, when, and how? (Each team member discussed what support he or she will need from the other team members.)
- define contingency plans? (The team discussed threats and how to manage them.)
- set expectations for CRM? ("Everyone makes errors. If …something that doesn't make sense to you, ask me.")
- ensure no questions or concerns? ("What have I missed? Anyone have any concerns?")

Once you have a plan, you must execute it using good CRM, to make sure that the plan is successful.

14.4 Act on the Plan

During the Act on the Plan phase, besides executing the plan as briefed, the team must constantly check how it is Exchanging Information, Communicating, Leading and Following, and Mutually Supporting. If team members are to maintain their situation awareness, they must have the time and working memory to perceive, comprehend, project, and exchange. Your team must manage distractions, workload, multitasking, and performance shaping factors (e.g., stress, fatigue). They must find ways to "buy time": find ways to have more time to think. Can you get to a safe or stable state that will give you some time to do a STAR? They must also find ways to increase margin. Finally, they must delay or even cancel non-priority tasks.

Your team members must check their situation awareness and mental models. First, you must explain your actions and decisions to your team members. Explaining allows them insight into your situation awareness and mental models. Second, team members need to pay attention to the actions of others. If someone is doing something that does not make sense, another team member must ask for an explanation of the unexpected actions. As team members actively listen to the explanation, they may need to change their situation awareness and mental models. If the explanation does not make sense to them, they must continue to ask questions. This requires a culture of psychological safety where asking questions is not only allowed, but expected, and the patience to answer them fully is expected of formal, informal, and situational leaders. Additionally, if someone looks overworked or distracted, a team member must support or back them up. The team realizes that old situation awareness is bad situation awareness, and situation awareness must constantly be built, maintained and, if necessary, rebuilt after busy or confusing periods. The team must call tag-ups (e.g., team huddles) to (re)build situation awareness just before an activity (e.g., just before implementing a contingency plan) or right after a busy time (e.g., handling an emergency procedure). Finally, team members must provide real-time feedback to each other to prevent, avoid or mitigate errors.

Summary Box 14.4
CRM Best Practices During Act on the Plan

Does your team… • manage distractions, workload, multitasking, and performance shaping factors? • buy time, and increase margin, if possible? • explain their actions and decisions? • pay attention to the actions of others? • speak up when things do not make sense? • actively listen to explanations, and modify their situation awareness and mental models? • use tag-ups to keep the team in sync? • provide feedback on CRM?

You have successfully executed your plan, but did you do it perfectly? Is there room for improvement? How do you make sure that you do better the next time? All that will be covered in the next chapter.

Chapter Debriefing

I want to call a quick STAR (Stop-Think-Act-Review): get off your email, stop your side conversations, and turn off the television. Let's see if you can expand upon these statements:

- Your plan must include goals and priorities, roles and responsibilities, information requirements, indications of threats and errors, and contingency plans, including critical data, triggers, and transitions.
- Your briefing guide must remind you to discuss CRM standards, expectations and best practices.
- During the task, the team must check for possible differences in situation awareness or mental models.

If this was an actual debriefing, we would ask you to expand further on each of these statements. Depending on your response, we would ask open-ended follow-up questions until we were sure you understood the material and had a plan to implement one or more best practices. We might ask, "What is a specific problem either developing or executing a plan that you experience on your job?" We would not be satisfied if you said, "We can't do contingency planning as well as we need to do." Again, we would ask open-ended follow-up questions until you might say, “We have a problem with team members determining when and how to go to a contingency plan.” We would then ask, “What can you do to fix that problem prior to your next shift?” We would then continue to ask open-ended follow-up questions until you might say, “I need to mention in the briefing what the triggers are and how we will transition to each contingency. During the shift, I need to assign at least one person to monitor each trigger. During the debriefing, we will discuss what about our mental models allowed us to not know about a trigger.” We might then ask, “How can you help other teams to prevent that error?” More open-ended questions until you might say, “We need to modify our briefing guide so that the teams discuss what data to check for, what limit would require a contingency, and how they would implement that contingency.”

CHAPTER 15

R STANDS FOR REVIEW

Chapter Briefing[125]

I want to call a quick STAR (Stop-Think-Act-Review): get off your email, stop your side conversations, and turn off the television. In this chapter, we will discuss the Review phase: using CRM to make sure that what we get is what we expect (ensuring good situation awareness and mental models), and that we do even better for the next phase or task. We will be successful if you can explain why you need to:

- stop, if something is better or worse than expected (Section 15.1);
- review prior to starting the next phase (Section 15.2.1); and
- review after a shift (Section 15.2.2).

The primary threat that you might experience is the introduction of a large number of concepts and terms, some of which you may have never encountered, and some of which you may think about in a different sense. We will therefore explicitly define and differentiate each term and concept. We also realize how busy you are. We will make sure that the chapter is short enough to be read in approximately thirty minutes. Finally, we provide Summary Boxes. The Summary Boxes serve two functions. First, they emphasize the take-home points in each section, and you can use them to check your understanding of those take-home points. Second, you can use them to determine if you and your team are implementing those take-home points. If a Summary Box does not make sense to you or you do not

---

[125] By now, you may feel that repeated use of the chapter briefing format is redundant. However, we believe that it is important to continue to emphasize that a good briefing builds mental models by discussing what is happening, what success looks like, and what threats or errors are possible and how you plan to prevent, avoid, or mitigate them. Hence, the repetitive nature is meant to cement this belief with an understanding that you will also immerse yourself in this book on an irregular and/or intermittent basis.

understand one or more take-home points, then review the related material before continuing to the next section.

Did I miss anything? Any concerns? Any questions? (Pause) No? Then, let's get started.

List of Abbreviations

CRM	Crew Resource Management
NICU	Neonatal Intensive Care Unit
RT	Respiratory Therapist
STAR	Stop-Think-Act-Review
STEP	Status-Team-Environment-Progress

The R in STAR stands for Review. As you act on your plan, you must make sure that what you are getting from your plan is what you expected. You review continuously as you monitor the situation (Section 15.1) but also between phases to make sure that you correct any CRM problems before starting the next phase (Section 15.2.1) and at the end of the task or shift to continuously improve (Section 15.2.2).

15.1 Review Continuously

As you are monitoring the situation, you are continuously checking for critical factors and critical data that you identified in the Think phase. Unfortunately, just reviewing for critical factors and critical data may not be sufficient. What if data that you deem not critical is different than expected? What do you do if you can overcome Expectation and Confirmation biases to notice it in the first place? Is this piece of data truly not significant, or might it represent a hole or gap in your situation awareness or mental model (i.e., it is critical data that you did not know about)? Until you can determine if any deviation is critical, or not, you should do a STAR, even a very brief one, to make sure that you know if your situation awareness or mental model might be wrong. Luckily, in a team, you have a diversity of situation awareness and mental models to help you decide.

As you review the situation, make sure that you look across all areas of STEP (Status-Team-Environment-Progress). You need to review the Status, first of your patient. What information tells you that the patient is doing well (or not), and how close is he or she to requiring a change in treatment? Second, you need to review the status of your tasks/procedures. You should review after every step in a task/procedure before you proceed to the next step. Your team needs to confirm that they are seeing and hearing what they are expected to see and hear. For example, if you administered a medication, did the patient respond as expected? If you changed a setting on a piece of equipment, does the user interface reflect that change, and is the patient responding in the manner in which you expected? Even a better-than-expected result may show that your situation awareness or mental model is wrong.

You need to review the Team, starting with the members of the team. Are they making numerous small mistakes, or slow to notice or react to information? You can also use third-party active listening: actively listening to the communication between team members. Do team members sound stressed? Asking a lot of questions of one another may be a sign of possible bad situation awareness or mental models. Teamwork, or, more specifically, the team's CRM, must also be reviewed. Are they passing on the right portion of their situation awareness to the right person at the right time, or are others having to pull that information? Are they using the right Communicating protocols, or are there a lot of questions to determine what information was passed? Are leaders building psychological safety and are followers inquiring, advocating, and being assertive if required, or are errors being hidden and recommendations not given or squashed? Are team members effectively backing each other up, or are you hearing or seeing "that's not in my job description" attitude?

You also need to review the Environment. Has anything changed that will affect your team? For example, you expected a quiet shift, but instead you have had to react to a series of problematic issues. How does that change your plan?

Finally, you need to monitor the Progress of your team. Is your team on schedule? Being behind schedule may indicate that either your situation awareness and mental model were wrong, or your plan was overly optimistic. In the preterm delivery scenario, the physician stated, "the natural history of surfactant deficiency is to worsen over the first 72 hours and then slowly resolve." What happens if it worsens more rapidly than expected, and is further complicated by infection? Is your situation awareness and mental model still correct? You should also assess any Times-to-Effect. You need to get the newborn to a Level 3 NICU as quickly as possible. Can that still be accomplished? Finally, you should assess any margins. Is a parameter approaching a trigger? Can you do something to increase margin? If not, are you ready to implement the contingency plan?

Whether S, T, E, or P, you need to review for the critical data (indications) that things are going well or that a threat or error is materializing. Any difference between what you expect and what you see, no matter how small or weak, may mean that you need to call a STAR to determine what is happening, and why. Beware of how any difference is explained away. Make sure that any explanation has sound technical basis and can be incorporated into your mental model without requiring mental convolutions, or without requiring you to accept something on blind faith. The Deepwater Horizon accident was caused, in part, because those working on the rig did not expect a change in pressure, and when it happened, a person of authority explained it as the "Bladder Effect".[126] The team accepted that explanation even though no one else had ever heard of it. Rather than treat an unexpected change in pressure as a sign of poor situation awareness or mental model, they explained it away (Deep Water 2011). If the explanation does not make sense to you, then someone's situation awareness or mental model is wrong. Do not progress until you determine whose.

Review is harder than you might assume. First, most people are can-do people who want to successfully complete the job assigned to them. They may believe that stopping to review may be perceived as a lack of knowledge, skill, or confidence. They may fear that stopping will put them behind schedule, despite the knowledge that should a suspected threat materialize, it will really put them behind schedule. Second, team members may possess a number of cognitive biases that prevents them from recognizing a variance (Kahneman 2011). Confirmation Bias refers to the tendency that people are more likely to see those things that tell them they are right than those things that tell them that they are wrong. Expectation Bias refers to the tendency that people are more likely to see those things that they expect than what they do not expect. Change Blindness refers to the tendency that people may not notice slow or unexpected changes. Finally, Normalization of Deviance refers to the tendency that minor violations of specifications, if accepted over a period of time, become the norm or accepted performance. (Vaughan 2016) The argument shifts from

[126] Also called The Gulf of Mexico oil spill, the largest marine oil spill in history, which began on April 20, 2010.

"prove that the deviance is safe" to "prove that it is unsafe". Normalization of Deviance was a cause of both the Challenger and Columbia Space Shuttle accidents (Bania 2010). There are technical ways to get around some biases, such as defeating change blindness, by setting limits on displays tightly enough to sound an alarm when the change exceeds a certain value. CRM also provides a means to mitigate these biases. The first way is the team; individual team members have different biases due to different mental models. Therefore, what one team member misses, another sees. This diversity of mental models allows the team members to see, hear, and feel most or all the things that are needed to accomplish their collective goals. The second way is planning for contingencies. When you accept that things might go wrong, you will be more vigilant and better able to detect deviations from the expected. Finally, by projecting future results, you will detect any differences between predicted and actual values and recognize that your situation awareness or mental model is not as good as is required. It is much more desirable to project a future state and notice any variances than to try to see and explain an unexpected state (e.g., "Is that what it is supposed to do?"). A statement in the briefing that reinforces your CRM expectations could be as simple as "If something we did or see is not as we expected, then we need to Stop and restart STAR".

Summary Box 15.1
Review After Every Step of a Task

Does your team…

- check that you get exactly what you expected for all areas of Status-Team-Environment-Progress (STEP)?
- treat any deviation as a sign of possible bad situation awareness or mental models?
- guard against cognitive biases, by soliciting feedback from team members?
- project what things should look like in the future?
- anticipate possible deviations from the expected course, and plan for contingencies?
- call a Stop-Think-Act-Review (STAR) if there is a deviation?

15.2 Review at the End

You should Review at every end: at the end of task or phase, and at the end of a shift or project.

15.2.1 Review at the End of a Task or Phase

You should review at the end of every major task. You should also review at the end of every phase, such as at the end of the Problem Definition, Course of Action Selection or Planning phase. This review serves multiple purposes. First, it checks to determine that the task or phase accomplished what was expected. Second, the review should discuss "How was our CRM? Did we communicate, build situation awareness, decide if differences in the situation affected our codified or naturalistic decision making, or set a climate for good CRM?" This review is not about fixing a specific error, but rather fixing the poor CRM that allowed it to happen. If you have poor CRM, fix it before you start the next phase or task. Third, the review explores the possibility that while you were defining the problem, selecting a course of action, or developing the plan, something changed in the situation or varied from your projection that might alter or even invalidate your Problem Definition, Course of Action Selection, Plan, and so forth. If it did, then you must go back to Stop and restart the STAR process.

15.2.2 Review at the End of a Shift or Project

Many teams do a review at the end of the shift or project as a debriefing. It is important to determine where your team succeeded, and where it failed, both in technical execution and in CRM, as a component of continuous improvement. The goal of any debriefing is to establish an accurate picture of the events that occurred, develop a comprehensive understanding of the situation, and determine whether the responses of the team were appropriate and executed in accordance with established guidelines. This should be done in a dispassionate, fact-based manner, and focused on the actions of the individual team members, how those actions contributed to the team's performance, and how team performance influenced the ultimate outcome (in healthcare, this is the quality of care delivered to the patient). Team members should leave a debriefing with strategies for replicating actions that facilitate successful human and system performance and avoiding those that are ineffective or harmful. Debriefings are about fixing problems, not assigning blame.

A debriefing should never be the final step in a task or project; rather it should lead to incorporation of the lessons learned into the organization's philosophies, policies, procedures, and practices. If your team relies on human memory or information locked in an electronic database to improve performance, then you will make the same mistakes over and over again. The Army's National Training Center says a debriefing (they call it an After Action Report) is not done until the improvements are implemented in procedures, training, and so on, and shown to fix underlying problems (Darling, Parry and Moore 2005).

Summary Box 15.2
Review at the End of Each Phase and After the Shift

Does your team…
- fix problems, not assign blame?
- ensure that results are exactly what you expected, and if not, conduct a Stop-Think-Act-Review (STAR)?
- combat cognitive biases by:
  - soliciting a diversity of mental models?
  - considering contingencies?
  - predicting changes?
- improve CRM prior to next task/phase?
- implement and validate improvements from the debriefing?

Chapter Debriefing

I want to call a quick STAR (Stop-Think-Act-Review): get off your email, stop your side conversations, and turn off the television. Let's see if you can expand upon these statements:

- Project what things should look like in the future.
- Check that you get exactly what you expected for all areas of Status-Team-Environment-Progress (STEP).
- Treat any deviation as a sign of possible bad situation awareness or mental model.
- Call a STAR if the deviation cannot be explained by your situation awareness or mental model.
- Review after each step in a procedure, and after each task and each shift.

If this was an actual debriefing, we would ask you to expand further on each of these statements. Depending on your response, we would ask open-ended follow-up questions until we were sure you understood the material and had a plan to implement one or more best practices. We might ask, "What is a specific Review problem that you experience on your job?" We would not be satisfied if you said, "We don't review as well as we need." Again, we would ask open-ended follow-up questions until you might say "We have a problem with team members being too fixated on their tasks that they miss other problems." We would then ask, "What can you do to fix that problem prior to your next shift?" We would then continue to ask open-ended follow-up questions until you might say, "In the briefing, we could discuss all the areas of STEP that need to be reviewed. During the task, we will mutually support each other to make sure that no one is fixated. In the debriefing, we will discuss how and why we missed information that did not match our expectations." We might then ask, "What can you suggest to help other teams?" More open-ended questions until you might say, "I need to work with management to modify our briefing guide so that each team member discusses what to review in terms of STEP to spot problems more quickly."

References

Klein, Gary A. Decision Making in Action: Models and Methods. Norwood, NJ: Ablex, 1995.

Taleb, Nassim. The Black Swan: The Impact of the Highly Improbable. New York. N.Y.: Random House, 2010.

PART 2B

OTHER TOOLS

Briefing[127]

I want to call a quick STAR (Stop-Think-Act-Review): get off your email, stop your side conversations, and turn off the television.[128] Here is what we will do in the next four chapters. We will discuss other tools that are both enabled by CRM, but also enable CRM. We will be successful if you can describe:

- the three decision making methods and how CRM enables each (Chapter 16);
- how conflict is managed by CRM and improves CRM (Chapter 17);
- how debriefings using self-discovery and self-correction improve CRM (Chapter 18); and
- how self-care is required if you are to be an effective member of a team (Chapter 19).

The primary threat that you might experience is the introduction of a large number of concepts and terms, some of which you may have never encountered, and some of which you may think about in a different sense. We will therefore explicitly define and differentiate each term and concept. We also realize how busy you are. We will make sure that the chapter is short enough to be read in approximately thirty minutes. Finally, we provide

---

[127] We will use the chapter briefing format throughout the book. You may feel the repeated use is redundant. However, we believe that it is important to continue to emphasize that a good briefing builds mental models by discussing what is happening, what success looks like, and what threats or errors are possible and how you plan to prevent, avoid, or mitigate them. Hence, the repetitive nature is meant to cement this belief with an understanding that you will also immerse yourself in this book on an irregular and/or intermittent basis. For more information on briefings and how this briefing embeds CRM concepts, see Section 14.2.

[128] For more information on STAR, see Chapters 11-15.

Summary Boxes. The Summary Boxes serve two functions. First, they emphasize the take-home points in each section, and you can use them to check your understanding of those take-home points. Second, you can use them to determine if you and your team are implementing those take-home points. If a Summary Box does not make sense to you or you do not understand one or more take-home points, then review the related material before continuing to the next section.

Did I miss anything? Any concerns? Any questions? (Pause) No? Then, let's get started.

List of Abbreviations

AFE	Amniotic Fluid Embolism
ANES	Anesthesia
Code	Code (resuscitation) team
DIC	Disseminated Intravascular Coagulation
DOC	Physician
ICU	Intensive Care Unit
L&D	Labor and Delivery
NUR	Nurse
OB	Obstetrics or Obstetrician

Let us start with a scenario that will show good and bad examples of decision making, managing conflict, debriefings, and self-care. We will use this scenario as we discuss these tools further in Chapters 16-19.

Personnel Involved in Scenario

Obstetric Team: OB DOC, OB NUR #1, OB NUR #2
Obstetric Anesthesiology: ANES DOC
Code Team: CODE DOC, CODE NUR #1, CODE NUR #2

A 29-year-old woman presented to L&D at 40 weeks, 5 days gestation for a scheduled induction of labor. She has been healthy, and her pregnancy has been uncomplicated to date. After cervical ripening with misoprostol followed by oxytocin to stimulate uterine contractions, she is in active labor and progressing well. Shortly after delivering a healthy male neonate, she complains of difficulty breathing. Within minutes she becomes unresponsive and goes into cardiac arrest. Only the obstetrician and two obstetric nurses are in the room at the time. OB DOC, who was managing delivery of the placenta, shouts "Call a code!" and proceeds to initiate chest compressions. OB NUR #1 runs to the front desk and tells the unit clerk to activate the Code team. OB NUR#2 searches for the self-inflating bag. When OB NUR #1 returns to the room, she asks OB NUR#2 what she is doing. Hearing that OB NUR #2 is looking for the self-inflating bag, OB NUR #1 reaches above the patient's headboard and pulls out the bag, a mask, and oxygen tubing from its container, connects the tubing to oxygen, and begins positive pressure ventilation. The Code team and the obstetric anesthesiologist arrive simultaneously.

After announcing their arrival, ANES DOC and CODE DOC begin shouting orders. OB DOC continues delivering compressions, but is also trying to provide pertinent patient history and give orders.

OB NUR#1: "Who is leading this code?"

CODE DOC, ANES DOC and OB DOC answer simultaneously: "I am."

CODE NUR#1: "We need to hear clear orders from one person, not three."

CODE DOC: "You are on my team; you take orders from me."

ANES DOC: "When is the last time that you resuscitated a pregnant patient?"

CODE DOC: "Never. But that doesn't matter, the algorithm is the same."

ANES DOC: "No, it is NOT."

CODE NUR #2: "You guys have to get this worked out NOW."

OB DOC (to OB NUR #2): "Take over chest compressions. Deliver 100 per minute."

OB DOC (to all): "We need to get on the same page here. Does anyone have prior experience with a pregnant patient in cardiac arrest?"

Everyone responds with "No" or shakes their head from side to side.

OB DOC (to all): "Okay, she was previously healthy, delivered, complained of difficulty breathing, then arrested, and is now bleeding out. My training says those are all signs of an amniotic fluid embolism. Does anyone have any other ideas?"

Everyone responds with "No" or shakes their head from side to side.

OB DOC (to all): "Then let's go with that as our working diagnosis, but be willing to revise it. Let's keep gathering data, and speak up if you have other thoughts. We all have jobs to do. I need to deliver the placenta and try to control her bleeding."
(to OB NUR #2): "Call the blood bank and activate the massive transfusion protocol."
(to ANES DOC): "You take over ventilation and intubate her."
(to CODE DOC): "You run the code and give orders to your team."

The three teams (Obstetric, Obstetric Anesthesia and Code) manage to coordinate their actions. After 20 minutes of advanced cardiac life support, the patient has a heart rate of 100 beats per minute but remains unconscious and mechanically ventilated. She is then transported to the ICU by some of the members of the Code team who, due to the need to continue their patient care responsibilities, will not be available for an immediate post-event debriefing. While such a debriefing ideally involves all members of the team(s) who cared for the patient, that is often not practical.

OB DOC: "I think we need to take 5 to 10 minutes now to debrief. First, does everyone here have the time?"

CODE DOC: "Yes, my colleagues can manage the transfer to the ICU."

ANES DOC: "I can be here until I get called again."

OB NUR #1: "She was my patient—so I don't have a current assignment."

CODE NUR#1: "I have time."

OB NUR#2 remains silent.

OB DOC: "We have limited time, so let's identify the two or three most important issues. We'll also need to review this in much more detail during our next monthly mortality and morbidity conference. To quickly review our ground rules: first, this conversation is protected under Code of Evidence 1157, so we can speak freely about what we saw and heard. Second, we will not discuss these events outside of this debriefing or a mortality and morbidity conference. Finally, I will speak with the patient's family and let them know what I know once we're finished here."

CODE DOC: "If you'd like me to accompany you, just let me know."

OB DOC: "Thank you, I will.
(to all) 'This is a technical performance debriefing, not a critical incident stress debriefing. I know that this was traumatic for everyone—if you don't believe that you are ready to debrief now, it's okay. Is everyone good to proceed?"

CODE DOC: "Yes."

ANES DOC: "Yes."

OB NUR#1: "I'm ready."

CODE NUR #1: "Me too."

OB NUR #2 remains silent.

OB DOC (to OB NUR #2): "It's okay if you need some time."

OB NUR #2: "Yeah, I've never seen this happen."

OB DOC: "Would you like to speak with the social worker or chaplain? Or is there someone else we can call for you?"

OB NUR #2: "Yes, I'd like to talk with the chaplain."

OB NUR #1: "I'll ask the front desk to call her."

OB NUR #2: "Thanks."

OB NUR #1 puts her arm around OB NUR #2 and escorts her from the room, returning within one minute.

OB DOC (to ANES DOC, CODE DOC, CODE NUR #1, CODE NUR #2): "Thanks for getting here so quickly. We don't see codes too often in L&D."

OB NUR #1 returns to the room.

OB DOC: "What was the likely underlying event?"

CODE DOC: "Sepsis? She was in DIC…"

ANES DOC: "It's rare, but I suspect an AFE, that is an amniotic fluid embolism."

OB DOC: "I agree, it was consistent with an AFE. So, what do we need to address?"

CODE NUR #1: "We need to discuss roles and leadership."

OB NUR #1: "Yeah, I agree. We had three people trying to lead the resuscitation."

CODE NUR #1: "Normally our team follows our leader's orders. But I was uncomfortable with a pregnant patient."

OB NUR #1: "Yeah, we usually follow the obstetrician's orders, but we very rarely have a patient arrest."

ANES DOC: "I can run a code on a pregnant patient, but I was the one who needed to manage her airway. I've seen AFEs before. I should have immediately intubated her."

CODE DOC: "I wanted to hear more background to help me understand what had happened. When that wasn't forthcoming, I went into my usual mode and took over."

OB DOC: "I've only run codes in simulations, never on a real patient. I knew this was an AFE, I knew she was hemorrhaging. But I was caught up doing compressions and trying to give you some history. I lost situation awareness and failed to deliver the placenta quickly and get the vaginal bleeding under control."

CODE DOC: "I saw that you were doing compressions and should have assigned a member of my team to immediately take over that task. That would have freed you up to manage the placenta and step back, think and provide some history."

OB DOC: "Okay, so what circumstances prevented us from doing what we needed to do?"

CODE NUR #1: "Our lack of experience with cardiac arrest in a pregnant patient."

CODE DOC: "Working in an unfamiliar environment."

OB NUR #1: "Having to immediately integrate the actions of three separate teams."

OB DOC: "Trying to think, talk, and carry out a manual task simultaneously. I was trying to prioritize what I was doing but it all seemed to be equally important. I certainly was task overloaded. Let me summarize. There were three teams who have never worked together in a situation none of whom had worked before: the OB team in a code, the Code team working on a pregnant woman, and the anesthesiologist needing to intubate this pregnant patient in the midst of relative chaos and conflict. In that stressful situation, all three physicians resorted to giving orders."

OB NUR #1: "Yeah, so how do we avoid those errors the next time that this happens?"

OB DOC: "I should have realized that role and leadership conflict was likely and have been quicker to first, announce that she was my patient, and second, assign roles. Of course, I was task overloaded."

ANES DOC: "Rather than waiting for directions, I can take over the airway as soon as I enter the room and intubate if necessary. That will free up the person who was at the airway for another task."

OB DOC: "I can immediately ask someone to take over compressions when they enter the room—anyone else should be able to carry out that task. That will then free me up to deliver the placenta, which is something that only I am trained to do. I can then also provide relevant history and help manage the bleeding."

CODE DOC: "I can clarify that I will lead the code but make it clear that I need input from the obstetric team. I can also direct members of my team to take over roles such as compressions."

OB NUR #1: "We should simulate these rare events and work on response times, role assignment, coordination, managing task workload and communication. We've never done that with all of our teams."

OB DOC: "We're almost at ten minutes, so we'll need to end this. Before we do, I'd like to know what facilitated the nurses' ability to speak up in the midst of this chaotic situation and ask for better leadership?"

OB NUR #1: "This was my patient, she was dying, and we weren't helping her. I needed to be her advocate and speak up."

CODE NUR #1: "As a member of the Code team, I have been in similar situations where leadership has been ineffective. As we were running here, I anticipated that could happen in this situation, so I was ready to call it out when I saw it. Plus, our team works and trains together frequently, so we've had time to break down issues of hierarchy.
(to CODE DOC): I've heard you say, 'Never let me hurt a patient,' so I know that I can speak up and not worry about any retribution."

At the end of this debriefing, CODE DOC seeks out a senior colleague who serves as a mentor to him at the hospital, explaining that he has a confidential clinical issue that he would like to review. After ensuring that he has invoked the same level of protected discussion as exists at a mortality and morbidity conference, he describes being called to resuscitate this pregnant woman and his initial insistence on leading the code. He states that only when he was asked if he had resuscitated a pregnant patient before, did he stop to question the appropriateness of his leadership in this situation. As he critiques his own performance, his mentor occasionally asks questions that elicit relevant context and stimulate even deeper levels of introspection. CODE DOC expresses his disappointment in his initial failure to recognize how the unique physiology of pregnancy created a situation unlike any he had experienced previously, and his dismay that he may have harmed the patient if the other members of the team had not challenged him. His mentor reinforces these insights, agreeing that he has learned a valuable lesson in recognizing the limits of his own knowledge and the value of teamwork, asking for help, and effective communication. While still unsettled by his actions, his discussion with his mentor has provided him with a better understanding of his weaknesses and strengths, making him both more resilient and determined to improve his performance.

While this debriefing was concluding, OB NUR #2 was meeting with the hospital chaplain. The chaplain asked her to talk about what happened and how she was feeling. She expressed the fact that she went into obstetrics because it is a field that celebrates the start of a new life and all the potential that new life holds. She stated that she had never cared for a patient who became so sick before today. This was obviously a traumatic event for her, so the chaplain consoled her as much as she could. The chaplain asked her if she wanted to see someone else, perhaps a psychologist or psychiatrist. OB NUR#2 said that she would think about it. The chaplain then asked her if she would like to go home rather than try to finish her shift. She said yes, she would like to leave, but worried that it would add to the workload of her colleagues and that nursing leadership might view her as "not strong enough" for a job in labor and delivery. The chaplain assured her that staffing was more than adequate and that no one would look down on her departure prior to the end of her shift. The chaplain also offered to speak with the charge nurse and let her know that she (the chaplain) recommended leaving early. OB NUR #2 agreed to that plan and thanked the chaplain for being so supportive. The chaplain told her that she would call her the next day to check in on her.

OB NUR #2 went home and napped. She set her alarm for dinner and ordered take-out to be delivered. After dinner she reviewed the events of the day in her mind and thought about what she could have done in a more effective manner, developing a short list of things to work on during simulations in labor and delivery. Although she vowed to do better in the future, she realized that even if she had performed her role perfectly, it would not have prevented an amniotic fluid embolism. She practiced yoga and spent additional time meditating, before taking a warm bath and going to bed earlier than usual. She then resolved to call the chaplain in the morning and ask for her suggestion for a referral to an appropriate mental health professional.

CHAPTER 16

MAKING DECISIONS

Chapter Briefing[129]

I want to call a quick STAR (Stop-Think-Act-Review): get off your email, stop your side conversations, and turn off the television.[130] In this chapter, we will discuss how a team uses CRM to make better decisions. We will be successful if you can explain:

- Codified Decision Making, and when to (not) use it (Section 16.1);
- Naturalistic Decision Making, and when to (not) use it (Section 16.2);
- Deliberate Decision Making, and when to (not) use it (Section 16.3);
- Risk, and how to evaluate it beyond likelihood and consequences (Section 16.4.1); and
- Uncertainty, as it applies to situation awareness and mental models (Section 16.4.2).

The primary threat that you might experience is the introduction of a large number of concepts and terms, some of which you may have never encountered, and some of which you may think about in a different sense. We will therefore explicitly define and differentiate each term and concept. We also realize how busy you are. We will make sure that the chapter is short enough to be read in approximately thirty minutes. Finally, we provide

---

[129] By now, you may feel that repeated use of the chapter briefing format is redundant. However, we believe that it is important to continue to emphasize that a good briefing builds mental models by discussing what is happening, what success looks like, and what threats or errors are possible and how you plan to prevent, avoid, or mitigate them. Hence, the repetitive nature is meant to cement this belief with an understanding that you will also immerse yourself in this book on an irregular and/or intermittent basis.

[130] For more information on STAR, see Chapters 11-15.

Summary Boxes. The Summary Boxes serve two functions. First, they emphasize the take-home points in each section, and you can use them to check your understanding of those take-home points. Second, you can use them to determine if you and your team are implementing those take-home points. If a Summary Box does not make sense to you or you do not understand one or more take-home points, then review the related material before continuing to the next section.

Did I miss anything? Any concerns? Any questions? (Pause) No? Then, let's get started.

NOTE
We realize how busy you are. We normally would make each chapter short enough to be read in approximately thirty minutes. Unfortunately, the subject matter in this chapter did not lend itself to that timeframe. If pressed for time, we suggest that you first read Section 16.4, which is new material. If you have more time, read Sections 16.1 and 16.2, which cover the two most common decision making methods more deeply. Finally, as time permits, read Section 16.3, which covers the decision making method where the most errors occur.

List of Abbreviations

ANES	Anesthesiology
CRM	Crew Resource Management
DOC	Physician
ED	Emergency Department
ISS	International Space Station
L&D	Labor & Delivery
NASA	National Aeronautics and Space Administration
NICU	Neonatal Intensive Care Unit
NTT	Neonatal Transport Team
OB	Obstetric
PED	Pediatric
STEP	Status-Team-Environment-Progress
TBD	To Be Determined
TT	Transport Team

Why is there a chapter on decision making since decision making is not a skill in our Crew Resource Management (CRM) model.[131] We do not consider decision making a CRM skill, since it is not a team skill. CRM does not diminish the leader's authority to be the final decision maker. It is, however, a follower's responsibility to provide the leader with all the information required to make that final decision.[132] In order to provide all that information, a follower must understand how the leader will make decisions. A follower must also know the threats and errors to decision making so that he or she can inquire, advocate, and assert if required.

This chapter is comprised of four sections. Section 16.1 provides additional information on Codified Decision Making. Section 16.2 discusses Naturalistic Decision Making. Section 16.3 focuses on Deliberate Decision Making, and Section 16.4 covers evaluating risk and uncertainty.

16.1 Codified Decision Making

Codified Decision Making—also called Rule-Based Decision Making—means that decisions have been codified in your company's philosophies, policies, and procedures. NASA's Johnson Space Center's flight controllers who operate the International Space Station have thousands of pages of codified decisions in multiple documents called Flight Rules. A codified decision has been pre-made, and you just have to follow it. There are 2 types of codified decisions: documented and briefed. An example of a documented codified decision is when your company writes down in a policy or procedure that if you see situation A, then do B. In our example, the decision to do a resuscitation was documented (in an algorithm). Codified decisions could also be incorporated in your training. When, how, and why to use the resuscitation algorithm could be taught in simulations. Codified decisions are documented in procedures, practiced in simulations and confirmed in briefings.

The second type of codified decisions is briefed codified decisions. Briefed codified decisions are decisions the team makes before the task or in the shift briefing. Modifying our scenario, let us suppose that the scenario started with a call from the ambulance that they were transporting a woman

---

[131] Decision Making is a skill in many CRM models.

[132] We are only addressing intra-team decision making, which is decision making in a team with a formal leader. We are not addressing inter-team decision making, or decision making between teams of equal rank and without a formal leader. In such inter-team situations, decision making is usually done by consensus.

in labor. The ED physician could have briefed the team before the ambulance arrived that if the baby had not crowned, they would send the woman to L&D; if the baby was crowning, they would hand over the woman to the Obstetric Team; and if the baby was delivered in the ambulance, they would hand the new mother over to the Obstetric Team, and the baby to the Pediatric Team. That statement in the briefing might have changed the codified decision in the hospital's policies and procedures.

The advantages of Codified Decision Making are that decisions have been made without the stress of being in the actual situation, and with the help of all the experts, information, and time. It is also the simplest and quickest form of decision making. It is best for new decision makers, in situations that require rapid response, where uniformity of response is required, where possible variations are limited, and entry conditions can be well defined. The main error in Codified Decision Making is applying a codified decision when the entry conditions are different than originally planned by leaders. You have to make sure that this is really Situation A, and not a situation subtly different for which the pre-made response does not work. In the preterm newborn delivery in the ED scenario, the decision to use the resuscitation algorithm is codified, as are the decisions about the interventions carried out during the resuscitation. The underlying assumption is that the algorithm can be used in the vast majority of cases when newborns require resuscitation. This is in contrast to the AFE scenario, where the Anesthesiologist realized that resuscitating a pregnant patient may require alterations to the adult resuscitation algorithm.

The problem with Codified Decision Making is that it is impossible to cover every possible situation. If the organization wants decision makers to apply Codified Decision Making properly, the codified decisions must state to what situations they apply and to which they do not, as well as the rationale. In our example, did the Resuscitation Algorithm specifically state when, how, and why to use it but also when not to use it? To improve Codified Decision Making, an organization must improve the codified decisions, which has value up to the point that the documentation becomes too unwieldy to use. An organizational error in using Codified Decision Making is to demand that teams follow codified decision (i.e., rules) even if their situation awareness shows that the situation is not the same as planned. There may be reasons for blindly following codified decisions, such as to prevent litigation, by saying "we followed the procedure". Unfortunately, using the codified decision in that situation might be wrong and actually increase damage done.

Summary Box 16.1
Codified Decision Making

Does your team use Codified Decision Making when… • the decisions are documented or briefed before the task. • the actual conditions of the situation match the entry conditions assumed by the organization's philosophies, policies, and procedures.

16.2 Naturalistic Decision Making

When experienced people see that the codified decision is not appropriate, they use the second decision making method: Naturalistic Decision Making (Klein, Orasanu, Calderwood, and Zsambok 1993), also called Experience Based Decision Making. Naturalistic Decision Making is how experienced people naturally make decisions. Naturalistic Decision Making assumes that you have experience dealing with this situation: the "Been There, Done That" means of decision making. In our scenario, the OB DOC asked if any team members had prior experience with a pregnant patient in cardiac arrest. Since no one did, Naturalistic Decision Making was not appropriate, and either Codified or Deliberate Decision Making should be used.

In Naturalistic Decision Making, it is important that the experiences are diverse, and not the same experience over and over (i.e., routine). An example of diverse experience is a physician who delivered a thousand babies of different gestation ages from mothers of different ages and health; routine experience is a physician who delivered a thousand full-term babies from mothers in excellent health. With diverse experience, you are more likely to identify how a situation is similar to, but different than, previous experience. How is the delivery of a 34-week premie of a 28-year-old mother of three similar, or different than, a full-term delivery to a 46-year-old mother with insulin-dependent diabetes? The differences could be in the health of the patient, the equipment available, who is on your team, or what operating room you are in (i.e., in any area of the Status, Team, Environment or Progress [STEP]). Ideally, experience should be personal, but people can get indirect experience through mentoring, or by listening to the stories of more experienced people. When the less experienced person sees a situation similar to a story mentioned during mentoring, he or she knows what to do.

The main error in Naturalistic Decision Making is that people who do not have diverse experiences think they recognize the situation. In reality, the situation is just different enough to invalidate their limited experience, or the story they heard during mentoring. A more inexperienced CODE physician may not realize that pregnancy is marked by unique changes in physiology that can complicate efforts at resuscitation. To improve Naturalistic Decision Making, you need to give decision makers more experiences with coaching or mentoring on spotting the subtle differences and how those differences affect their mental models built from previous experiences.[133]

NOTE: More experiences without effective coaching or mentoring could result in the unseasoned team member taking the wrong action but getting lucky that it worked in that very specific case. Unfortunately, that person has learned that wrong action and may not be so lucky next time. Experience with mentoring help people develop deeper, broader, and more refined mental models as they incorporate new knowledge. With better mental models, people can determine if they perceive subtle differences (Level 1 Situation Awareness) and how those differences might affect the current and future situation (Level 2 and 3 Situation Awareness).

Also, a word of warning: be careful that your experience is priming you to do the right thing as opposed to the most comfortable. Is your experience telling you what you should do, and not just telling you to perform a task in the same way you always have?

Summary Box 16.2
Naturalistic Decision Making

Does your team use Naturalistic Decision Making when…

- the decisions are based on decisions made in past experiences or mentoring.
- diverse experiences allow you to determine if, and how, this situation varies from previous experiences and how that affects the current decision.

[133] This is called deliberate feedback. See *Cambridge Handbook of Expertise and Expert Performance* by Ericsson for more information.

16.3 Deliberate Decision Making[134]

Deliberate Decision Making (also called Analytical or Classical Decision Making) is required when there are no rules (Codified Decision Making) or experience (Naturalistic Decision Making) to guide your actions. Deliberate Decision Making is also required when you need to justify your decision to management, who will ask you if you considered other options or courses of action. In Deliberate Decision Making, you look at two or more courses of action and evaluate them against various discriminating factors to determine the best course of action. The usual discriminating factors are some forms of benefits, or what good things you get from the course of action; costs or what resources such as personnel, money, time, or other activities you can no longer perform because you are doing this course of action (i.e., lost opportunities); and risks or the chance that something bad will happen and possibly cause damage. In Codified Decision Making, your organization decided the tradeoffs between benefits, costs and risks. In Naturalistic Decision Making your experience told you what was the best tradeoff. In Deliberate Decision Making, your explicit analysis of benefit versus cost versus risk will decide the best tradeoff.

Deliberate Decision Making requires both time and data. Therefore, in emergency situations, where less time or data is available, leaders usually rely more on Codified Decision Making or Naturalistic Decision Making. Unfortunately, if neither Codified Decision Making nor Naturalistic Decision Making is available, and time is short, the team may be forced to look at fewer options, use fewer discriminating factors, or do fewer levels of analysis in an effort to shorten how long it takes to do Deliberate Decision Making. Unfortunately, as a team does this, it increases the risk of missing something. Again, we emphasize using the diversity of your team's mental models to help ensure that you do not miss anything truly crucial.

Before we dive deeper into Deliberate Decision Making, here is a comparison of the three decision making methods.

[134] The author would like to acknowledge Robert H. Smith, formerly of United Space Alliance Shuttle Upgrades, for his mentoring on how to use Deliberate Decision Making.

Table 16-1
Comparison of the Three Decision Making Methods

Codified Decision Making	Naturalistic Decision Making	Deliberate Decision Making
The scientific method codifies what sections to include in documenting research studies.	Experience makes it easier to decide what benefits research participants might glean from this study, because you have seen what benefits past participants have experienced.	When starting a research study involving complex sets of variables you have never measured before, you have to deliberate more in order to choose an appropriate set of analyses.
Laundry detergent directions codify which amounts and temperatures should be used to wash which garments.	Experience washing bright white shirts with new red socks in hot water makes it easier to decide what water temperature to use when washing new garments for the first time.	When you need to buy a new dryer with a gas hookup but have only purchased electric dryers in the past, you are more likely to need time to deliberate and compare pros and cons of buying different brands (with different features) before purchasing one.
A recipe codifies what beans to use when making Texas Chili.	Experience makes it easier to decide exactly how much chili powder to use for your taste preferences. You must decide, however, how much your experience making Hungarian Chili applies to making Texas Chili.	When you try to mimic the Texas Chili you ate at the State Fair last week, but have no recipe to guide you, you have to make an educated guess about which chili peppers were used to achieve the flavor profile you liked.

Diving deeper to demonstrate all aspects of Deliberate Decision Making, this Deliberate Decision Making scenario might play out over minutes, if not hours. Our example is where the neonate must be transported to a Level 3 NICU. The Pediatric physician might consider only one discriminating factor and that might be the earliest arrival time at a Level 3 NICU. Other possible factors—other benefits, costs, or risks—might not be considered. Let's make up some numbers to illustrate Deliberate Decision Making, other possible courses of action, and other factors.

Table 16-2
Looking at Only the Earliest Estimated Time of Arrival

Courses of Action	Use Neonatal Transport Team (NTT#1) from nearby NICU	Use own Hospital Transport Team (TT)	Use air TT	Use Neonatal Transport Team (NTT#2) from NICU farther away
Estimated Time of Arrival	4-5 hours (due to other tasks)	Unknown until they determine if extra personnel can be called in.	Up to 12 hours (due to inclement weather).	9 hours (due to round trip travel times).

Unfortunately, if the physician did not specifically state by when the newborn was required to be in a Level 3 NICU, we cannot be sure if Air Transport or NTT#2 were viable course of actions. So, it was not much of a Deliberate Decision Making trade study: The first choice is NTT #1, with possible back-ups of transport by your team if people can be brought in, air transport if the weather unexpectedly improves in the next 9 hours, or NTT#2.

To make for a better Deliberate Decision Making example, let us assume that the physician stated that the neonate can be made stable for 12 hours. That makes two courses of action (Air TT and NTT #2) viable, with the possibility of a third (Own TT). Let us also add two more discriminating factors: Shortest Time Enroute (benefit) and Team Training and Experience (enabling factor).[135]

Table 16-3
Adding One Benefit and One Cost

Courses of Action	NTT#1	Own TT	Air TT	NTT#2
Estimated Time of Arrival	4-5 hours	To Be Determined. Need extra personnel.	Up to 12 hours	9 hours
Shortest Time Enroute	1 hour	1 hour	15 minutes	4 hours
Team Training and Experience	Trained and experienced in neonatal transfers.	Trained and experienced in neonatal care, but not transfers.	Trained and experienced in general transfers.	Trained and experienced in neonatal transfers.

The next step in Deliberate Decision Making is scoring the courses of action versus the discriminating factors. Let us assume we will use a 9 (Best) - 5 - 3 - 1 (Worst) scoring system.[136] Since we cannot be sure if transport by our team is even possible, disregard it for now. Our example might look like:

[135] Enabling factors are those factors, that, if present, allow a wider choice of courses of action.
[136] 7 is specifically excluded to force a bigger differentiation between Courses of Action. To force even greater differentiation, some scoring schemes use only 9-3-1.

Table 16-4
Adding Scoring

Courses of Action	NTT#1	Air TT	NTT#2
Estimated Time of Arrival	9	1	3
Shortest Time Enroute	5	9	1
Team Training and Experience	9	5	9
Totals	23	15	13

But is each discriminating factor equally important? Let us assume that earliest Estimated Time of Arrival is three times and Team Training and Experience two times as important as Shortest Time Enroute. Multiplying the scores by these weightings, we get:

Table 16-5
Adding Weighting

Courses of Action	NTT #1	Air TT	NTT #2
Estimated Time of Arrival (w=3x)	27	3	9
Shortest Time Enroute	5	9	1
Team Training and Experience (w=2x)	18	10	18
Totals	50	22	28

Deliberate Decision Making says that you pick the course of action with the highest total. That only further strengthens the decision to go with NTT #1 but moves NTT #2 to the second choice.

Let us add some more complications. For purposes of exploring other possible trade study scenarios, what if the NTT#1 was not available; your own TT would be available as soon as personnel arrive in 1 hour; and weather is scheduled to improve in 9 hours. What would the trade-offs look like, then?

Table 16-6
Complicating the Decision

Courses of Action	Own TT	Air TT	NTT#2
Estimated Time of Arrival	2 hours (1 hour for extra personnel to come in + 1 hour trip to the Level 3 Neonatal Intensive Care Unit).	No earlier than 9 hours	9 hours
Time - Shortest Time Enroute	1 hour	15 minutes	4 hours
Team skill	Trained and experienced in neonatal care, but not transfers.	Trained and experienced in general transfers.	Trained and experienced in neonatal transfers.

Scoring and weighting the Courses of Action might look like:

Table 16-7
Scoring and Weighting the New Situation

Courses of Action	Own TT	Air TT	NTT#2
Estimated Time of Arrival (w=3x)	9 (27)	1 (3)	1 (3)
Shortest Time Enroute	5	9	1
Team Training and Experience (w=2x)	5 (10)	1 (2)	9 (18)
Total	42	14	22

This trade study says that using your own transport team is the best idea but may also show a problem with Deliberate Decision Making. Although Deliberate Decision Making looks objective (comes up with a definite number), it really is subjective. It depends on the discriminating factors you pick, and, how you score and weight them. Depending on scoring and weighting, you might get an answer that "doesn't feel right". When that happens, some teams change the scores or ratings to get an answer that "feels right". What if your experience told you that NTT #2 was the best course of action? You might decide that your scores and weighting were wrong and adjust them. Doing that, you can probably get NTT #2 and Own TT to have the same score, and when that happens you can either find additional factors, employ "eeny meeny miney mo", or just pick the course of action you always wanted anyway.

In essence, a major problem with Deliberate Decision Making is the subjectivity of the ratings. How much difference in arrival time is required to get a 9 versus a 5? Is arrival time really three times more important than enroute time? It is a good idea to get an agreement on discriminating factors, scores, and weighting with the final decision maker, so that your choices do not get second-guessed. Another problem is finding discriminating factors without strong correlation. Correlation means that two factors are related to each other. For example, when buying a house, you could use discriminating factors of cost, square footage, number of bedrooms, and number of bathrooms. But houses that have the most square footage usually have the most bedrooms and bathrooms, so the house with a 9 in square footage will usually get high scores for number of bedrooms and bathrooms. That is a strong positive correlation. Discriminating factors with strong positive correlation are essentially redundant and can and should be eliminated. It turns out cost may have a strong negative correlation, meaning, the house with the most square footage (score = 9) would cost the most (score =1). The challenge is finding discriminating factors with at most moderate correlation (i.e., a high score in one factor does not automatically mean a high or low score in other factors).

An alternate scoring approach might be assigning a plus or minus (versus assigning a numerical value) to the various factors—a plus if the course of action is better for that factor, or a minus, if worse—and then picking the course of action with the most plusses (maximizing) or the one with the least minuses (minimizing).

Summary Box 16.3
Deliberate Decision Making

Does your team use Deliberate Decision Making when you…

- have no rules or experience relevant to the current situation.
- need the optimal answer or need to justify the answer to superiors.
- have the time and data.
- can find discriminating factors with as little correlation as possible.
- can work with the final decision maker to determine factors, scoring and weighting.

NOTE: If you are changing factors, scores, or weights to get the answer you want, then you are not doing effective Deliberate Decision Making.

16.4 Risk and Uncertainty

16.4.1 Risk

Some people conflate risk and uncertainty, but they are different and distinctive. Let's discuss risk first. Risk describes the likelihood (how probable) and consequences (how bad) of a threat or error. Let us use an example from the International Space Station (ISS). [137] When a Multiplexer/Demultiplexer (essentially, a computer) fails on the ISS, the Mission Control Center has two possible courses of action on how to replace it:

[137] Our apologies to our Mission Control Center friends for this modified, simplified scenario for illustration purposes.

- Course of Action #1: Just like you would do if your computer at home failed, the astronauts could unplug the failed computer and plug in a new computer. This would take minutes, so Course of Action #1 is fast and easy.
- Course of Action #2: Perform long, complex procedures to power down major portions of the ISS before replacing the computer and another set of long, complex, procedures to power up the ISS. This would take hours, so Course of Action #2 is slow and difficult.

Without looking at risk, it seems fairly obvious that the Mission Control Center should go with Course of Action #1.

Let us look at the risks of each course of action. There are many books on how to analyze risk. We will cover the two aspects most pertinent to STAR: first, any analysis must look at how effective any mitigations are and how easy any contingency is to implement, and second, any analysis must look at all areas of STEP. Any analysis of risk must start with the most likely risk and the worst possible risk (sometimes referred to as the worst case scenario). The primary risk with Course of Action #1 is the worst-case scenario: since the astronauts are unplugging and plugging into a hot (electrically powered) outlet, there is a very small likelihood of the astronaut receiving an electrical shock, with a result of injury or even death.

The entire purpose of Course of Action #2 is to get into a configuration where the astronauts are not unplugging and plugging into a hot outlet. The long, complex procedures remove power from the outlet. Course of Action #2, however, is not without risk. Long, complex procedures are inherently error-prone (most likely risk); and in the hours that major portions of the ISS are unpowered, there are a number of other failures that, were they to occur, would endanger the ISS (worst-case scenario).

There is one other important difference between the two Courses of Action. In Course of Action#1, most actions are done by the crew, probably by two astronauts who received their technical and CRM training possibly years ago. In Course of Action #2, those long, complex procedures are done by mission controllers, probably consisting of team of teams totaling dozens of people who received more technical and CRM training more recently.

Table 16-7
The First Layer of Risk Analysis

	Likelihood	Consequences
Course of Action #1: Unplug/Plug	Very low	Very bad
Course of Action #2: Power Down/ Power Up	Moderate	Moderate

Because some risk analysis goes only so far, you might still like Course of Action #1 since the likelihood of the threat is very low. What if our risk analysis went a little deeper? Let us consider the possibilities of mitigations (ways to prevent, avoid or lessen the likelihood) and contingencies (is there a Plan B if the risk materializes?).

Mitigations for Course of Action #1 are relatively few: the crew will go over the procedure and any safety concerns before starting. Mitigations for Course of Action #2 consists of two things. First, there are more eyes to check for possible errors before they happen (i.e., more Mutually Supporting team members). Second, another purpose of those long complex procedures is to configure the various systems so that the likelihood and consequences of any future failures are reduced.

The primary contingency for Course of Action #1 for any injuries too serious to be handled on the ISS is to return the astronaut to Earth. For Course of Action #2, there are multiple contingencies (i.e., procedures) to cover any errors or additional failures.

Table 16-8
The Second Layer of Risk Analysis

	Likelihood	Consequences	Mitigations	Contingencies
Course of Action #1	Very Low	Very bad	Very few	One
Course of Action #2	Moderate	Moderate	Several	Multiple

Now Course of Action #1 is not as obvious, especially since it seems if you select Course of Action #1, there are very few ways to mitigate any risk and only one possible contingency plan. As mitigation and contingency options approach zero, a course of action becomes essentially all-in: either the course of action works, or you must live with the full consequences of the risk. All-in courses of action should be reserved for only those situations when you are very, very, sure that the risks are very, very, low. For Course of Action #2, there are several ways to prevent, avoid, or lessen likelihood as well as consequences of risks and multiple contingencies. But again, since the likelihood of the risk for Course of Action #1 is very low and you do have a contingency if that risk materializes, maybe you are still leaning toward Course of Action #1.

Before selecting a course of action, you might want to know the effectiveness of the mitigations and the ease to implement a contingency. You would like mitigations that are effective and contingencies that are easy, fast, or cheap to implement. If the Course of Action #1 mitigation and contingency were easy to implement, then Course of Action #1 may appear even more attractive. Unfortunately, the Course of Action #1 contingency of returning the injured astronaut to Earth is not easy, fast or cheap. To bring one astronaut back to Earth requires a crew of three in the returning capsule, which results in the loss of three highly trained astronauts from the ISS. Also, depending on the position of the orbit over the Earth, it might be several hours before the crew can re-enter, which is a potentially dangerous delay for an injured astronaut. There is another consideration: how risky the contingency is. For Course of Action #1, re-entry is one of the riskiest things an astronaut must do.[138]

[138] The other two very risky things are launch and space walks.

Before leaving the discussion on risk, we need to mention that any analysis must include all areas of STEP.

Table 16-8
Analysis Using Status-Team-Environment-Progress (STEP)

	Course of Action #1: Unplug/ Plug	Course of Action #2: Power Down/ Power Up
Status: International Space Station (ISS)	Chance of an additional failure during the procedure is very, very, low.	Chance of an additional failure during the long complex procedure must be mitigated and contingencies considered.
Task	Fast and simple. The procedure affects only a small portion of the ISS.	Long and complex. The procedure affects many ISS systems.
Team: Team Members	Two people who have been together for months.	Dozens of people in ad hoc team-of-teams structure.
Teamwork	Trained in CRM months/years previously; little opportunity to practice/receive feedback on CRM while on ISS.	Level of CRM training varies by team. Team in Mission Control Center trained in CRM months/years previously, but with more opportunities to practice/receive feedback on CRM.
Environment	Primarily on-board ISS, with more stressors.	Primarily in the Mission Control Center, with fewer stressors.

Progress: Schedule	Due to short duration, little effect on ISS operations.	Due to long duration, greater effect on ISS operations, possibly requiring some tasks to be delayed or cancelled.
Progress: Times-to-Effect/Margin	Due to short duration, no/few times-to-effect/margin.	Depending on what systems are powered off, there may be some decrease in margins (e.g., equipment left without cooling).

All of these areas of STEP must be considered in a risk analysis.

16.4.2 Uncertainty

Uncertainty is another challenge. We want to address one specific uncertainty: uncertainty in your situation awareness, or everyone perceiving everything that they need to perceive (Level 1 Situation Awareness), and comprehending and projecting properly (Levels 2 and 3 Situation Awareness)? Starting with Level 1 Situation Awareness uncertainty, remember that in Bottoms-Up Situation Awareness, what you perceive determines what mental models you activate. If you do not perceive the right information, you will not activate the right mental models, and a wrong mental model will bias what information you seek, and what you comprehend and project. Even if you activate the right mental models, Level 1 Situation Awareness uncertainty says that if you input bad information into a perfect mental model, you will get bad comprehension and projection. Level 1 Situation Awareness uncertainty is usually represented by missing, unreliable, conflicting, ambiguous, or lagging information. How confident are you in the information you have? You could set as your first goal obtaining more or better information, similar to a physician ordering more tests. Just be aware that a common pitfall is "paralysis by analysis", therefore, determine how long you can seek more information based on a time-to-effect and have someone monitor that time.

Uncertainty in Levels 2 and 3 Situation Awareness are essentially uncertainty in your mental models: are you confident that your education, experiences, self-discovery, and self-correction have developed a good mental model. By good, we mean it is deep (with a thorough understanding of the subject), broad (it covers all areas of STEP), refined (it is able to discern subtle differences in circumstances and how that affects the situation) and without holes or errors. Without that good mental model, even if you input total and perfect information, you will get bad comprehension and projection. Looking back at your history, how often have you been wrong about what is happening or will happen? Be aware that there is an excellent chance that you overestimate the fidelity of your mental model. It is human nature to remember all the times you were right and forget the times you were wrong. Finally, when dealing with complex situations and complex systems (e.g., major illness in a patient with pre-existing conditions), no one can ever have a perfect mental model. You can never know for sure if a patient will improve, or not.

Here are some actions that you can take to reduce the uncertainty in your situation awareness. You can decrease workload, distractions, and stress to give your team more cognitive resources to perceive, comprehend, and project. Another option is to "Do-a-little, Learn-a-little" in which you make your best guess based on what limited data is available, then try the least risky action and see what happens. You may have to do this several times, but the incremental results will, hopefully, help you converge on the right mental model. Finally, and most importantly, you can always use the diversity of your team—maybe someone is perceiving, comprehending, or projecting something that you do not—and use active listening and the "Power of And" to build better situation awareness.

Going back to our Mission Control Center example on how to respond to a failed computer, for Course of Action #1, how certain would the crew's mental model be if they were never trained on the specific procedure and the general training they had may have been years ago? For Course of Action #2, the Mission Control Center had more people with more and diverse information, and recently checked mental models to rely on. So, although Course of Action #1 is very fast and the risk of injury is very low, the lack of a mitigation coupled with a single costly, risky contingency plus the fact that the Mission Control Center has more diverse mental models and more information, means that the Mission Control Center leader may pick Course of Action#2, unless there are some extenuating circumstances.

The extent of any risk analysis that you can and need to do is based on the level of risk and the amount of time and data that you have. As available time and data decrease, a leader is forced to rely more on Codified or

Naturalistic Decision Making. Even when time is short, however, your team can ask itself the questions in the following Summary Box to make sure that you are not missing something crucial (and of course, actively listen to your team's diverse mental models):

Summary Box 16.4
Risk and Uncertainty Analysis

Does your team evaluate…
• risks of possible threats and errors in all areas of Status-Team-Environment-Progress (STEP)?
• each risk's likelihood and consequences?
• each risk's possible mitigations and contingencies?
• the effect of missing, unreliable, conflicting, ambiguous, or lagging information?
• the depth, breadth, and refinement of its mental models?

There is a fourth decision making process, which is how to make a decision when you are facing a "Black Swan" problem (Taleb 2010), a problem so unexpected that there are no procedures, no practices, no experience, and no mental models, and for which you cannot readily devise even one possible course of action. Think United Flight 232! The crew was faced with a never-imagined problem that seemingly had no solution: controlling an airliner with no hydraulics, and, therefore, no way to change direction or altitude.[139] Using CRM, they developed a solution that had never been seen or trained before. Although CRM is a needed tool for the team to handle this type of situation, we did not consider this decision making process, because it is very rare that any team will ever be in that situation and therefore beyond the scope of this book.

---

[139] Imagine driving across town and suddenly realizing that your car has no steering and no brakes. You and your three passengers have to figure out how to steer and stop your car. Without any rules, experience, or known options, you determine that you can steer left (or right) by opening the two left (or right) doors, increasing the drag on that side. You determine that you can slow down by opening all four doors. Now, all you have to do is get across town and park in a parking spot with cars on either side. That was the miracle of United Flight 232's "Black Swan" decision making, enabled by CRM. There are many excellent articles about United 232. Here is one from *Popular Mechanics*:
https://www.popularmechanics.com/flight/a10478/the-final-flight-of-united-232-16755928/

All three decision making models, Codified, Naturalistic and Deliberate, assume a defined leader (someone who makes the final decision). In healthcare (and in our scenarios), there are often multiple teams working together, with each team leader being co-equal with the other team leaders. When a team-of-teams forms, there is often no established structure or process to determine who has the ultimate decision making authority (i.e., how to designate the "leader-of-the-leaders"). When decisions do need to be made in these situations, there may be conflict, as each team leader tries to force his or her decision on the other teams. This conflict must be managed. Managing conflict is the subject of the next chapter.

Chapter Debriefing

I want to call a quick STAR (Stop-Think-Act-Review): get off your email, stop your side conversations, and turn off the television.[140] Let's see if you can expand upon these statements:

- When to (not) use Codified Decision Making.
- When to (not) use Naturalistic Decision Making.
- Determine discriminating factors, with as little correlation as possible.
- Evaluate risk beyond likelihood and consequences.
- Evaluate uncertainty in terms of knowing what to perceive and how and why events happen.

If this was an actual debriefing, we would ask you to expand further on each of these statements. Depending on your response, we would ask open-ended follow-up questions until we were sure you understood the material and had a plan to implement one or more best practices. We might ask, "What is a specific decision making problem that you experience on your job?" We would not be satisfied if you said, "Our risk assessment isn't very good." Again, we would ask open-ended follow-up questions until you might say, "We have a problem with our risk assessment being too shallow, considering too little." We would then ask, "What can you do to fix that problem prior to the next shift?" Again, we would ask open-ended follow-up questions until you might say, "Our risk assessment needs to consider such things as the number of contingencies, and the ease or difficulty in executing a contingency." We might then ask, "How might you help other

---

[140] See Chapters 11-15 for information on STAR.

teams?" More open-ended questions until you might say, "I will work with management to modify the organization's risk assessment process."

CHAPTER 17

MANAGING CONFLICT

Chapter Briefing[141]

I want to call a quick STAR (Stop-Think-Act-Review): get off your email, stop your side conversations, and turn off the television. Here is what we will do in the next chapter. We will discuss how managing conflict facilitates and strengthens CRM. We will be successful if you can identify:

- Eight common causes of conflict (Section 17.1);
- The key elements of an effective plan to address an instance of conflict (17.2); and
- The important parts of a script for stating the conflict in order to resolve it (Section 17.2).

The primary threat that you might experience is the introduction of a large number of concepts and terms, some of which you may have never encountered, and some of which you may think about in a different sense. We will therefore explicitly define and differentiate each term and concept. We also realize how busy you are. We will make sure that the chapter is short enough to be read in approximately thirty minutes. Finally, we provide Summary Boxes. The Summary Boxes serve two functions. First, they emphasize the take-home points in each section, and you can use them to check your understanding of those take-home points. Second, you can use them to determine if you and your team are implementing those take-home points. If a Summary Box does not make sense to you or you do not

[141] By now, you may feel that repeated use of the chapter briefing format is redundant. However, we believe that it is important to continue to emphasize that a good briefing builds mental models by discussing what is happening, what success looks like, and what threats or errors are possible and how you plan to prevent, avoid, or mitigate them. Hence, the repetitive nature is meant to cement this belief with an understanding that you will also immerse yourself in this book on an irregular and/or intermittent basis.

understand one or more take-home points, then review the related material before continuing to the next section.

Did I miss anything? Any concerns? Any questions? (Pause) No? Then, let's get started.

List of Abbreviations

ANES	Anesthesiology
CODE	Code (resuscitation) Team
CRM	Crew Resource Management
DOC	Physician
ED	Emergency Department
ICU	Intensive Care Unit
NUR	Nurse
OB	Obstetric
STATE	Share-Tell-Ask-Talk-Encourage

Conflict is a disagreement or an opposition of interests or ideas. In simple terms, what you want, believe, or perceive does not match what others want, believe, or perceive. Most of us seek to avoid overt conflict because it is often emotionally taxing. We also frequently find a different path to achieve what we want without having to invest the time or the emotional labor into resolving conflicts. However, avoiding conflict may risk harming ourselves, our teams, and our patients by leaving information underground that would otherwise have been exchanged and used to improve our situation awareness. Team members often hesitate to offer mutual support or communicate contradictory information to avoid conflicts and thereby debilitate the leader's decision-making ability and the team's ability to self-correct or avoid errors.

Recognizing the eight common causes of conflict will help you to constructively resolve conflicts when they inevitably arise. While the priority order of steps necessary to resolve conflict well may differ depending on the amount of time available to make a decision and the decision-making model in use by your team, the causes of conflict (Section 17.1), and the best practices for resolving them remain the same (Section 17.2).

17.1 Eight Common Causes of Conflict

The first logical steps in resolving conflict are to identify the problem and then identify what caused the conflict. What do you desire, versus those who conflict with you? Why are you dissatisfied? Bell (2002) identified six reasons for conflict in the workplace: conflicting needs, conflicting styles, conflicting perceptions, conflicting goals, conflicting pressures, and conflicting roles. Hart (2000) added two more common causes of conflict that seem especially relevant in healthcare: different personal values, and an absence of clear policies or standards of behavior. The table below provides a listing of the eight common causes, along with examples of each. These causes will become "muscle memory" for you even more quickly if you come up with your own examples for each one and use these causes to structure simulation-based training scenarios or mental rehearsals for yourself.

Table 17-1
Eight Common Causes of Conflict

Cause	Definition	Example
Conflicting Needs	More than one person needs the same limited resource (e.g., space, time, supplies, attention, funding) to accomplish something.	Three nurses need the same wheelchair to discharge multiple waiting patients.
Conflicting Styles	Two or more approaches are applicable to the same situation, task, etc. but only one may be applied at a time.	One charge nurse prefers admission files alphabetized; the other charge nurse at the same station prefers them ordered by room number.
Conflicting Perceptions	People have different views of, or information about, the same event.	The mother of a patient gives one nurse very different background information about the patient's accident than the patient volunteered to the physician on rounds earlier. When the CODE and ANES physicians disagree on whether the resuscitation algorithm is the same for a pregnant patient in our scenario.

Conflicting Goals	People have different priorities for accomplishing similarly important or dependent responsibilities.	The hospital must discharge patients quickly to meet demand for beds, but the unit is concerned that patients may not be truly stable enough to be safely discharged.
Conflicting Pressures	People are demanding multiple things or accomplishments from the same person, group, or team at the same time.	Four patients code in the Emergency Department at the same time. When the team must deal with a delivery, resuscitation, and code simultaneously in our scenario.
Conflicting Roles	People are asked to do something without clear responsibility or sufficient authority to do it.	Both the primary and on-service physician are asked to authorize a change in the treatment course. When the OB, CODE and ANES physicians all think they are leading the code in the scenario.
Different Personal Values	Varying levels of salience given to broad desirable goals that motivate each person's philosophy on life and how to live it (and that may lead to different approaches to caring for a patient).	Members of the hospice team differ as to whether a transition to comfort care is a reasonable option to be offered to the family members of a critically ill, heavily sedated, patient in the Intensive Care Unit.
Predictability of Policies	There is no clear and current standard of operation or organizational policy such that two or more people must guess what is desired by the organization in a given situation.	An oncologist sees a one percent chance of survival as a reasonable chance, while the intensivist does not and wishes to withdraw life-sustaining treatment.

Determining the most likely cause of the conflict is half the battle. The other half relies on presenting your theory about the cause to those involved in a way that supports discussion and subsequent coordination (of priorities, roles, tasks, procedures, relationships, etc.). Part of practicing good CRM is understanding how mismatches in CRM skills drive these eight types of conflicts, and vice versa. For example, different Level 1 Situation Awareness can stem from, and contribute to, conflicting perceptions. Different mental models may lead team members to conflicting goals. In such cases, resolving the conflict may be largely about articulating the missing CRM skills so that team members can decide what behavior within that skill should be applied. This is frequently part of the self-correction process that teams go through during debriefings, as they discuss why mental models were different and what information changed their situation awareness. However, in time-pressured situations, instances when it is not clear who has final decision-making authority, or when debriefings are severely constrained, your ability to quickly sort through the eight common causes of conflict to pick the one most salient cause becomes crucial to preventing errors.

17.2 Addressing the Primary Cause of Conflict

Productively engaging in meaningful conflicts with our teammates is vital to CRM. Teams that resolve conflicts productively outperform teams that avoid conflict. Teams that manage conflict well have higher team member satisfaction (and thus long-term viability of the team continuing to work together) and make more efficient and effective decisions compared to teams that do not manage conflict well or at all (De Witt, Greer, and Jehn 2012). Cooperation without conflict resolution (i.e., going along without resolving conflicts in priorities, processes, and roles) leads to mediocre, or even substandard, patient care (Marshall and Robson 2005). Poor conflict management behavior impacts not only those directly involved in the conflict, but also all of those who see it or hear about it. Interestingly, great conflict resolution behavior positively impacts not only the health and well-being of those directly involved in the conflict, but also the psychological safety and trust within the surrounding organization.

First and foremost, in dealing with conflict, you will have to honestly evaluate how much of an impact the conflict has, and then, decide how much time you have to actually address the conflict. Do not confuse this step with deciding how much time the team has to make a decision about a particular patient, test, or issue during clinical practice. There will be times when the conflict is straightforward and must be resolved in seconds in order to stabilize a patient. In these cases, you will have to rely on your team's implicit or explicit mental models of leadership and decision-making authority to address the surface-level aspects of the conflict at a minimum. However, the majority of conflicts, even those that arise during time-critical operations, usually have a much deeper root cause that should still be addressed as time permits.

As many conflicts are capable of quickly generating vigorous emotional responses, you stand a better chance of addressing causes well when you take a mental timeout to calm yourself first and plan what to say. Calming yourself can be as simple as doing a ten-count breathing exercise (e.g., if pressed for time), but if the emotional turmoil is substantial enough, it may also require a longer cooling off period and series of consultations with impartial colleagues. Simply put, resolving the conflict may first involve planning on how to do just that. The key is to first get yourself to a place where you can think more broadly than "this should not have happened" or "they should have done this, not that". If thoughts of the conflict are still triggering blaming or shaming thoughts, then you are likely not composed enough to address the multi-faceted causes of most team conflicts, nor will you be able to fairly coordinate CRM. Good plans are not made in a reactive instant. Finding a few minutes or more to carefully list and prioritize your options for constructively addressing the conflict is a good idea, and your willingness to find those minutes is also a cue you can use to confirm that you are now calm enough to do so. A good plan to address a conflict has three key elements:

1. You have articulated an idea about the cause of the conflict and have chosen the one most important topic or instance of that conflict to address, as in our Amniotic Fluid Embolism scenario when CODE Nurse #1 recognized that there were conflicting roles and asked the three physicians to identify who was giving the orders.
2. You have planned a specific and reasonable time and place to address that topic or instance when the people involved are most likely to be willing and able to discuss it, as the OB physician did when asking if everyone had the time to do the debrief.
3. You have thought of ways to keep yourself and others focused on that one instance of conflict (i.e., not all ten instances over the last month) and to discuss resolutions that rely on changeable behaviors (i.e., how to confirm understanding in the future)—as the team did during their discussion on how to avoid errors next time.

Whether you initiate the discussion, or, are simply participating in a discussion to manage a conflict, you best support CRM when you also follow a script that encompasses best practices summarized by Patterson, Grenny, and McMillan (2002) in the STATE format[142]:

- Share your facts first. Facts are what you saw, heard, smelled, tasted, and the information and tools upon which you relied in the situation that you are addressing—as the OB physician did by stating the patient was previously healthy, had delivered, then complained of difficulty breathing, arrested, and was then hemorrhaging.
- Tell your story or your idea about the cause based on your understanding of your facts. The goal of your story should be to expand shared understanding, not to prove a point, as the OB physician did by recalling that previous training indicated an amniotic fluid embolism.
- Ask for others' understanding of the facts, as the OB physician did by asking if anyone else had any ideas about a possible diagnosis.
- Talk with an open mind, and do not disguise your beliefs or opinions as fact. Admit you might not have the whole picture but that you are interested in building a better one, as the OB physician did by stating the team needed to stay willing to revise their working diagnosis.
- Encourage the testing of your idea about the cause with constructive criticism, as the OB physician did by asking the others to speak up if they perceived new or conflicting data. The more others see that you want to come to a better understanding of the conflict's causes the more willing they will be to discuss and adapt resolutions (as the CODE Nurse#1 articulated during the debrief in our scenario).

You can say as little as five sentences to cover all the STATE elements, in as little as thirty seconds, with some practice. From our scenario, the OB physician stated,

> "Okay, she was previously healthy, delivered, complained of difficulty breathing, then arrested and is now bleeding out. (State) My training says those are all signs of an amniotic fluid embolism. (Tell) Does anyone have any other ideas?" (Ask)
> Everyone responds with "No" or shakes their head from side to side.

---

[142] DESC is another format to address conflicts. See Section 8.3

"Then let's go with that as our working diagnosis but be willing to revise it. (Talk) Let's keep gathering data, and speak up if you have other thoughts. (Encourage)

Managing conflict to support CRM gets better as you and your teams have more practice addressing conflicts productively. For the first few times that you address a conflict with a team, it helps to outline a STATE script and refer to it during discussions. In time-pressured situations, you may also need to vary the order of STATE by starting with E to encourage the testing of all ideas, and letting the team know that there is a strict time limit for sharing facts in this situation. When managing conflicts to achieve time-critical decisions, there are two additional specific best practices that help: 1) assign the order in which the team members will speak to share facts (e.g., the person who has the greatest amount of first-hand observations of the patient will speak first), and, 2) assign a team member to monitor the patient and appoint a timekeeper to watch the clock to inform the rest of the team when patient status or time restrictions dictate that an action absolutely must be taken.

Finally, for complicated conflicts, even the most experienced conflict management consultants recognize that time-outs or multiple debriefings over time must sometimes be implemented. In such cases, the team should agree as to when and where to pick up the discussion, in order to reduce the emotional burden of resolving it. The biggest win is when every team member walks away from the discussion with a little better understanding of the cause of the conflict, even if there are not yet any foreseeable resolutions. Those understandings allow you to compensate for a few more of the blind spots in your situation awareness, or exchange additional information that bridges a mental model gap. How a team practices CRM and in turn performs is always negotiable, and those negotiations happen as you address conflicts in the moment of conflict and in subsequent debriefings.

Summary Box 17.1
Best Practices for Resolving Conflict in a Team

- Determine which of the 8 common causes of conflict are most relevant to your team's current conflict: Conflicting Needs, Styles, Perceptions, Goals, Pressures, Roles, Personal Values, or Policies.
- A plan to resolve the conflict must address the primary cause of the conflict, feature a reasonable time and place to discuss it as a team, and remain focused on discussing changeable behaviors.
- Using the STATE script to discuss a conflict will facilitate efficient and effective resolution of the conflict—share the facts first, tell the story of your understanding of those facts, ask for others' understanding of the facts, talk with an open-mind, and encourage the testing of your idea about the conflict's cause.

Chapter Debriefing

I want to call a quick STAR (Stop-Think-Act-Review): get off your email, stop your side conversations, and turn off the television.[143] Let's see if you can answer these questions:

- What is the most likely cause(s) of conflict in your team or organization?
- How much time do you really have to address the cause of the conflict? Do you need to limit yourself to the surface level for now or adjust how you STATE the issue? Does the team need you to name an order for sharing facts? How will you maintain situation awareness on all areas of STEP if you must address the conflict in real time?
- What script will you use to STATE the conflict?
    - What facts will you Share to support your idea that this is the cause?
    - How will you order these facts to Tell the story of how you understand what these facts mean?
    - How will you Ask for others to share their understanding of the facts?
    - How will you Talk so that others know you are not misrepresenting your beliefs as facts?

[143] See Chapters 11-15 for information on STAR.

    - How will you Encourage others to question your understanding of the facts?
- How will you stay focused on discussing what behaviors you can change to address it?
- Will it be easier to discuss the non-time-critical aspects of the cause later or in intervals?
    - If so, what is the plan for agreeing on when and where to pick up the discussion or debrief the conflict?

If this was an actual debriefing, we would ask you to expand further on each of these statements. Depending on your response, we would ask open-ended follow-up questions until we were sure you understood the material and had a plan to implement one or more best practices. We might ask, "What problem in conflict management do you see in your team?" We would not be satisfied if you said, "Managing conflict between specialties isn't as good as we need." Again, we would ask open-ended follow-up questions until you might say, "We have a problem with a team member thinking his or her approach is the best." We would then ask, "What can you do to fix that problem prior to your next shift?" We would then continue to ask open-ended follow-up questions until you might say, "In the briefing, I will discuss the STATE format. During the shift, I need to mentor my team on how to use the STATE format. In the debriefing, we will discuss how we could have better scripted our STATE statements." We would then ask, "That will help your team better explain their perspective in a conflict. How will you help other teams to better explain their perspective?" More open-ended questions until you might say, "I need to work with management to better train the use of conflict management tools."

References

Bell, Art (2002). Six ways to resolve workplace conflicts. San Francisco, CA: University of San Francisco.

de Wit, Frank R., Lindred L. Greer, and Karen A. Jehn. "The Paradox of Intragroup Conflict: A Meta-Analysis." Journal of Applied Psychology 97, no. 2 (2012): 360–90. https://doi.org/10.1037/a0024844.

"Conflict in the Workplace by Monica A. Frank, Ph.D.." Excel At Life. Accessed October 30, 2021. https://www.excelatlife.com/articles/conflict_at_work.htm.

Marshall, Pam, and Rob Robson. "Preventing and Managing Conflict: Vital Pieces in the Patient Safety Puzzle." Healthcare Quarterly 8, no. sp (2005): 39–44. https://doi.org/10.12927/hcq..17660.

Patterson, Kerry, Ron McMillan, and Joseph Grenny. Crucial Conversations: Tools for Talking When Stakes Are High. New York etc.: McGraw-Hill, 2002.

CHAPTER 18

DEBRIEFING[144]

Chapter Briefing[145]

I want to call a quick STAR (Stop-Think-Act-Review): get off your email, stop your side conversations, and turn off the television.[146] In this chapter we will discuss debriefing, with the goal of fixing team interactions (i.e., CRM) using self-discovery and self-correction. We will be successful if you can:

- define what a debriefing using self-discovery and self-correction is (Section 18.1);
- describe the reasons for conducting a debriefing (Section 18.1);
- list the characteristics of a good debriefing (Section 18.2); and
- list at least two debriefing errors seen in your organization/culture (Section 18.3).

The primary threat that you might experience is the introduction of a large number of concepts and terms, some of which you may have never encountered, and some of which you may think about in a different sense. We will therefore explicitly define and differentiate each term and concept.

---

[144] A debriefing is not a CRM skill. It is, however, a required tool in order to perform CRM properly, and to perform at a higher level. Without a debriefing, your team will never practice self-discovery and self-correction. Without self-discovery and self-correction, your team will eventually make an error, then fail to handle it properly, and that may result in an accident.

[145] By now, you may feel that repeated use of the chapter briefing format is redundant. However, we believe that it is important to continue to emphasize that a good briefing builds mental models by discussing what is happening, what success looks like, and what threats or errors are possible and how you plan to prevent, avoid, or mitigate them. Hence, the repetitive nature is meant to cement this belief with an understanding that you will also immerse yourself in this book on an irregular and/or intermittent basis.

[146] For more information on STAR, see Chapters 11-15.

We also realize how busy you are. We will make sure that the chapter is short enough to be read in approximately thirty minutes. Finally, we provide Summary Boxes. The Summary Boxes serve two functions. First, they emphasize the take-home points in each section, and you can use them to check your understanding of those take-home points. Second, you can use them to determine if you and your team are implementing those take-home points. If a Summary Box does not make sense to you or you do not understand one or more take-home points, then review the related material before continuing to the next section.

Did I miss anything? Any concerns? Any questions? (Pause) No? Then, let's get started.

List of Abbreviations

AFE	Amniotic Fluid Embolism
ANES	Anesthesiologist
CRM	Crew Resource Management
DOC	Physician
NUR	Nurse
OB	Obstetric
STEP	Status-Team-Environment-Progress

The best of the best teams, in various industries, debrief what went well and poorly for both their technical actions and their Crew Resource Management (CRM) actions. Since this book is about CRM, the rest of this chapter will deal with a specific technique to debrief CRM actions. The best teams realize that they need to continue to refine, deepen and adapt their CRM skills, therefore they value feedback. They debrief their CRM at the end of every shift or task, even if everything went well. A debriefing might take as little as 2-5 minutes. A debriefing can be done by CRM skill (e.g., How were our Leading and Following skills today?) or by event (e.g., How did our CRM help or hurt us when we had multiple physicians issuing orders?).

In too many organizations and for too many teams, the debriefing is led by the team leader. A leader-led debriefing is where the team leader says, "You did this wrong; fix it by doing…". Regardless how knowledgeable and experienced the leader is, no one person can see and know everything, especially the tasks that other team members must accomplish and how they must do so. As a leader skilled in CRM, you know that everyone's mental models are different based on their role, experience, and goals. Hence, you will not know how to fix their mental model problems. A leader-led debriefing is often incomplete and possibly wrong.

What type of debriefing are we advocating? We are advocating a much more powerful method of debriefing—a debriefing using self-discovery and self-correction. You will learn about our method of debriefing and the reasoning behind it in Section 18.1, what constitutes a briefing in Section 18.2, and common errors and remedies in Section 18.3.

NOTE
Although our goal is for your team to conduct debriefings using self-discovery and self-correction, performing such debriefings requires your team to meet three conditions:

1) the team is experienced (i.e., the team is not in technical training);
2) the team is familiar with CRM in a manner similar to you after you have finished this book, and you have had a chance to practice and receive feedback on your CRM skills; and
3) the team is familiar with and comfortable doing self-discovery and self-correction.

Until (and only until) your team meets all these conditions, you will need to use an intermediate tool, called Facilitated Debriefings, which can be found in Appendix B.

18.1 What is Our Concept for Debriefing and Why Do It?

Before we get started, we need to make something clear. It is important to note that there is a difference between a technical performance debriefing and a critical incident stress debriefing. Technical performance debriefings serve to dispassionately assess individual, team, and system performance during a real or simulated event. In contrast, critical incident stress debriefings are conducted to provide psychological support after "an event that has the potential for people to experience significant physical, cognitive, emotional and behavioral reactions immediately after the incident or days, weeks, months and even sometimes years later." (Tompkins 2000) Most of what has been published in the healthcare literature about debriefing blurs the border between these two types of debriefings. Many healthcare authors describe reaction, description, analysis, and summary phases of a debriefing. Such a model implies that psychological distress after a real or simulated clinical scenario is a frequent occurrence and that those being debriefed are not able to effectively participate in that debriefing without first having an opportunity to "ventilate" pent-up emotion. This runs counter to the manner in which debriefings are conducted in other industries. Moreover, within healthcare, Henricksen, Altenburg, and Reeder (2017) examined the expression of psychological distress in 3,900 subjects undergoing debriefing after simulated clinical scenarios. They found that less than one percent of the subjects were perceived to manifest signs of significant distress, indicating that such responses are quite rare. In this book, debriefing refers to a technical performance debriefing. In the scenario, the OB physician specifically stated that the debriefing would be a technical performance debriefing.

NOTE: If your debriefing primarily discusses the emotional impact of the task, or you do not debrief when events turn out well, then your debriefings do not match the standards set in the military, space, commercial aviation, and other high-risk occupations in the oil and gas, maritime, or nuclear power industries (Sawyer and Deering 2013).

So, what do we mean by the term debriefing? In our concept, team members discuss among themselves what the team did right and wrong in their team interactions, and then determine how they should improve. The purpose of our debriefings, therefore, is for the team members to examine their team interactions (self-discover) and to figure out how to fix any problems (self-correct). The main problem with team interactions, which we call their CRM Mental Models, is that the mental models may be different for different team members, incomplete in places or insufficiently defined in others. In other words, the team wants to improve their CRM Mental Models to be more correct (no gaps or errors), more complete (covering all aspects of STEP) and more refined (adaptable to different situations). At the end of a debriefing every team member has better complementary mental models on what information to pass to whom and when (improved Exchanging Information), how (improved Communicating), how to enable CRM (improved Leading) while inquiring, advocating, and asserting if required (improved Following), and how to back up and support each other (improved Mutually Supporting).

Our debriefing concept is advantageous in five ways. First, it relies on an adult learner's own motivation to improve. Second, your team is required to think about their problems and how to fix them. They, therefore, must process knowledge more deeply which means that they will retain that knowledge longer, and will be able to draw upon the knowledge more readily and effectively in the future. Third, because they are addressing holes in their own mental models, the fixes are to their existing mental model, rather than a 'foreign' mental model imposed by the leader. Fourth, because they came up with the fixes themselves, they more readily buy into the fixes. The fifth and the most important advantage is the fact that your team develops a habit of self-discovery and self-correction, and, hopefully, continues this practice after every task or shift.

Summary Box 18.1
The Reasons to Conduct a Debriefing Using Self-Discovery and Self-Correction

A debriefing using self-discovery and self-correction…
• relies on adult learners' motivation to learn and improve; • requires your team members to process deeper, retain longer and recall easier; • develops fixes to team members' existing mental models, instead of a 'foreign' mental model; • creates more buy-in to the fixes; and • develops a habit of self-discovery and self-correction.

18.2 What Are the Characteristics of a Good Debriefing?

Your team must discuss the following:

- Team interactions: The goal of a debriefing is to improve the team members' mental model of interactions: how best to exchange information, communicate, lead, follow, and mutually support one another. To best cover interactions, team members must address (i.e., interact with) each other directly, and discuss how they were affected by the actions of others.
- What they were thinking: To improve mental models, the team needs to analyze the rationale underlying the decisions that they made. They then need to talk about how their mental models allowed a bad decision to be made, and how they would need to change their mental models to eliminate that deficit. In the debriefing of the AFE scenario, the physicians needed to discuss why each one thought that he or she needed to take charge.
- Context: Context determines how a CRM skill will be applied. They need to discuss what enabled or impeded their success,

including the why and how (i.e., why and how the Environment (E in STEP) affected the outcome). Since context changes, they need to discuss how they might handle things differently in a different situation. The context in the AFE scenario consisted of three physicians dealing with a maternal arrest following a delivery. A slightly different case that they might want to discuss is a situation where the ANES physician arrives late: how would the Obstetric (OB) and CODE physicians have handled that? Or what if the cause was sepsis (versus an AFE), how would that have changed Leading and Following? The point is to not find a solution that is restricted to one context. Try to identify how you will find the right solution depending on the context.

- An action plan to improve team performance: It is not enough for the OB physician to say, "I need to improve my situation awareness." Instead, the OB physician should say, "I need to realize that as compressions take up more and more of my attention, I become fixated. I need to take a second to step back, even just mentally, to consider the whole situation. I could also include in my shift briefing that I need the OB nurses to help me by pointing out when they think I might be losing situation awareness." Hopefully a nurse could also say, "I realize that as important as doing my own tasks are, I have a responsibility to support my team and ensure they are not making errors. In the shift briefing, I could ask how I can better support my team if we get busy or distracted."

Summary Box 18.1
What You Want Your Team to Discuss in a Debriefing

Does your team discuss…
• their interactions?
• what they were thinking?
• the context?
• their action plans?

18.3 Debriefing Errors[147]

Unfortunately, it is not that easy to conduct a debriefing using self-discovery and self-correction. Here are some common errors and how to avoid or mitigate them.

- Not establishing psychological safety. In the scenario, a physician tried to establish psychological safety in several ways by stating:
    - the debriefing was covered under Code of Evidence 1157 to ensure confidentiality and encourage discussion.
    - none of topics covered would be discussed anywhere else (other than in a formal morbidity and mortality conference) to address concerns that people might talk behind their backs.
    - in addition, the CODE physician stated in a previous shift, "Never let me hurt a patient", thereby admitting potential fallibility and indicating a need for input from team members.

With insufficient psychological safety, you will see one of two problems. The first problem is that some healthcare professionals find it easier to point out team weaknesses, as this often diffuses responsibility from one or a small number of individuals to the more nebulous "team". When that happens, no one person needs to accept responsibility for failure, nor are individuals called out by name (i.e., instead the "royal we" is used). Psychological safety is required for an individual to admit an error, and then for the team to discuss, if there was a team interaction problem that caused it.[148] Why did he or she not get the right information? Was it an error in Exchanging Information (e.g., no one knew to pass that information to that person at that time)? The second problem is the opposite: a team member is fearful of reprisals for pointing out the error of another, especially the error of a superior. Each individual only discusses his or her personal errors. In our scenario, each team member was initially discussing individual errors (I did…) and individual fixes (I need to …). It wasn't until a nurse summarized the situation that they started talking about the team interaction problem of Leading and Following. Fearing to point out the errors of others is mitigated by the superior stating in the briefing and

---

147 According to Hollnagel, many errors are not due to personal flaws but caused by organizational or structural faults. If different people in the same situation make the same error, it is not a human problem; it is a system problem.

148 In a debriefing, we are not addressing individual technical errors (e.g., someone not knowing how to intubate). Correcting individual technical/manual skills is the sole responsibility of the healthcare professional manifesting that weakness.

reinforcing in the debriefing that he or she needs their inputs to improve his or her CRM. In the scenario, the CODE physician admitted to reverting to his/her usual mode under stress, and the OB physician admitted to losing situation awareness. Regardless, the goal of the debriefing is not to assign blame, but to find ways as a team to improve CRM skills to prevent errors from recurring.

- Discussing only errors committed by the team. It is equally important to discuss what the team did right so that they understand what they did right, why it was right, how it was right, and how to improve or adapt the next time (Halamek, Cady, and Sterling 2019). In the AFE scenario, the OB physician wanted to ensure that the team understood why the nurses knew to be assertive.
- Not understanding the difference between skill and luck. Just because a positive outcome occurred does not mean that the team performed at a high level. To think the outcome was based on skill may be a fallacy and sets the team up to commit errors in the future. Do not debrief based on the outcome, but rather on the quality of the team's use of CRM skills.
- Hindering team member participation by providing your analysis or evaluation before the team members complete theirs. Giving your opinions turns the debriefing into a 'you-led' debriefing which defeats the concept of self-discovery and self-correction. If you tell them what they did wrong and how to improve, they do not have to think.
- Accepting a poor or incomplete analysis (e.g., one that is too broad or too general). "Our CRM was bad" is not an analysis. Since different CRM problems have different remedies, you must delve deeper. "Our CRM was bad because our communicating was bad because we didn't use the right format" provides insight into what to correct.
- Accepting a specific, incomplete, or wrong solution. While stating a specific fix to a specific error is required, it will not help your team when they are in a somewhat different situation. The team must address the generic error and the discussion should produce a generic solution. It is not sufficient to say "Next time, let us use Format *X*" because in another situation Format *X* may not be correct. The generic error is using wrong formats, and the generic solution is how to determine what is the right format. During the debriefing of the AFE scenario, the teams could have come up with more generic errors and solutions.

- Allowing Hindsight Bias to influence analysis.[149] Hindsight Bias will lead to simple, linear, context-specific fixes, assuming it was obvious how a missed threat led to poor Exchanging Information, which led to Communicating errors, which led to poor decisions, which eventually allowed an accident to occur. But in real time, all the team had were vague indications that something was not right. During the debriefing, the team needs to identify and address the holes in its mental models that led to poor Exchanging Information, errors in Communicating, and poor decision making. Concentrate the debriefing there: what, why, and how did CRM behaviors let the threat materialize, and how to fix CRM behaviors, both specifically and generally.
- Permitting the debriefing to take too long, meander, or be skipped entirely because there is not enough time. When time is short (isn't it always!) then set a time limit and pick only the one or two most important CRM topics to discuss. If you debrief all the time, you can catch other problems in another debriefing. In the AFE scenario, the OB physician said to cover only the two or three most important issues, and, later, mentioned when they reached the 10-minute point that was proactively set.

Summary Box 18.2
Debriefing Errors and Remedies

Do you…
- discuss only what went wrong? Know that you should also discuss what went right to reinforce the practices that allowed the team to do the right thing.
- take over and turn it into a 'you-led' debriefing? Remember, a debriefing is about the team self-discovering and self-correcting.
- accept incomplete, wrong, too specific or broad analysis or solutions? Your team must fix the immediate problem, but also have the tools to do the right thing when the situation is slightly different.
- not do a debriefing because there was no time? When time is short, set a time limit and discuss only the most important CRM problems.

---

149 A cognitive bias caused by taking a retrospective perspective on an issue that leads to thinking that those involved should have been able to anticipate the chain of events that occurred.

Unfortunately, in some organizations and cultures, the transition from leader-led debriefings to debriefings using self-discovery and self-correction is too large to make in single leap. A tool to help make that transition over time as the team gets used to self-discovery and self-correction is a Facilitated Debriefing. For more information on Facilitated Debriefings, see Appendix B.

Chapter Debriefing

I want to call a quick STAR (Stop-Think-Act-Review): get off your email, stop your side conversations, and turn off the television.[150]. Let's see if you can expand upon these statements:

- Psychological safety is required to conduct a debriefing using self-discovery and self-correction.
- Debriefings using self-discovery and self-correction are powerful because they rely on an adult's motivation to improve, require deeper processing, build on existing mental models, have more buy-in, and build the habits of self-discovery and self-correction.
- Debriefings must discuss team interactions, thought processes, context, and action plans.
- Debriefing must discuss both errors and effective actions.
- Do not take over and turn a debriefing into a 'you-led' debriefing.
- Do not accept analyses or solutions that are incomplete, wrong, too broad, or too specific.
- When time is short, set a time limit and debrief only one or two of the most important CRM issues.

If this was an actual debriefing, we would ask you to expand further on each of these statements. Depending on your response, we would ask open-ended follow-up questions until we were sure you understood the material and had a plan to implement one or more best practices. We might ask, "What is a specific debriefing problem that you experience on your job?" We would not be satisfied if you said, "Our debriefings don't cover CRM as well as we need." Again, we would ask open-ended follow-up questions until you might say, "We have a problem with team members only covering the 'what we did wrong' and not the why or how." We would then ask, "What can you do to fix that problem for the end of your next shift?" We would then continue to ask open-ended follow-up questions until you might

[150] See Chapters 11-15 for information on STAR.

say, "In the briefing, I need to remind the team that we just do not want to fix problems, but also to reinforce the good things we do. During the shift, I need to document at least one instance of the team doing the right thing. In the debriefing, I need to ask open-ended questions to get the team to discuss the thought processes and context for both good and bad behaviors." We would then ask, "How will you help other teams do better?" More open-ended questions until you say, "I need to work with management to change our debriefing guide to discuss the thought processes and context behind good and bad behaviors."

References

Halamek, Louis P., Robert A.H. Cady, and Michael R. Sterling. "Using Briefing, Simulation and Debriefing to Improve Human and System Performance." Seminars in Perinatology 43, no. 8 (2019): 151178. https://doi.org/10.1053/j.semperi.2019.08.007.

Henricksen, Jared W., Catherine Altenburg, and Ron W. Reeder. "Operationalizing Healthcare Simulation Psychological Safety." Simulation in Healthcare: The Journal of the Society for Simulation in Healthcare 12, no. 5 (2017): 289–97. https://doi.org/10.1097/sih.0000000000000253.

Sawyer, Taylor Lee, and Shad Deering. "Adaptation of the US Army's after-Action Review for Simulation Debriefing in Healthcare." Simulation in Healthcare: The Journal of the Society for Simulation in Healthcare 8, no. 6 (2013): 388–97. https://doi.org/10.1097/sih.0b013e31829ac85c.

Sawyer, T, D Loren, and L P Halamek. "Post-Event Debriefings during Neonatal Care: Why Are We Not Doing Them, and How Can We Start?" Journal of Perinatology 36, no. 6 (2016): 415–19. https://doi.org/10.1038/jp.2016.42.

Tompkins, Mimi. "Facilitating a Critical Incident Stress Debriefing." Essay. In Facilitation and Debriefing in Aviation Training and Operations, edited by R. Key Dismukes, 93–104. Burlington, VT: Ashgate, 2000.

CHAPTER 19

CARING FOR YOURSELF

Chapter Briefing[151]

I want to call a quick STAR (Stop-Think-Act-Review): get off your email, stop your side conversations, and turn off the television.[152]. Here is what we will do in the next chapter. We will discuss how caring for yourself, or self-care, enables CRM. We will be successful if you can explain:

- how self-care enables CRM (Section 19.1);
- the four parts of self-care to monitor (Section 19.2); and
- how an individual manages self-care to support CRM (Section 19.3).

The primary threat that you might experience is the introduction of a large number of concepts and terms, some of which you may have never encountered, and some of which you may think about in a different sense. We will therefore explicitly define and differentiate each term and concept. We also realize how busy you are. We will make sure that the chapter is short enough to be read in approximately thirty minutes. Finally, we provide Summary Boxes. The Summary Boxes serve two functions. First, they emphasize the take-home points in each section, and you can use them to check your understanding of those take-home points. Second, you can use them to determine if you and your team are implementing those take-home points. If a Summary Box does not make sense to you or you do not

---

[151] By now, you may feel that the repeated use of the chapter briefing format is redundant. However, we believe that it is important to continue to emphasize that a good briefing builds mental models by discussing what is happening, what success looks like, and what threats or errors are possible and how you plan to prevent, avoid, or mitigate them. Hence, the repetitive nature is meant to cement this belief with an understanding that you will also immerse yourself in this book on an irregular or intermittent basis.

[152] For more information on STAR, see Chapters 11-15.

understand one or more take-home points, then review the related material before continuing to the next section.

Did I miss anything? Any concerns? Any questions? (Pause) No? Then, let's get started.

List of Abbreviations

CRM	Crew Resource Management
DOC	Physician
NUR	Nurse
OB	Obstetric

Many of you work in healthcare because you value compassion and helping others. However, along the way, you may lose sight of why it is important to show yourself compassion and what denying yourself compassion costs your team and your patients. Demanding, stressful, and seemingly meaningless tasks, as well as the morally distressing experiences inherent to healthcare, can chip away at your personal satisfaction with your work and can drag you into compassion fatigue. Your satisfaction with your ability to help people protects you from stress, depression, and burnout (Neff, Knox, Long, and Gregory 2020). Your compassion is a resource you rely on, and self-care is all about refueling that resource by treating yourself with compassion first. Just as before every commercial flight, flight attendants remind you to put on your oxygen mask before assisting others in the event the cabin depressurizes, in healthcare, you must see to your own basic functional needs before you can safely and effectively support your team members and help your patients. In this chapter you will learn how self-care enables CRM (Section 19.1), the four parts of self-care to monitor (Section 19.2) and how individuals manage self-care to support CRM (Section 19.3).

19.1 How Self-Care Enables CRM

Caring for yourself is not a luxury, and it is not selfish. There are many definitions of self-care in popular literature. To keep it simple, practical, and operational, we will focus on the definition used to train astronauts and special forces. Self-care is your own efforts to keep yourself self-satisfied and productive under demanding circumstances. In a teamwork setting, this includes managing your own stress and interactions with others when in difficult conditions. This also includes finding ways to put stressful or frustrating events into perspective and preventing them from interfering with performance. Self-care is a skill based on knowing yourself accurately, and it can be learned and strengthened with practice.

In a teamwork context, positive and negative thinking tends to be contagious. Therefore, controlling your thoughts is fundamental to self-care. You have the opportunity and power to generate positive thinking and reduce negative thinking in your team members as well as yourself. You have likely read some version of this sentiment on a motivational poster or meme before now. However, the posters often leave out how to "flick the switch" from negative to positive thinking. There are two steps to "flick the switch": 1) develop realistic expectations and goals for yourself, and 2) identify ways for yourself to monitor and manage your stress. Since you are constantly thinking and thus cycling between positive and negative thoughts, you are continuously in charge of your "switch" and will keep rotating through these two steps to adjust your expectations and manage your stress. Good self-care is based on continuous self-reflection (i.e., your willingness to think about your own nature, purpose, context, and roles within your teams). Granted, not all of us like self-reflection, and doing too much unfocused self-reflection can actually be bad for your health and performance. The key to doing better self-care is to do a very focused self-reflection. You focus your self-reflection on the four parts of self-care that frequently impact CRM and, therefore, teamwork.

19.2 The Four Parts of Self-Care

Of the four parts, the most popularly discussed is 1) managing stress. Equally important, though seldom mentioned, are 2) metacognition, or, thinking about how you think, 3) fundamental physical care of yourself, and 4) maintaining resilience. All these parts directly impact your ability to practice CRM. If you do not get enough sleep, you are a lot less likely to engage in any metacognition, and you will fail to notice that you are not exchanging information you have that is important to the whole team. If you are still processing a stressful argument with a colleague or patient's family, you might fail to perceive an important aspect of the situation and, consequently, build poor situation awareness. Those are obvious examples that many of you have experienced. Unfortunately, many of you have also never received any formal training on how to do self-care, and your CRM practice suffers until you gain enough trial-and-error experience and mentorship to figure it out. Table 19.1 lists each of the four parts of self-care with a practical definition and some practical actions to support each one (Barnett, Baker, Elman, and Schoener 2007; Cook-Cottone 2015; Borges 2019; Skovholt, Grier, and Hanson 2001; Nagoski and Nagoski 2020). Some of these may prove familiar, some you may already do (or at least know you should do), but even if all of them are familiar, your ability to help your team will still benefit from regularly reviewing the basics of self-care (especially if you are willing to do a self-audit of your self-care on a regular basis).

Table 19-1
The Four Parts of Self-Care

Self-Care Part	Definition	Practical Actions to Support It
Managing Stress	Dealing with the emotional and physiological responses to exposures to stressors.	• Acknowledge and accept all your emotions as valid. Just acknowledging and naming them helps process them. • Finish dealing with the stress (rather than just the stressor) by doing something to physically increase your heart rate and release physiological tension too. • Prioritize what things you can say “no” to when your plate gets too full. • Meditate or practice moments of mindfulness (i.e., just seeing, hearing, smelling, tasting, feeling what is right here right now without making judgments about it). The OB NUR #2 did this by practicing yoga. • Take advantage of the positive feeling of “flow” by doing something you are good at, or interested in, for a few minutes when you need a break. Or do something that truly gives you joy. • Make a “done” list instead of or in addition to a “to-do” list. • Rehearse stressful events and tasks by visualizing them ahead of time and planning how you want to respond to the most likely difficulty. Then, rehearse or role play them with a trusted colleague, if possible. • When you do experience a trauma, talk or write about it to process it as soon as possible (stressors that you let simmer too long grow out of control). • Seek social support early and often and call for professional help before emotional pain becomes unmanageable. (Both the CODE physician and the OB NUR #2 sought support at the end of the AFE scenario.)

Metacognition	Thinking about how you think. In terms of self-care especially, thinking about how you think about yourself and understanding your own behaviors, reactions, and motivations (e.g., mental self-care).	• Identify your personal preferences (these change over time and exposures) and take stock of how they are shaping your behavior. (The CODE physician did this during discussion with a mentor, and the OB NUR #2 did this at home after her shift ended.) Are there ways you can improve your satisfaction with your actions and reactions? For example, would you be more confident that you could handle a conflict well if you waited a ten-count before refuting each proposed solution? • Ask those you trust how they perceive your behavior when you are not sure what others think about your preferred reactions and responses. (The CODE physician sought his mentor's perception during their discussion.) Often it is easier to see how you can be more effective through others' eyes. Just be careful to ask them to describe how they see or interpret your behaviors first (and not how to fix them). • Think about what knowledge, skills, and abilities you have, and how those relate to the demands you are facing right now. Think about how to recruit help to close any gaps. • Think about your individual performance and define what you should keep doing to increase your odds of success, and what you should stop doing to reduce your odds of error. • Pay attention to how you talk to yourself in times of stress and seek to reframe overly negative self-talk into productive (and more realistic) self-talk. • Identify moments where you should have called halt because you were too hungry, angry, lonely, or tired (HALT) to be rationale and plan how to call HALT next time. (The OB NUR #2 called HALT when she napped and ate dinner.)

Physical Care	Taking care of your basic biological needs: respiration, hydration, sleep, sustenance, shelter, and social support.	• Schedule necessary medical care, including preventative care. • Exercise to a level of fitness that allows you to meet your daily demands. • Practice good sleep hygiene by going to bed and getting up at consistent times, reserving the bed primarily for sleeping, stopping stimulants five hours before bed, not eating or drinking or using electronic screens an hour before bed, and giving yourself eight hours in a comfortable bed (i.e., dark enough, quiet enough, warm/cool enough to fall asleep easily). (The OB NUR #2 practiced physical care with a bath and early bedtime.) • Eat well enough and often enough to keep your blood sugar levels from impairing your performance. • Establish a safe place for yourself and a backup shelter so you are not scrambling to find shelter should anything go wrong with your home before work (e.g., this makes it easier to be more physically resilient through natural disasters and domestic upheavals). • Do something every week to seek and give affection to strengthen the relationships that matter most to you.

Maintaining Resilience	Showing yourself some compassion to keep your limited emotional, mental, and physical well-being fueled.	• Recognize when you are faced with emotionally taxing work. For example, work that involves a lot of one-way caring for someone or caring despite limited resources. • Remember that willpower and attention are limited commodities and allocate accordingly (e.g., in the middle of a divorce, or buying a house, is not really a good time to start a new job also). • Plan moments of enjoyment. Create or schedule time in your day to do something that brings you joy or allows you to engage in creative expression. • Nurture a spiritual or communal connection that restores your faith in life or your purpose in living. • Make a list of all the difficult challenges you have survived (and refer to it when you wonder if you can trust yourself to survive this next one). • Find someone with admirable self-care skills and emulate them.

Not everyone is a planner, but if you are, then creating a self-care plan is immensely helpful. If you are not much of a planner, then you will need at least to make sure you know your answers to three key questions:

1. What will you do for self-care? When in doubt, stick to the basics, and add certain self-care activities to your calendar. Some examples are getting enough sleep, exercising regularly, eating healthfully, spending time with loved ones, and engaging in a relaxation activity.
2. What stressful events are challenging you? Knowing these is often enough to kick your sub-conscious mind into protective gear. By answering this question, you will be attuned to when anxiety is likely to hit and have some idea about how you want to handle it (even if you did not have time to make a detailed plan).
3. Whom can you reach out to if you need more help? Identify people in your life who you trust and can talk to about the good and bad that may happen. Identify who you can call if you are feeling overwhelmed, anxious, or sad. This may include colleagues, loved ones, a coach, teacher, mentor, or mental health professional.

While you may not always need to plan your self-care explicitly, remember that the basis of great self-care is taking the time to do self-reflection, so that you can keep improving your self-awareness.

Summary Box 19.1
Self-Refection Keys to Self-Care for CRM

- Managing stress includes minding your positivity and negativity. What is your self-talk like, mostly positive or mostly negative, right now? What expectations or goals need adjusting to your current reality?
- Metacognition matters. When was the last time you gave yourself space and time to think about your self-care and how to enhance it?
- Physical fitness depends on developing healthy habits. What are your strengths and weaknesses? On whom can you rely, and will you feel safe relying on them when you need help or support (including encouragement)?
- Maintaining resilience is based on planning to show yourself compassion. What one thing can you do to strengthen your self-care? What is your plan to do it?

19.3 Preparing to Do Self-Care Well

With practice, preparing to do self-care takes less and less time. One way to further enhance your skill and speed up your self-reflection is to engage your most trusted colleagues, friends, and family in helping you talk through your actual, observable, self-care behaviors. There are four general things to talk about with others. Alternatively, you can also use these "Talk Abouts" as personal thought exercises (i.e., metacognition prompts) to warm yourself up to think about self-care before, or after, a shift or event.

Table 19-2
Four Talk Abouts

Talk About	Discuss
A past time when your self-care impacted others, either positively or negatively.	What behaviors/impacts did you notice? What did others notice? What did you do? How did it turn out? What would you do again and what would you do differently if faced with similar stress on your team today?
How your typical behavioral patterns and preferences impact your self-care.	What types of things run you down the most (or the most quickly)? What types of things put you in a bad mood most quickly? What types of things make your blood pressure spike? Of these things, which can you control, avoid, or mitigate as they threaten your teamwork today? How do others know you are stressed? How do you react when you are told that you look overworked or fatigued? What kinds of help do you like from your team members when this happens? How do you prefer to recruit that help?

How you react to someone else's failure to do self-care.	Have you been in a situation where someone's failure to do self-care negatively impacted performance? What was that like? What did you do? How do you react when a team member looks overworked or over-tired? What are the warning signs that you notice? What help are you best prepared to offer to protect both your own and the team's performance?
How you could keep enhancing your self-care.	How often are you reflecting on how well you take care of yourself? How positive or negative is your self-talk during adverse events, right now? Are there expectations that you need to adjust to better fit the reality your team faces right now? Are there better ways to monitor and manage your stress right now? How effective is your current self-care? What are your relative strengths and weaknesses when it comes to self-care? What easy actions can you take to strengthen self-care this month? Who or what self-care resources can you likely rely on this month? For which one might you need substitutions or alternatives?

Even the most self-aware person dedicated to perfecting self-care will have bad days. This is not about perfection. This is about creating a trend of getting more skilled about taking better care of yourself, so that you can look forward to working on teams and keep performing through new challenges. The only way to lose is to quit entirely. There are, however, many ways to win at self-care spectacularly. We encourage you to find your own way and obtain personal satisfaction with your efforts to continuously enhance this skill. Most importantly, remember that self-care is not selfish. Just as you cannot help anyone else put on their oxygen mask on the airplane if you do not put yours on first, you also cannot help your team practice CRM unless you practice good self-care first. Self-care is a gift you give to every member of every team you ever work on, because it supports your ability to do good CRM and enables you to save lives.

Chapter Debriefing

I want to call a quick STAR (Stop-Think-Act-Review): get off your email, stop your side conversations, and turn off the television.[153] Let's see if you can answer these questions:

- How are you today? Can you name and acknowledge the emotions you are experiencing?
- What do you want to do to keep yourself satisfied through your current stressors?
- What warning signs can you use to identify when self-care is needed to avoid negatively impacting CRM?
- What warning signs can you use to identify when your self-care is beginning to actually negatively impact CRM?
- How do you prefer to support and be supported by others in your own self-care to protect your ability to do good CRM? How will you recruit help when needed?
- How will you recognize and handle threats to your physical energy and mental well-being that are likely to impact your teamwork?
- What re-energizes you right now, and what is your plan to take advantage of that?
- What new or additional self-care resources can you try out or rely on?

If this was an actual debriefing, we would ask you to expand further on each of these statements. Depending on your response, we would ask open-ended follow-up questions until we were sure you understood the material and had a plan to implement one or more best practices. We might then ask, "How is your self-care?" We would not be satisfied if you said, "My self-care isn't as good as I need." Again, we would ask open-ended follow-up questions until you might say "I dwell on minor errors that I make." We would then ask, "What can you do to fix that problem prior to your next shift?" We would then continue to ask open-ended follow-up questions until you might say, "I should write down my feelings and share my feelings with my mentor." We would then ask, "What can you do to help others with their self-care?" More open-ended questions until you might say, "I need to work with management to better emphasize that self-care is crucial to our ability to care for others."

---

[153] See Chapters 11-15 for information on STAR.

References

Barnett, Jeffrey E., Ellen K. Baker, Nancy S. Elman, and Gary R. Schoener. "In Pursuit of Wellness: The Self-Care Imperative." Professional Psychology: Research and Practice 38, no. 6 (2007): 603–12. https://doi.org/10.1037/0735-7028.38.6.603.

Borges, Anna. The More or Less Definitive Guide to Self-Care. New York: The Experiment, 2019.

Cook-Cottone, Catherine P. Mindfulness and Yoga for Self-Regulation: A Primer for Mental Health Professionals. New York: Springer Publishing Company, 2015.

Nagoski, Emily, and Amelia Nagoski. Burnout: The Secret to Unlocking the Stress Cycle. New York, NY: Ballantine Books, 2020.

Neff, Kristin D., Marissa C. Knox, Phoebe Long, and Krista Gregory. "Caring for Others without Losing Yourself: An Adaptation of the Mindful Self-Compassion Program for Healthcare Communities." Journal of Clinical Psychology 76, no. 9 (2020): 1543–62. https://doi.org/10.1002/jclp.23007.

Skovholt, Thomas M., Tabitha L. Grier, and Matthew R. Hanson. "Career Counseling for Longevity: Self-Care and Burnout Prevention Strategies for Counselor Resilience." Journal of Career Development 27, no. 3 (2001): 167–76. https://doi.org/10.1177/089484530102700303.

PART 3

ORGANIZATION AND CULTURE

Briefing [154]

I want to call a quick STAR (Stop-Think-Act-Review): get off your email, stop your side conversations, and turn off the television.[155] Here is what we will do in the next two chapters. We will discuss how you can influence your organization to implement CRM, and how you can tell how well your organization is implementing CRM. We will be successful if you can describe:

- several methods to influence your organization to implement CRM (Chapter 20); and
- several methods to evaluate how well CRM is embedded into your organization (Chapter 21).

The primary threat that you might experience is the introduction of a large number of concepts and terms, some of which you may have never encountered, and some of which you may think about in a different sense. We will therefore explicitly define and differentiate each term and concept. We also realize how busy you are. We will make sure that the chapter is short enough to be read in approximately thirty minutes. Finally, we provide Summary Boxes. The Summary Boxes serve two functions. First, they emphasize the take-home points in each section, and you can use them to check your understanding of those take-home points. Second, you can use

---

[154] We will use the chapter briefing format throughout the book. You may feel the repeated use is redundant. However, we believe that it is important to continue to emphasize that a good briefing builds mental models by discussing what is happening, what success looks like, and what threats or errors are possible and how you plan to prevent, avoid, or mitigate them. Hence, the repetitive nature is meant to cement this belief with an understanding that you will also immerse yourself in this book on an irregular and/or intermittent basis.

[155] For more information on STAR, see Chapters 11-15.

them to determine if you and your team are implementing those take-home points. If a Summary Box does not make sense to you or you do not understand one or more take-home points, then review the related material before continuing to the next section.

Did I miss anything? Any concerns? Any questions? (Pause) No? Then, let's get started.

CHAPTER 20

INFLUENCING YOUR ORGANIZATION

Chapter Briefing[156]

I want to call a quick STAR (Stop-Think-Act-Review). Get off your email, stop your side conversations and turn off the television. Here is what we will do in this chapter. We will discuss how to influence your organization to support you and your team's practice of CRM. We will be successful if you can describe:

- the sources of power an individual has in spreading the practice of CRM, regardless of authority (Section 20.1);
- what is a grassroots or viral model for changing the CRM culture (Section 20.2); and
- how an individual can influence an organization to support CRM (Section 20.3).

The primary threat that you might experience is the introduction of a large number of concepts and terms, some of which you may have never encountered, and some of which you may think about in a different sense. We will therefore explicitly define and differentiate each term and concept. We also realize how busy you are. We will make sure that the chapter is short enough to be read in approximately thirty minutes. Finally, we provide Summary Boxes. The Summary Boxes serve two functions. First, they emphasize the take-home points in each section, and you can use them to check your understanding of those take-home points. Second, you can use

---

[156] By now, you may feel that repeated use of the chapter briefing format is redundant. However, we believe that it is important to continue to emphasize that a good briefing builds mental models by discussing what is happening, what success looks like, and what threats or errors are possible and how you plan to prevent, avoid, or mitigate them. Hence, the repetitive nature is meant to cement this belief with an understanding that you will also immerse yourself in this book on an irregular and/or intermittent basis.

them to determine if you and your team are implementing those take-home points. If a Summary Box does not make sense to you or you do not understand one or more take-home points, then review the related material before continuing to the next section.

Did I miss anything? Any concerns? Any questions? (Pause) No? Then, let's get started.

List of Abbreviations

CRM	Crew Resource Management
SBAR	Situation-Background-Assessment-Recommendation
STAR	Stop-Think-Act-Review

Until your senior management embraces CRM and implements a top-down plan to embed CRM into your organization's philosophies, policies, processes, and practices, you may be forced to try a bottom-up approach to influence your organization. In this chapter, you will learn what sources of power you have to influence your organization (Section 20.1), the viral model you can use (Section 20.2), and how you can pitch CRM to gain support (Section 20.3).

20.1 Sources of Power

Most healthcare professionals hold multiple roles in multiple organizations simultaneously. You likely work in a complicated system of healthcare with conflicting cultures, policies, directives, and standards of care. This makes a vast, unified implementation of any team skill or practice especially difficult. Thus, you will not be able to rely on authority or position to encourage the implementation of CRM in your organization(s). If you wait for leadership to require it, or even for your colleagues to largely agree and authorize it by committee for the good of all patients, you will likely burn out with frustration before you see anyone else intentionally practice CRM.

Chances are, that to some degree, you will need to apply the grassroots or viral model of CRM implementation and influence others by explicitly practicing good CRM. You may need to actively cultivate enthusiasm for CRM until enough of your colleagues adopt it. Even if you already work for an organization that believes in or requires the implementation of CRM, applying this viral model of spreading CRM will create a culture that self-perpetuates and continuously improves how CRM is applied.

The key to doing so is focusing on your influence rather than your authority. You do not need anyone to give you permission to reduce medical errors and other threats to patient safety and well-being, but it is a lot easier to do so with everyone's buy-in. Influence is based on the sources of power that you have available to you. Let's take a closer look at six well-known sources of power (Feldman 1985), some simple examples of using each source of power to influence the adoption of a CRM tool (e.g., briefings, debriefings, STAR), and the pros and cons associated with each source.

Table 20.1
Sources of Power

Source of Power	Example	Pros	Cons
Authority: power derived from a formal position or title	The Section Chief requires all physicians to do a STAR (Stop-Think-Act-Review) with the whole care team prior to changing any documented treatment plans.	+ Quick to implement. + Not likely to be openly rejected by those without authority.	- Requires having an official position or title. - Keeps all responsibility with the wielder/fails to develop others' responsibility. - Often inspires only passing or fleeting compliance.
Reward: power related to your ability to give (or withhold) rewards	A colleague publicly praises a resident for contributing vital information during a debriefing.	+Quick to implement. +Helps develop the rewarded person and others learn from the story of it. +Influence has longevity.	-Must be implemented immediately, and publicly, to be effective. -Embarrassing to some people and/or in some cultures.
Coercive: power based on punishing or reprimanding non-compliance	A physician reprimands a nurse for a sloppy handover and requires the nurse to recite SBAR (Situation-Background-Assessment-Recommendation) and then repeat the patient handover, using SBAR.	+Highly memorable.	-Must be implemented immediately, and privately, after the behavior to be effective. -Requires a relationship of trust to exist first. -Perceived punishments often cause backlash or resistance. -Can be demoralizing.

Expert/ Credibility: power based your demonstrated knowledge	A doctor who serves on the hospital's quality assurance council summarizes the evidence for implementing self-discovery/self-correction debriefings to the unit.	+Usually very comfortable for all involved in and across many cultures. +Memorable. +Influence has longevity.	-Takes time to build credibility/expertise. -Requires continuous building of expertise to maintain. -Easy to lose if wielded too much or too carelessly.
Referent/ Attractive: power acquired from building interpersonal fondness, trust, or respect	A respected nurse tells the team about a time that summarizing back the physician's directions before implementing them helped prevent a deadly error or saved a patient.	+Highly Memorable. +Quickly and widely spreads.	-Takes time to earn respect. -Requires humility, empathy, and explicit awareness of good practices. -Horrific stories may demoralize or paralyze the team (beware of fear-mongering). -Must be diligent in protecting the privacy of patients and healthcare professionals.
Informational/ Means-Control	The charge nurse restricts the team to discussing only very specific information about each patient, in the exact same order, each time as a Communicating protocol for the unit.	+Helpful for maintaining attention in the face of multiple distractions or conflicting powers.	-Control is easy to misuse/ abuse by refusing to share information. -May make it hard for younger or more junior members of a team to assert a relevant concern.

Authority, Reward, and Coercive powers are the least effective sources of power, as they influence healthcare professionals to meet (or appear to meet) only the explicit minimum standards dictated, rewarded, or punished. Informational/Means-Control power is the most frequently misused. Many people misinterpret Informational Control to mean that they should hoard information in order to maintain or enhance power. Informational Control as a source of power is about sharing information wisely (well-packaged, formatted, concisely, clearly, and timely [as discussed in Chapter 8 on Communicating]) and requiring information to be prioritized in order to produce a manageable cognitive workload. Expert and Referent powers take longer to establish, and require more humility, to maintain responsibly; but they are much more effective at motivating and inspiring others to change their behaviors. The bottom line is that the more sources of power to which you have access, then the more influence you will have because you can tailor the amount of power you apply from each source to fit your team, your situation, and your objectives. You may not have any legitimate authority yourself, but you may find an opportunity to cultivate some by networking with others who do. Any team member may build all the sources of power to at least some degree. A few words of caution, though, in order to honor the Hippocratic Oath and avoid causing harm, you must first honestly, humbly, and persistently practice self-awareness before cultivating power and exerting influence. For example, you may get what you want in the short-term by withholding information to maintain or enhance your Informational/Means-Control power, but ultimately you will destroy some trust and long-term credibility in the process (and potentially extinguish a team's willingness to practice or improve CRM in the process). Using tactics associated with a source of power that is not congruent with good CRM behaviors will eventually destroy your credibility. Power and influence are best wielded to enhance a group or organization's CRM capability and culture. If you facilitate CRM well, the group/team will feel responsible for all the good outcomes and believe that they can continue to improve CRM.

Summary Box 20.1
Harnessing Sources of Power

Do you harness all sources of power to help your team implement CRM?
• What formal leaders, authority figures, or policies/rules can you point to that sponsor, advocate, or support CRM to give you legitimate power? • Who can you discover doing CRM well and how can you praise them to enhance your reward power? • When, with whom, and how can you constructively correct individuals in private to improve CRM behaviors? • What expertise about implementing CRM can you learn, borrow, or contract that your team will recognize as credible? • How can you humbly, compassionately, and positively model CRM with your team so that you possess referent power? • What processes, information, or resources do you already control that allow you to support the team doing CRM well?

20.2 The Viral Model of Influence

With practice, spotting and leveraging your sources of power becomes second nature. Once you are comfortable with influencing CRM at this level, then you may truly benefit from implementing a viral model to accelerate and amplify your individual influence over the broader unit, section, organization, system, etc.

There are three primary phases in implementing a viral model of organizational development: 1) thoroughly infiltrate the host (your organization) with mentions of CRM, 2) share an infectious enthusiasm for CRM, and 3) influence your organization's CRM health (i.e., how individuals in it learn about, implement and improve CRM). That is the simple overview of the viral model. Now, let us break that down into practical steps that any individual can implement in order to influence an organization.

Table 20.2
Viral Model of Spreading CRM: Steps, by Phase

Phase	Steps
Infiltrate: Get the information, understanding, and partners you will need in order to convincingly pitch CRM.	A. Find the pain points or strategic opportunities that will make CRM look attractive to the organization. This is what Kotter (2014) calls, "creating a sense of urgency." Why CRM? Why now? What is in it for each of the stakeholders? This step requires active inquiry, reading, attending meetings just to listen, and asking mentors and colleagues questions about what pain points and opportunities are obvious to them. B. Find and network with the other CRM champions, advocates, and sponsors who are also interested in spreading the practice. These will be your fellow "Knights of the Round Table" or "coalition."
Infect: Model CRM and inspire others to try it to maximize its spread in your organization.	C. Use your coalition to brainstorm, articulate, and polish a pitch about how CRM answers those pain points that you discovered. You may even choose to have multiple pitches, each tailored to lead with the most important benefit for each type of stakeholder. D. Use your pitch(es) to recruit an army of stakeholders interested in thinking about how to systemically and intentionally build CRM skills. You will need a diversity of perspectives to build a CRM model that is tailored to your organization (anything less will fail to gain buy-in). This will become your core working group "of those who advocate CRM here."

Influence: Change conversations, policies, procedures, standards, training, and management's perspective to better support CRM throughout the organization.	E. As a working group, identify and prioritize some quick wins to pursue. What aspects of CRM are easy to highlight on rounds, at a lunch meeting, during a tour, in a simulation, etc.? What policy debates or procedure re-writes might be easily influenced by questions about CRM right now? What training is easy to inject CRM into already? Who is best positioned to go after these wins right now? F. Amplify each win by collecting stories about how and why CRM helped, celebrating/praising publicly all of those who made it possible, and publishing, or publicizing, these wins. Note, that it is far easier for most people to amplify others' wins and have them amplify yours in return, than it is to convincingly brag about your own achievements in spreading CRM. G. Keep looking for opportunities to go after bigger, bolder wins. As you influence colleagues to achieve minor wins in implementing some aspect of CRM, more will become interested and find ways to extend those wins to major policies and initiatives across more areas of the organization. You may even have enough interest at this point to recommend that management start a top-down approach to fostering CRM, removing barriers to practicing CRM in your organization. The most important thing to remember is that this is a viral model, and you cannot sustain the organizational practice of CRM without continuously seeking to improve CRM and infecting new generations with a desire to influence how CRM is practiced in your organization.

Obviously, implementing a viral approach takes some time and patience. Psychologically speaking, we all tend to resist considering even good ideas (change is uncomfortable) and practicing new behaviors (even when those behaviors are good for us). The beauty of the viral model is that it can spread when others are exposed to it (via reading about it, hearing a description of it, or seeing it practiced).

The momentum of influence can appear fitful at times, but it is always self-perpetuating once it has taken root. But it is a culture change, and changing a culture takes time. In smaller, more change-eager organizations, you may see obvious evidence of your influence in as little as a year, but more likely it will be two to three years before you see tangible evidence of change. In large, historic, or highly change-resistant organizations, it will likely require at least five years before you see obvious evidence of your influence. One strategy for driving changes is to first practice with a smaller representational group of your organization (such as your own team, unit, or department) before attempting to expand application of the viral model to your whole organization or system.

Summary Box 20.2
Preparing to Influence Your Organization as an Individual

Do you know…
Infiltrate:
- What are the pain points in your organization that CRM will alleviate?
- What strategic opportunities or organizational goals exist that CRM will accelerate?
- Who already knows or cares about CRM issues or practice?

Infect:
- Who are all the CRM stakeholders?
- How will you connect to those who already care about CRM, and get them to explain or show others how it benefits them?
- Who is likely to buy-in and help you talk about how to make CRM a more systematic, intentional, organizational practice?

Influence:
- What quick wins are your stakeholders willing and able to help you achieve in practicing or implementing CRM a little more right now?
- How can you help your stakeholders amplify each CRM win?
- How can you keep looking for bigger wins and ways to improve CRM continuously?

20.3 Pitching CRM

While business and psychology books abound with ways to build and deliver effective pitches, elevator speeches, narratives, visions, etc., your pitches for CRM will work best if you honor a few recommendations that are universal to many evidenced-based methods of influence (Grenny, Patterson, Maxfield, McMillan, and Switzler 2013):

1) Perfect and practice your pitches as a coalition. All members of the coalition must be at least nominally comfortable with the elements of each pitch. Everyone will need a safe space to practice putting it into their own voices, without losing or corrupting the essentials of the message.
2) Build pitches that are short, clear, inclusive, positively phrased, and memorable. Pitches that viscerally engage a pain point or desired goal are memorable. Pitches that tell a story can also be memorable.
3) As newspaper editors used to tell journalists, "Don't bury the lead." Your pitch should start with the most remarkable, sensational element as the headline. The first sentence of your pitch must make folks want to read or learn more, in case that is the only thing that they have time to see or hear in that moment.
4) Persist in both pitching and perfecting your pitches. The relevance of even the best pitches may change over time, and you may have to change the sources of power that your pitch relies on over time to keep influencing others to support CRM.

Here are a few example pitches (that adhere to these principles) from some of our attempts to virally spread CRM in various organizations:

- "Implementing facilitated debriefs reduced the simulations we needed to get everyone to do this consistently before the Joint Commission inspectors arrived."
- "[Our main competitor] cut their medical error rates in half by having team leaders state the Communicating protocol they would use at the start of each shift."
- "Nutrition eliminated $2.7 million worth of waste after teaching their interns how to assert and advocate in their CRM training."
- "The whole unit's job satisfaction ratings increased after one workshop on building situation awareness. One of the charge nurses even told Human Resources that she decided to delay her

retirement a little longer, because she wanted to see how the unit changed after that."

- "Sharing their CRM Behaviorally Anchored Rating Scale reduced the number of conflicts between Intensive Care and Oncology. They agree more often now about how to communicate treatment options to the patient."
- "Fellows thought more highly of us after adding good CRM behaviors to our selection criteria. Even the applicants we did not choose rated our selection process as "Very Fair" and "Highly Professional."
- "Medical errors and employee attrition significantly decreased each month after we integrated CRM into our training."

Summary Box 20.3
Pitching CRM effectively

Are your CRM pitches…
• comfortable for you to share on the fly?
• memorable?
• focus on a hot-button benefit, first and foremost?
• kept relevant?
• rely on the appropriate sources of power to influence doing CRM?

Another key to influencing your organization is the ability to recognize the signs that you are achieving the change that you are championing. For that reason, we will talk more about how you can evaluate the state of CRM in your organization in the next chapter.

Chapter Debriefing

I want to call a quick STAR (Stop-Think-Act-Review): get off your email, stop your side conversations, and turn off the television.[157] Let's see if you can answer these questions:

- How can you use all sources of power to implement CRM?
- How can you use the viral model of Infiltrate, Infect and Influence to spread CRM?
- What is one CRM pitch that you will use to spread your message about the benefits of CRM?

---

[157] See Chapters 11-15 for information on STAR.

If this was an actual debriefing, we would ask you to expand further on each of these statements. Depending on your response, we would ask open-ended follow-up questions until we were sure that you understood the material and had a plan to implement one or more best practices. We might ask, 'What is a specific problem implementing CRM that you experience on your job? 'We would not be satisfied if you said, "We are not embracing CRM is quickly as we need." Again, we would ask open-ended follow-up questions until you might say "Upper and middle management seem very lukewarm to CRM." We would then ask, "What can you do to fix that problem?" We would then continue to ask open-ended follow-up questions until you might say, "We need to develop our CRM pitches to focus on a hot-button benefit first and foremost." We would then ask, "Who will you work with to develop those pitches?"

References

Feldman, Robert S. Social Psychology: Theories, Research, and Applications. New York: McGraw-Hill, 1985.

Grenny, Joseph, Kerry Patterson, David Maxfield, Ron McMillan, and Al Switzler. Influencer: The New Science of Leading Change. New York, NY: McGraw-Hill, 2012.

Kotter, John P. Accelerate: Building Strategic Agility for a Faster Moving World. Boston, MA: Harvard Business Review Press, 2014.

CHAPTER 21

EVALUATING YOUR CRM CULTURE

Chapter Briefing[158]

I want to call a quick STAR (Stop-Think-Act-Review): get off your email, stop your side conversations, and turn off the television. Here is what we will do in the next chapter. We will discuss how to determine if CRM has fully taken root in your organization. We will be successful if you can identify at least one instance in your organization where CRM is or is not evident in your:

- organization's philosophies, policies, and procedures (Section 21.1); and
- team's practices (Section 21.2).

The primary threat that you might experience is the introduction of a large number of concepts and terms, some of which you may have never encountered, and some of which you may think about in a different sense. We will therefore explicitly define and differentiate each term and concept. We also realize how busy you are. We will make sure that the chapter is short enough to be read in approximately thirty minutes. Finally, we provide Summary Boxes. The Summary Boxes serve two functions. First, they emphasize the take-home points in each section, and you can use them to check your understanding of those take-home points. Second, you can use them to determine if you and your team are implementing those take-home points. If a Summary Box does not make sense to you or you do not

[158] By now, you may feel that repeated use of the chapter briefing format is redundant. However, we believe that it is important to continue to emphasize that a good briefing builds mental models by discussing what is happening, what success looks like, and what threats or errors are possible and how you plan to prevent, avoid, or mitigate them. Hence, the repetitive nature is meant to cement this belief with an understanding that you will also immerse yourself in this book on an irregular and/or intermittent basis.

understand one or more take-home points, then review the related material before continuing to the next section.

Did I miss anything? Any concerns? Any questions? (Pause) No? Then, let's get started.

List of Abbreviations

BARS	Behaviorally Anchored Rating Scales
CRM	Crew Resource Management
STAR	Stop-Think-Act-Review

In Chapter 20, you learned how to influence your organization to embed CRM. In this chapter, you will learn how to evaluate your organization's progress to embed CRM. In Section 21.1, you will learn organizational hallmarks, and in Section 21.2, you will learn the hallmarks at the team level.

21.1 Organizational Hallmarks of an Effective CRM Culture

On a very broad level, an effective CRM culture builds CRM into the very fabric of the organization so that even the organization's vision and mission reference achieving safety and quality through teamwork. CRM must be part of the organization, and each department and team within the organization will include CRM metrics in their dashboards for measuring performance. Those metrics are tied to relevant, observable outcomes from exchanging information well (e.g., 99% of the time, the unit communicates the status of every bed to dispatch before noon), communicating successfully (e.g., every nurse on shift follows the protocol for orienting patients to the floor), leading and following responsibly (e.g., one or more clarifying questions is asked during every patient update), and mutually supporting one another (e.g., the unit has gone 320 days without having to unexpectedly work in a short-staffed manner).

Another hallmark of an effective CRM culture is a coordinated effort by the organization and every member in it to spread CRM throughout the local community and all associated professional organizations. In the most basic terms, your organization becomes a massive influencer, because it is known for the safety and quality it has obtained by integrating CRM into its existential blueprint. Such success further enables you and your organization to influence public perceptions and policies about teamwork in healthcare.

In an effective CRM culture, senior management serve as CRM champions, and advocates for working across professional and departmental boundaries to maintain a strong common understanding of CRM, as well as how to practice and improve it continuously. Additionally, all managers and administrators "walk about" to see how teams are implementing CRM. This is a very focused version of "management by walking around", where managers personally visit teams implementing CRM. Effective "walking about" has four main characteristics:

1. The "walk about" is scheduled and planned, so that managers and leaders get to see a broad sample of teams practicing CRM and get to hear about all the challenges that teams practicing CRM encounter in the organization. The purpose of the walk about is to support, not surprise, teams. It is also not about evaluating or grading a team's CRM; rather it is an effort to see how CRM is implemented, and what issues teams are having at the organizational level.
2. Those walking about include key executive leaders such as the Chief Executive Officer, Chief Operating Officer, Chief Medical Officer, and Chief Nursing Officer, as well as directors, managers, supervisors, and team leaders.
3. Those walking about collect specific information about the progress of CRM in practice by asking questions such as:
   - How do you see CRM being practiced on your team?
   - What aspects of CRM need to be fixed?
   - Who should I acknowledge for supporting or doing great CRM?
   - Do you have everything you need to practice CRM?
4. The information collected while walking about is documented because leaders in an effective CRM culture also analyze and act upon that information. The organization maintains a formal feedback program for the information obtained, which also allows everyone to fix what needs to be corrected and publicize success stories.

In an effective CRM culture, there are non-attributable ways for everyone to document challenges and failures so that the organization has a database to build CRM case studies and simulations (this may be separate from or related to the preservation of information collected while walking about). Even more importantly, walking about feeds into an attributable way of recognizing strong CRM behavior, with both formal and informal rewards.

Another hallmark of an effective CRM culture is the incorporation of CRM into all forms of training. In fact, CRM culture is most immediately influenced by training in healthcare (Hefner et al. 2016). CRM training must be provided to all healthcare professionals, and other staff, involved in direct patient care. Not all training is created equal, so we want to mention a few hallmarks of good CRM training:

- Training is customized to your organization's specific CRM behaviors. No one outside the organization provides the behavioral anchors for the CRM model upon which your training is based. Your organization does the work to define it and agree on the behaviors that exemplify each competency in the CRM model that you are using (i.e., the behaviors in your organization that exemplify Exchanging Information, Communicating, Leading and Following, and Mutually Supporting).
- The training is interdisciplinary and continuous. No one in the organization is ever finished with CRM training.
- There are some short CRM dedicated lessons but, more importantly, CRM skills training is embedded in technical training. Instructors train both technical and CRM aspects as an integrated whole. Simulations challenge both technical and CRM skills simultaneously.
- The training is skills-based (i.e., you learn the behaviors that constitute skillful performance), and it is predominantly experiential (i.e., filled with opportunities for practice and immediate feedback).
- The transfer of training is measured in terms of what CRM behaviors teams exhibit in practice at your organization before, during, and after participating in the training.
- Refresher training is provided at regular intervals (determined by the actual rate CRM behaviors start to decay or become neglected at your organization) to ensure the CRM culture that you built continues.
- CRM training is also provided to new team members. Healthcare employee turnover averaged 19% in 2019 (NSI Nursing Solutions 2020). Each one of those new employees requires CRM training to equip them with the same CRM skills, vocabulary, and expectations that the rest of your teams already possess.

The last hallmark of an effective CRM culture is the use of artifacts that encode the organization's CRM norms for practical posterity and training:

- Behaviorally Anchored Rating Scales (BARS) specify examples of observable bad, good, and great CRM behaviors in your organization so that anyone can gauge his or her own performance at any time as well as provide feedback to others upon request in a structured and valid way. All evaluations (formal and informal) include CRM behaviors.
- All technical checklists mention key CRM behaviors.
- Standard operating procedures include CRM behaviors.
- Standard Communication protocols are based on CRM expectations.
- The Policy Manual includes teamwork and CRM behavioral guidelines.
- CRM skills are included in job descriptions, as well as in the guidelines for hiring and promotion.
- Tools (e.g., decision-making tools such as STAR [Stop-Think-Act-Review] or briefing and debriefing guides) include CRM skills.

21.2 Team Hallmarks of an Effective CRM Culture

How can you tell if your organizational CRM hallmarks have filtered down to your team? Two of the most important team hallmarks are your briefings and debriefings include CRM topics. The briefing embeds CRM best practices. It can also help less experienced team members by helping build their situation awareness and mental models by discussing what is happening, what success looks like, what threats or errors are possible and how you plan to prevent, avoid, or mitigate them. A briefing brings together the entry conditions, goals, risks, critical data, critical factors, and so forth, from the Problem Definition phase with the approved course of action that covers how each will be met. The briefing also includes each team member's roles, responsibilities, and tasks; coordination and communication plan; and possible contingencies. Debriefings of CRM occur frequently, involve the entire team, and focus explicitly on CRM behaviors and how to improve those behaviors in the future. Debriefings should occur even when all outcomes were positive. A mistake that many organizations and teams make is debriefing only negative outcomes. Quality, safety, and performance benefit even more from debriefing what worked well, why it went well, and how to make sure it goes well again next time even in a different situation. You can think of this like coaching a sports team: you cannot coach a team to win a championship by coaching only after a loss or by focusing only on what not to do. When CRM debriefings are the norm, you will notice that each team member makes recommendations to improve CRM. Each individual team member considers how individual actions impact the team, and the team considers how their actions impact the patient, the family, the unit, the department, the organization, and the community. Individuals within the team volunteer feedback about what they can do, and say, to help the team anticipate and respond to challenges in the future. Because of debriefings and the foresight they produce, there are fewer surprising events that require immediate reaction. Teams have anticipated those events and have taken action to prepare for them. Teams have discussed how to prepare for challenging situations such as high census/high acuity periods and take care of themselves and each other so that no one's cognitive workload is overwhelmed, and situation awareness is sustained. Finally, debriefings are spontaneous and habitual in an effective CRM culture, as opposed to a less mature CRM culture where they are driven by team leaders and only at formal checkpoints.

A later-stage hallmark of a mature CRM culture is an abundance of high-performing teams exhibiting excellent CRM skills. CRM mastery resulting in higher performance on one team breeds more CRM mastery and higher performance on more teams. We like being on competent teams, and competent teams attract more members. There is a relationship between team cohesion and competent performance such that more of one often leads to more of the other (Matheiu et al. 2015). This kind of team cohesion is not as much social cohesion (e.g., how well team members know each other personally) as it is behavioral cohesion (e.g., how well we understand what being a member of this team means and how to do the most important tasks together). CRM helps teams become more cohesive, and perform better, by making the behavioral requirements of teamwork explicit and easy to understand. Because debriefings and CRM tools (e.g., BARS) make competent teamwork explicit, individuals across the organization start with similar mental models about teamwork, which is an important boost in behavioral cohesion over organizations without a CRM culture.[159] CRM empowers "plug-and-play" ad hoc teams to perform well even when they are composed of members who do not know one another or have much experience working together (a common occurrence in healthcare as members flex across units and shifts).

[159] See Section 2.5 for more information about CRM as a Teamwork Mental Model.

In summary, there are seven hallmarks of an effective CRM culture and associated cues that you can use to gauge and celebrate progress in how your organization is embracing CRM.

Summary Box 21.1
Hallmarks of an Effective CRM Culture

	Hallmark	Your Cues
1	Vision-Mission Clarity	Does your organization's philosophies, policies, and processes support CRM? Do your metrics tie to observable CRM skills, or measure the behaviors that are best practices of those skills? Do you have obvious CRM advocates and champions across professional and departmental boundaries?
2	CRM Spread	Do you influence how other organizations practice CRM? Do you influence public perceptions and policies on teamwork in healthcare?
3	CRM Walk About	Do managers, executives, and other formal leaders walk about asking questions about how CRM is happening every week? Do you document and act on information about how to improve CRM obtained from walking about the organization? Do you recognize and reward good CRM behaviors?
4	CRM Training	Is CRM training continuously done by everyone? Are all four core skills represented in our training? Is CRM training embedded in all technical training?
5	CRM Artifacts	Do you have CRM Behaviorally Anchored Rating Scales (BARS)? Is CRM an explicit part of your Standard Operating Procedures? Is doing CRM the policy? Do your job descriptions include CRM responsibilities and skills? Do you have visible CRM tools or include CRM in visible tools (e.g., decision-making algorithms or briefing guides)?

6	Debriefing, including CRM skills	Do you do debriefings after every major event, including events that ended well, in order to facilitate replication of good CRM? Do individuals, regardless of formal leadership roles, initiate and participate in debriefing?
7	Many High-Performing Teams	Do you have a lot of high-performing teams doing excellent CRM? Are you able to interchange or “plug-and-play” team members and still perform well?

Chapter Debriefing

I want to call a quick STAR (Stop-Think-Act-Review): get off your email, stop your side conversations, and turn off the television.[160] Let’s see if you can answer these questions:

- How does my organization’s philosophies, policies and processes incorporate CRM?
- Does our management walk about observing and asking about CRM?
- How is CRM embedded in our technical training?
- How is CRM documented in artifacts such as Standard Operating Procedures and guides?
- How do our debriefings include good and bad CRM examples?
- Do ad hoc teams show strong CRM behaviors?

If this was an actual debriefing, we would ask you to expand further on each of these statements. Depending on your response, we would ask open-ended follow-up questions until we were sure you understood the material and had a plan to implement one or more best practices. We might ask, “How well is CRM embedded in your organization?” We would not be satisfied if you said, “CRM is not embedded as we need.” Again, we would ask open-ended follow-up questions until you might say, “We have a problem where CRM is still considered an add-on subject, if you have time after discussing technical subjects.” We would then ask, “What can you do to fix that problem?” We would then continue to ask open-ended follow-up questions until you might say, “We need to modify our training, Standard

[160] See Chapters 11-15 for information on STAR.

Operating Procedures and debriefings to specifically address how CRM enables successful completion of technical tasks." We would then ask, "Who will you work with to modify the training, Standard Operating Procedures, and debriefing guide?"

References

Hefner, Jennifer L., Brian Hilligoss, Amy Knupp, Judy Bournique, John Sullivan, Eric Adkins, and Susan D. Moffatt-Bruce. "Cultural Transformation after Implementation of Crew Resource Management: Is It Really Possible?" American Journal of Medical Quality 32, no. 4 (2016): 384–90. https://doi.org/10.1177/1062860616655424.

"2020 NSI National Health Care Retention & RN Staffing Report." NSI Nursing Solutions. Accessed October 30, 2021. https://www.nsinursingsolutions.com/Documents/Library/NSI_National_Health_Care_Retention_Report.pdf.

Mathieu, John E., Michael R. Kukenberger, Lauren D'Innocenzo, and Greg Reilly. "Modeling Reciprocal Team Cohesion–Performance Relationships, as Impacted by Shared Leadership and Members' Competence." Journal of Applied Psychology 100, no. 3 (2015): 713–34. https://doi.org/10.1037/a0038898.

APPENDIX A

USING A BEHAVIORALLY ANCHORED RATING SCALES (BARS) CHART

A Behaviorally Anchored Rating Scales (BARS) is a list of Unacceptable, Acceptable, and Outstanding behaviors for a set of skills.[161] In our example, a BARS is a list of observable behaviors required to perform the Crew Resource Management (CRM) Skills of Exchanging Information, Communicating, Leading and Following, and Mutually Supporting. BARS, as we use it, is not a 'scoring' system. Instead, BARS is simply a tool to document the observed behaviors in one of the three columns. During a shift/task, some Exchanging Information (or other CRM skill) behaviors by the team will be Unacceptable, some Acceptable, and, hopefully, a few will be Outstanding. Determining a 'score' is not relevant to determine what CRM behavior to improve prior to the next shift. During the debriefing, you fix any Unacceptable behaviors, and hope to turn any Acceptable behaviors to Outstanding.

A BARS chart is normally used during training and evaluations (i.e., as performance assessments of your CRM skills). We propose you use it for formative reasons (i.e., as a tool for individuals and the team as a whole to find ways to change and improve CRM behaviors). We want you to use BARS as a…

1. quick reference of CRM behaviors. The goal is to remind you and your team on what CRM is and how to do it.
2. list from which you can pick one to three behaviors that you can discuss in your briefing. The behaviors can be based on either past performance problems, or skills that will be the most required for

[161] Could be Unsatisfactory, Satisfactory, and Outstanding; or Below, Meets, or Exceeds Expectations. The point is that BARS lists examples of behaviors that need improvement, that show proficiency and that show mastery of CRM.

the task or shift. The goal is to improve their CRM mental models at the start of a task or shift.

3. list from which you can pick one to three behaviors that you can discuss in a mini-debriefing prior to starting the next phase of a task or shift (e.g., at the end of the Planning Phase, prior to the start of the Execution Phase). The goal is to fix any CRM problems during a task or shift. This mini-debriefing can be short; one to five minutes should be sufficient.
4. checklist for any behaviors that need to be debriefed at the end of the task or shift. The goal is to fix any CRM problems prior to the next task or shift.

Reasons 3 and 4 require you and your team to take note of instances when the team did Unacceptable, Acceptable, or Excellent behaviors. As you take note of the instances, you will notice that you and your team did some unacceptable behaviors, some acceptable behaviors, and maybe a few excellent behaviors for the same CRM skill. For example, in Communicating, you and your team failed to use the proper format two times, did use the proper format three times, and planned the proper format of a complex phase of the task one time. You should note how your team's behaviors changed over the task or shift. Did your team start off with the Unacceptable behaviors and worked themselves to Acceptable, and even Excellent behaviors? That is exactly what you want: your team is self-correcting their CRM. Or did your team start off with the Acceptable behaviors but during the shift, their CRM behaviors degenerated to Unacceptable? If your team can do good CRM, but stops it mid-task or shift, there may a cultural or leadership issue: they believe that you do not care if they do CRM or, worse, believe that you do not want them to do CRM. If there is no trend toward improvement or degeneration (i.e., they are as likely to do Unacceptable and Acceptable behaviors at the beginning of the shift as at the end), then there may a CRM mental model issue. Your team's grasp of CRM is not sufficient for them to differentiate between Unacceptable and Acceptable behaviors. If that is true, you will need to use the debriefing, and the next task or shift briefing to build up their CRM mental model.

Our notional BARS is meant to be applicable to a general population. To really make it work for you, you may need to replace the broad, generic behaviors with behaviors specific to your culture, team, and task. The specific behaviors should reflect both best practices but also "how we do it around here". A few words of caution as you make those changes:

1. Make sure that you list observable behaviors. You should be able to say, "I saw …" or "I didn't hear …". For example, "I saw you provide back-up to Chris during that procedure." or "I didn't hear you use the right format.". Your team cannot argue with what you saw or heard. They can argue if you state opinions, such as "You were complacent" or "You weren't paying attention.". Even saying "You did a good job" is not helpful. Unless you can mention a specific behavior, they do not know what to fix or what to continue doing.
2. You need to tie the behaviors to "how we do it around here" to have "face validity", so that it makes sense and seems doable to the people in your organization. Unfortunately, in some organizations, there is too much difference between "how we do it around here" and best practices (scientific validity). That may be a culture problem that you must work before trying to implement a CRM program.
3. Be careful not to start "CRM Skills Creep" where, over time, you add a fifth or sixth skill. Although there are CRM models that have six to eight skills that include "Planning", "Decision Making", "Problem Solving", or "Resilience", you will see two problems:
    a. There comes a point where there are just too many skills to remember all of them. Your CRM model is not easy to use or remember.
    b. The bigger problem is your skills may no longer be independent. Independent means one mistake can be easily isolated to a failure to do one CRM skill. For example, if you failed to
        - provide the right information, it is the skill Exchanging Information.
        - speak clearly, it is the skill Communicating.
        - inquire when you did not understand a decision, it is the skill Following.
        - listen to a recommendation, it is the skill Leading.
        - offer or accept assistance, it is skill Mutually Supporting.

For those CRM Models with 6-8 skills, you and your team may have a difficult time deciding to which category to assign an error. Was it Problem Solving or Adaptability or Planning? When you may consider the error Problem Solving, Chris considers it Adaptability, and Pat thinks of it as Planning, it will be more difficult to develop a clear CRM mental model.

Also, because each type of error requires a different remedy, by mischaracterizing an error, you may apply the wrong remedy.

We suggest that you stay with these four CRM skills and just better define observable behaviors specific to your culture, team, and task. Do not add any CRM skills without the assistance of a CRM expert and, then, beware that any CRM expert will advocate their own CRM model.[162] Any major change to a CRM model requires a great deal of time and effort as you will have to re-educate your team on the new model, modify tools and training, and of course, add new skills to your briefing and debriefing.

[162] Yes, we see the hypocrisy in that statement. Ideally if you had the time, expertise, and determination, your organization would do a Team Cognitive Task Analysis to determine the exact CRM behaviors required and group them with labels (e.g., is it Situation Awareness or Exchanging Information?) that make the most sense to your organization.

Table A-1.
A Notional Behavior Anchored Rating Scales (BARS) Sheet
Yours Should Be Based on Your Culture and Tasks.

CRM Skill	Unsatisfactory Behaviors (did not do CRM)	Satisfactory Behaviors (did CRM)	Outstanding Behaviors (planned for CRM)	Example behaviors observed during task/shift
Exchanging Information: Passing the right information to the right person at the right time (and vice versa)	Did not give the right info, based on Status and Environment mental models Did not give the info to the right person, based on Team Mental Model Did not give the info at the right time, based on Progress Mental Model Did not state Exchanging Information expectations	Gave the right info, based on Status and Environment Mental Models Gave the info to the right person, based on Team Mental Model Gave the info at the right time, based on Progress Mental Model Stated Exchanging Information expectations	Briefed unique Exchanging Information requirements Set up synch points to update situation awareness Discussed potential threats and errors to Exchanging Information, and their indications and implications Determined what to pass to next team to build their situation awareness	Did not push Status-Task information @ 1h 30 m Did not state Exchanging Information expectations during briefing Gave a complete STEP update @ 3h 5m Gave margin update when situation changed Did quick tag-up to make sure all information included in handover Did a quick debriefing to assure that their Exchanging Information was correct before starting the next phase.

			Did a real-time review of the Exchanging Information process	
Communicating: exchanging information using the right format and terminology clearly, concisely, etc. and ensuring the information was understood through 3-way communication and active listening.	Used jargon or improper terminology or protocols Used inappropriate communication style or approach based on audience Communicated too little or too much for the listener to understand the situation Failed to provide confirmation to the sender that the message was understood Failed to notice signals that the receiver did not understand	Used proper terminology and protocols Changed communication style, approach, and content based on audience Communicates proper amount and level Provided confirmation (e.g., repeat in own words, etc.) that message was understood Noticed signals that the receiver may not understand; used additional methods to ensure understanding	Developed communication plan, including any modified terminology and protocols Planned out required communication and had it vetted and waiting prior to need	Did not confirm understanding (2 times early) Confirmed understanding (3 times later) Used wrong format Noticed that receiver was having a hard time understanding and modified format and terminology Developed a Communication Plan Practiced difficult communication protocol for a time-critical, safety-critical task

Leading: developing psychological safety, setting CRM expectations, and ensuring every team member had situation awareness and the right mental models.	Found fault/blame, rather than fixes Did not model CRM behaviors Did not set CRM expectations	Monitored performance; provided mentoring Found fixes, rather than assigning blame/fault Explained expected CRM behaviors and standards	Set up psychological safety in briefing Codified CRM behaviors in the plan/procedures	Framed response of an error as "You did..." Leader did not admit to an error Framed response to an error as "Why did you..." Asked open ended questions to understand a recommendation (did not accept it in the end but explained why)
Following: following directions but inquiring when unsure and advocating and asserting if required	Did not ask questions when unsure Did not offer recommendations with rationale	Asked questions when unsure Offered recommendations with rationale	Planned out recommendation and had it vetted	Set up planned STARs Practiced recommendation with a team member to make sure rationale was sufficient

Mutually Supporting: Providing task support by requesting or accepting back-up behaviors; providing social support; and providing feedback	Did not offer backup Did not request backup Did not help team member combat Performance Shaping Factors Did not provide peer feedback in a psychologically safe manner	Offered backup Requested backup Helped team member combat Performance Shaping Factors Provided peer feedback in a psychologically safe manner	Used briefing to set CRM expectations for Mutually Supporting, and build mental models to enable task assistance Planned back-up for error-prone, time-critical, or safety-critical tasks Planned ways to prevent or avoid Performance Shaping Factor Developed format to provide real-time peer feedback	Refused backup support when offered: "I don't need your help" Provided feedback in a derogatory manner: "You screwed up by…" Provided words of encouragement when a team member made an error: "Everyone makes that error at least once." Provided feedback to fix a team member's situation awareness and mental model: "What you haven't seen yet is..." Set up back-up: "Chris, when we get to this portion, you need to help Pat by …"

APPENDIX B

FACILITATED DEBRIEFINGS

What is a Facilitated Debriefing?

Facilitated Debriefings are debriefings of a team's technical and CRM actions and behaviors where the facilitator, ideally the team leader, asks a series of open-ended questions to get the team to determine for themselves what they did right and wrong (i.e., self-discover), as well as why, and how to improve (i.e., self-correct). The team members do the majority of the talking, while the facilitator ensures that the debriefing covers all major areas and issues, interjects with probing questions or comments if required to guide the discussion, and ensures that the debriefing is efficient and effective. (McDonnell, Jobe and Dismukes 1996)

How is a Facilitated Debriefing different than the debriefing concept in Chapter 18, especially since both rely on self-discovery and self-correction? The difference is a team fully trained, knowledgeable about CRM, and familiar and comfortable with self-discovery and self-correction does not need a designated facilitator. Rather, as the debrief continues in such a team, various team members may ask open-ended questions, make sure all areas are covered, and/or ensure the debriefing is efficient and effective. In other words, the role of facilitator flows between team members as required.

Why Do a Facilitated Debriefing?

In organizations and cultures where they do leader-led debriefings, the transition to debriefings discussed in Chapter 18 may be too large a leap to make at once. Instead, a Facilitated Debriefing is a bridge where the facilitator decreases his or her role as the team gets used to doing their own self-discovery and self-correction. Eventually, the facilitator is not needed, and the team can conduct their own debriefings.

Summary Box B.1
What is a Facilitated Debriefing and Why Do It?

What is a Facilitated Debriefing? • The leader acts as a facilitator asking open-ended questions to encourage the team to self-discover and self-correct. Why do a Facilitated Debriefing? • As a bridge between leader-led debriefing to the eventual goal of a team debriefing themselves using self-discovery and self-correction.

Establishing Psychological Safety

The first and most important thing you must do to ensure a quality Facilitated Debriefing is to establish psychological safety. Psychological safety exists when team members believe that they can admit to an error without fear of retribution. Without psychological safety, team members will not be willing to admit their errors. One way to establish psychological safety is for you as a leader to first admit to an error. In the amniotic fluid embolism (AFE) scenario, the CODE DOC admitted to reverting to his/her usual mode under stress, and the OB physician admitted to losing situation awareness. A more difficult problem to solve occurs when team members are reluctant to highlight an error made by a teammate. This reluctance may be due to a fear of retaliation, or of being ostracized. Again, you can help the team overcome that fear by admitting an error that you made and emphasizing that you need their inputs in order to improve. In the AFE scenario, psychological safety was built in several ways:

- the debriefing was covered under Code of Evidence 1157, to eliminate the potential for discovery in a U.S. court of law.
- it was emphasized that the topics of discussion would not be discussed in any other venue except a formal mortality and morbidity conference, therefore those participating in the debriefing would not need to be concerned about others 'talking behind their backs'.
- the CODE DOC stated in a previous shift, "Never let me hurt a patient", indicating that s/he was aware that s/he might make a mistake and therefore needed input from other members of the team.

You can also emphasize that pointing out errors is not about assigning blame, but rather helping the team perform better.[163] This changes "You did this wrong" to "This is something you can do to improve.". Of course, you then have to be supportive when a team member admits to an error.

It is important to note that there is a difference between a technical performance debriefing and a critical incident stress debriefing. Technical performance debriefings serve to dispassionately assess individual, team, and system performance during a real or simulated event. In contrast, critical incident stress debriefings are conducted to provide psychological support after "an event that has the potential for people to experience significant physical, cognitive, emotional and behavioral reactions immediately after the incident or days, weeks, months and even sometimes years later." (Tompkins 2000) Most of what has been published in the healthcare literature about debriefing blurs the border between these two types of debriefings. Many healthcare authors describe reaction, description, analysis, and summary phases of a debriefing. Such a model implies that psychological distress after a real or simulated clinical scenario is a frequent occurrence, and that those being debriefed are not able to effectively participate in that debriefing without first having an opportunity to "ventilate" pent-up emotion. Moreover, within healthcare, Henricksen Altenburg, and Reeder (2017) examined the expression of psychological distress in 3,900 subjects undergoing debriefing after simulated clinical scenarios and found that <1% were perceived to manifest signs of significant distress, indicating that such responses are quite rare. In this book, a Facilitated Debriefing refers to a technical performance debriefing. In the AFE scenario, the OB physician specifically stated that the debriefing would be a technical performance debriefing.

Explaining to Your Team What a Facilitated Debriefing Is

How you actually start a CRM Facilitated Debriefing depends on two factors: how familiar your team is with the concept of Facilitated Debriefings, and how familiar they are with CRM. If your team is unfamiliar with Facilitated Debriefings, you must take steps to introduce them to your new role as a facilitator and their new role as active participants in the debriefing. In introducing your new role as a facilitator, you will have to

[163] According to Hollnagel, errors are not due to personal flaws, but caused by organizational or structural faults. If different people in the same situation make the same error, it is not a human problem; it is a system problem.

address the fact that you will not lead the debriefing, will not tell them what they did wrong, and will not tell them how to fix those problems. This may require a huge change in culture at your institution. Instead, you will help them identify topics, ensure that all issues are addressed, and make sure that the debriefing is efficient and effective. You can say that in a Facilitated Debriefing, you will talk little and solely in the form of open-ended questions. You can also say that as your role has changed, so has theirs. They will do most of the talking. They will need to analyze each situation and how they interacted with each other, evaluate how things turned out, and determine what they would do differently as individuals and a team, both in that specific situation but also in other situations. In the first Facilitated Debriefing, it is possible that you may have to illustrate the process by admitting a specific error that you made (which also helps establish psychological safety), its impact on the team effort, and its specific fix. You can then generalize to the CRM skill that was used and how you would adapt that skill to a different situation. In the AFE scenario, the OB DOC admitted to fixating on doing compressions (specific error) and indicated that asking the OB NUR to do the compressions would have remedied this error (specific fix). The generalized skill is maintaining situation awareness during stress, and the generalized fix is asking for help. In the team environment, there is also the generalized skill of Mutually Supporting and the generalized fix is offering and accepting physical/task support to reduce stress/workload (e.g., the CODE physician realizing that his/her team could support the OB team).

Setting the Right Level of Facilitation

The second factor in how you start a Facilitated Debriefing is how familiar your team is with CRM. Depending on your team's CRM knowledge, you will have to determine the level of facilitation (i.e., how involved you are as a facilitator). For teams that are well versed and practiced in CRM, your involvement may be minimal. Your sole input may be the initial open-ended question "How did we do today?" As long as your team addresses every major issue, and comes up with good solutions, you have little need to talk. The more experienced the team members, the more they can set the agenda, raise issues, and initiate discussions. Even the most experienced team, however, may have a CRM blind spot, which requires you to be more involved (i.e., to provide guidance in that one area). They may miss an important issue, develop a solution that is too limited to a specific situation, or implement a strategy that does not reflect best practices. If so, you are still responsible to ask open-ended questions to guide them to a deeper level of understanding.

What if your team is brand new to CRM? Then you will be the most involved. That does not mean you will revert to a leader-led debriefing where you tell them what they did wrong and how to fix it. Instead, it means that you must ask open-ended questions specific to what you need the team to discuss. As you actively listen to their answers, you must come up with additional open-ended questions to force them to drill down to not only the specific CRM error and its solution, but also the general class of CRM error and adaptive fixes. Instead of saying, "How did we do today?", you may have to say, "Our Leading and Following wasn't as good as we needed in the first few minutes. What did or didn't we do that made our Leading and Following bad? How can we do better next time?" If that does not produce the answer that you wanted, you might have to ask, "Why didn't we predict what was going to happen?" Keep asking questions until they figure out what they did wrong. Then do the same thing until they figure out how to improve. It is possible that even the most inexperienced team may have some expertise in CRM that requires you to be less involved. For example, you may have to ask multiple follow-up questions to get them to fully address their Exchanging Information issues, but if they did a good job of addressing their Communicating issues, your contribution may be only to mention a best practice that they did not know.

More than likely, your team's experience with CRM is between generally highly experienced and quite inexperienced. In this case, you may pick a general topic area and ask an open-ended question to get them started, actively listen to their answers to determine the exact level of facilitation required, and ask follow-up questions to ensure that they express a level of detail sufficient to derive the correct solution. Teams with an intermediate level of experience require the greatest flexibility by the facilitator who must constantly change the level of facilitation based on the team's expertise in that specific topic.

Over time, as your team becomes more familiar with dealing with CRM skills, you will ask fewer questions, and they will start talking among themselves and identifying their own errors (self-discovery) and their own fixes (self-correction). Hopefully, they will get so accustomed to debriefing their CRM skills, they won't even realize that they are doing it. In the AFE scenario, the teams did not require a facilitator because they were all comfortable talking about what went right and wrong. Even so, the nurse had to act as a de facto facilitator to move the team members from talking about individual errors and fixes, to the more general team problem of ambiguous leadership roles.

Summary Box B.2
How to Start a Facilitated Debriefing

Do you…
• establish psychological safety?
• brief your team on the Facilitated Debriefing concept, their role as participants and your new role as a facilitator?
• change the facilitation level and the number and specificity of open-ended questions based on their CRM experience and answers?

What You Want Your Team to Discuss During a Facilitated Debriefing

In a Facilitated Debriefing, you want to guide your team to discuss the following:

- Team interactions: The goal of a team debriefing is to improve the team members' mental model of interactions: how best to exchange information, communicate, lead and follow, and mutually support. To best cover interactions, you need to help team members address each other directly, and discuss how they were affected by the actions of others.
- What they were thinking: Another goal of a debriefing is to improve mental models, therefore, the team needs to analyze the rationale underlying the decisions that they made. They then need to talk about how their mental models allowed a bad decision to be made and how they would need to change their mental models to eliminate that deficit. In the scenario debriefing, each physician should discuss why each thought he or she needed to take charge.
- Context: Context determines how a CRM skill will be applied. They need to discuss what enabled or impeded their success, including the why and how, i.e., how the critical factors affected the outcome.[164] Since contexts change, they need to discuss how they might handle things differently in a different situation. The context for the scenario was three physicians dealing with a code

[164] See Chapter 12 for more information on critical factors.

during a delivery. A slightly different case they might want to discuss is what if the anesthesiologist was late in arriving: how would the OB and CODE physicians have managed that? Or what if the cause was sepsis (versus embolism), how would that have changed Leading and Following? The point is to not find a solution that is restricted to only one context. Try to identify how you will find the right solution depending on the context.

- An action plan to improve performance: It is not enough for the OB physician to say, "I need to improve my situation awareness." Instead, the OB physician should say, "I need to realize that as the compressions take up more and more of my attention, I become fixated. I need to take a second to 'step back', even just mentally, to consider the whole situation. I could also include in my shift briefing that I need the Obstetric nurses to tell me when they think I might be losing situation awareness." You may need to ask a series of open-ended questions to get them to that point. Finally, when debriefing formal teams, you may be responsible for tracking those action plans to make sure that your team members accomplish them.[165] If a team member has committed to changing his or her briefing to include more Mutually Supporting behaviors, track his or her performance. If he or she is getting better, then congratulations are due; if not, then, provide more mentoring. Also, if during your debriefing, a CRM error was caused by a poorly written procedure or inadequate training, you are responsible for not only working with your organization to change the procedure or training but checking that the changes actually prevented the error.

Summary Box B.3
What You Want Your Team to Discuss in a Facilitated Debriefing

Does your team discuss… • their interactions? • what they were thinking? • context? • action plans?

[165] With ad hoc teams, you will not be able to track team member performance. Instead, you will need to remember that an error made by this team member may be made by the next team. You need to track common threats and errors.

Facilitation Errors

Unfortunately, it is not that easy to conduct a Facilitated Debriefing. Here are some common errors that facilitators make and how to avoid or mitigate them.

- Not establishing psychological safety. In the AFE scenario, the leader tried to establish psychological safety in several ways by stating:
    - the debriefing was covered under Code of Evidence 1157 to eliminate the potential for discovery in a U.S. court of law.
    - it was emphasized that the topics of discussion would not be discussed in any other venue except a formal mortality and morbidity conference; thus, those participating in the debriefing would not need to be concerned about others 'talking behind their backs'.
    - the CODE physician stated in a previous shift, "Never let me hurt a patient", indicating that he or she was aware that he or she might make a mistake, and therefore needed input from other members of the team.

With insufficient psychological safety, you will see one of two problems. The first problem is some healthcare professionals find it easier to point out team weaknesses, as this often diffuses responsibility from one or a small number of individuals to the more nebulous 'team'. When that happens, no one person needs to accept responsibility for failure, nor are individuals called out by name (i.e., instead the 'royal we' is used). Psychological safety is required for an individual to admit an error, and then for the team to discuss if there was a team interaction problem that caused it[166]. Why did he or she not get the right information? Was it an error in Exchanging Information? Did no one know to pass that information to that person at that time? The second problem is the exact opposite: a team member is fearful of reprisals for pointing out the error of another, especially the error of a superior. So, each individual only discusses his or her personal errors. In the AFE scenario, each team member was initially discussing individual errors ("I did…") and individual fixes ("I need to…"). It wasn't until a nurse highlighted this that they started talking about the team interaction problem of Leading and Following. Fearing to point out the errors of others is

---

[166] In a debriefing, we are not addressing individual technical errors (e.g., someone not knowing how to intubate). Fixing individual technical problems is the sole responsibility of the healthcare professional.

mitigated by the superior stating in the briefing, and reinforcing in the debriefing, that he or she needs their input to improve his or her CRM. In the scenario, the CODE physician admitted to reverting to his/her usual mode under stress, and the OB DOC admitted to losing situation awareness. Regardless, the goal of the debriefing is not to assign blame, but to find ways as a team to improve CRM skills to prevent that error again.

- A natural tendency is to discuss only errors committed by the team. It is equally important to discuss what the team did right, so that they understand what they did right, why it was right, how it was right, and how to improve or adapt the next time (Halamek, Cady, and Sterling 2019). In our scenario, the OB DOC wanted to make sure that they knew why the nurses knew to be assertive.
- Good teams understand the difference between skill and luck. Just because a positive result occurred does not mean that the team performed at a high level. To think the outcome was based on skill may be a fallacy and sets the team up for errors in the future. Do not debrief based on the outcome, but rather on the quality of the team's use of CRM skills.
- Avoid unwittingly hindering team member participation by providing your analysis or evaluation before the team members complete theirs. That turns the debriefing into a leader-led debriefing, rather than facilitated debriefing and defeats the concept of self-discovery and self-correction. If you answer their questions, they don't have to think. Don't answer for them when they don't immediately respond to your question. Use silence, or pauses, to elicit their response (Halamek, Cady, and Sterling 2019). Realize that silence is as uncomfortable for the team members as it is for you; eventually someone will speak up. You may have to wait 10 to 15 seconds to allow team members to process your question and formulate a response.
- Accepting a poor or incomplete analysis. It could be too broad or general an analysis. "Our CRM was bad…" is not an analysis. Since different CRM problems have different remedies, you must guide them to delve deeper. "Our CRM was bad because our communicating was bad, because we didn't use the right format." provides insight into what to fix.
- Accepting a specific, incomplete, or wrong solution. While stating a specific fix to a specific error is required, it will not help your team when they are in a somewhat different situation. Your follow-up questions must address the generic error and the discussion

should produce a generic solution. It is not sufficient to say "Next time, let us use Format X…" because in another situation Format X may not be correct. The generic error is using wrong formats, and the generic solution is how to determine what is the right format. Even in our scenario, the teams could have come up with more generic errors and solutions. An inexperienced team may also come up with an incomplete solution. If so, you could engage them in a discussion about a best practice that could be used in such a situation. When teams provide a wrong answer, and your open-ended questions aren't helping them self-discover and self-correct, as a last resort, you may need to temporarily abort attempts at further facilitation and simply tell them what error was made and how to avoid or correct it.

- Hindsight Bias.[167] Hindsight Bias will lead to simple, linear, and context-specific fixes, assuming it was obvious how a missed threat led to poor Exchanging Information, which led to Communicating errors, which led to poor decisions, which eventually allowed an accident to occur. But in real time, all the team had were vague indications that something was not right. You need the team to address holes in the team's mental models that permitted the missed threat, poor Exchanging Information, a Communicating error, and poor decision-making. Concentrate the debriefing on that: what, why and how did CRM behaviors let the threat materialize, and how to fix it specifically and generically.
- Let the debriefing wander off topic or drag on. One reason a facilitated debriefing will wander is the facilitator is not involved enough (i.e., too hands off) for the knowledge and experience level of the team members. If the team members are struggling to find the right answers or are "spinning their wheels" covering the same material, then the facilitator should be more involved and ask more detailed, specific questions. In the scenario, the Obstetric physician said to cover only the two or three most important issues, and later mentioned when they reached the 10-minute point. The debriefing doesn't have to be long. If time is short, just cover the one or two biggest CRM issues. If you debrief all the time, you can catch other problems in another debriefing.

[167] A cognitive problem whereby looking into the past, permits the thought that it should have been obvious to determine the chain of events.

Summary Box B.4
Facilitated Debriefing Errors and Remedies

Do you…
• discuss only what went wrong? Also discuss what went right to reinforce the practices that allowed the team to do the right thing. • answer for them when they do not immediately come up with an answer? Use silence up to 10-15 seconds to prompt discussion. • accept incomplete, wrong, too specific or broad analysis or solutions? Your team must fix the immediate problem but also have the tools to do the right thing when the situation is slightly different. • let the debriefing wander or drag out? Change the level of facilitator involvement based on the team's familiarity with Facilitated Debriefings and CRM.

An Example of a Facilitated Debriefing

Let's start with an example of a bad Facilitated Debriefing. This is what we call the "50,000 foot answer", an answer so high level as to have no value. Although the following is a blatantly exaggerated example, you will see subtler variations of this in teams and leaders with low experience in Facilitated Debriefings and CRM. For this example, we will use a modified version of the Elaine Bromiley case study (McClelland, Smith 2016) with the change that good CRM prevented her death.

NOTE: F = Facilitator, DOC = Physician, NUR = Nurse

F: "What did we do wrong?"
DOC: "We lost track of time."
F: "What do we need to improve?"
DOC: "We need to keep better track of time."
F: "Right. Next topic."

Instead of that answer, debriefings should go from specific action, impact, and desired behavior (a-i-d) to generic desired action, and adaptive behavior (A-I-D):

F: "What did we do wrong?"
DOC: "We lost track of time."
F: "What circumstances led to that?"
DOC: "We were having trouble with the intubation (specific action). That caused us to fixate on that and we lost

track of the length of time that the patient's oxygen saturations were low (specific impact)."

F: "What happened that got us over the fixation?"

DOC: "The nurse reminded us, very forcefully, that we were taking too long. (Looks at nurse) Thank you. (specific desired behavior)"

F: "What generic CRM skill are you referring to?"

DOC: "Keeping my Total Situation Awareness. I need to keep track of more than just what task I am working on."

F: "Nurse, how did you know that it is okay to be so forceful?"

NUR: "In the shift briefing the physician stated that I was responsible for keeping track of time and preventing anyone from fixating. (Generic action) I guess that is part of Mutually Supporting."

Facilitation Best Practices

Here are best practices on how to conduct a Facilitated Debriefing:

- In the briefing, tell them that they will be debriefing using a facilitated debriefing and they will be expected to participate. This informs them that they will need to look for and note possible errors. This has an additional benefit of causing them to be better at STAR's Review phase, because they will be more attuned to look for a difference between expected and actual results.
- Ask open-ended ('what', 'how' and 'why') questions to encourage team member participation, deeper discussion, and discovery of their own answers. If a question can be answered by 'yes', 'no' or a single word, it is not an open-ended question. By definition, an answer to an open-ended question will take time to develop, and the answer will be in the form of a sentence or two.
- Actively listen to their answers to determine follow-up questions to force them to think deeper about the cause of the error and how best to fix it. It may take two or more follow-up questions to get to that level.
- Rather than answer a question from a team member, redirect questions and comments back to the team. For example, if a team member asks, "What should I have done?", you should respond with "What do you think you should have done?" or "What does the rest of the team recommend that she do?" The second question

has the effect of engaging the entire team in the Facilitated Debriefing and increasing the pool of possible solutions.

- Because engaging all team members in the discussion often results in the most robust discussion of problems and solutions, you may have to find a way to encourage quiet team members to actively participate. You can direct questions to them, but that may be interpreted as "putting them on the spot" and elicit fear that their responses could be wrong or even worse, unintelligent. This may actually cause them to become even less communicative. Another strategy to engage quiet team members is to ask them to comment on the response provided by another team member. That allows the quiet team member to a) simply agree or disagree with the response, b) explain their rationale for doing so and c) add to that team member's response if they so choose.

Summary Box B.5
Facilitated Debriefing Best Practice

Do you…
• tell them you will be doing a Facilitated Debriefing and their role to find problems and solutions?
• ask open ended questions?
• actively listen to determine follow-up questions?
• redirect questions, rather than answer them?

Appendix B. Debriefing

Again, your attention. Can you elaborate on the following statements?

- Ask open-ended questions to force your team to self-discover and self-correct.
- Psychological safety is required to conduct a Facilitated Debriefing.
- Change your level of facilitation (involvement) based on your team's knowledge of Facilitated Debriefing and CRM.
- A Facilitated Debriefing should discuss team interactions, thought processes, context, and action plans.
- Actively listen to team member responses to determine follow-up questions.
- Redirect questions rather than answer them.
- Engage the entire team in discussion.
- Don't hinder team member participation.

- Discuss both errors and effective actions.
- Don't accept analyses or solutions that are incomplete, wrong, too broad, or too specific.
- Don't let the debriefing wander off topic or become unnecessarily prolonged.

If you are having trouble expanding upon these statements, go back to the respective section and re-read the material.

References

Halamek, Louis P., Robert A.H. Cady, and Michael R. Sterling. "Using Briefing, Simulation and Debriefing to Improve Human and System Performance." Seminars in Perinatology 43, no. 8 (2019): 151178. https://doi.org/10.1053/j.semperi.2019.08.007.

Henricksen, Jared W., Catherine Altenburg, and Ron W. Reeder. "Operationalizing Healthcare Simulation Psychological Safety." Simulation in Healthcare: The Journal of the Society for Simulation in Healthcare 12, no. 5 (2017): 289–97. https://doi.org/10.1097/sih.0000000000000253.

McClelland, G, and MB Smith. "Just a Routine Operation: A Critical Discussion." Journal of Perioperative Practice 26, no. 5 (2016): 114–17. https://doi.org/10.1177/175045891602600504.

"Facilitating LOS Debriefings: A Training Manual." Accessed October 30, 2021. https://humansystems.arc.nasa.gov/flightcognition/Publications/Final_Training_TM.pdf.

Tompkins, Mimi. "Facilitating a Critical Incident Stress Debriefing." Essay. In Facilitation and Debriefing in Aviation Training and Operations, edited by R. Key Dismukes, 93–104. Burlington, VT: Ashgate, 2000.

APPENDIX C

INDEX CARDS OF A LEADER SETTING THE TEAM CLIMATE FOR CRM

"BREVITY IS THE BROTHER OF BRILLIANCE."
ANTON CHEKHOV

Be On Time.
Be Courteous.
Be Succinct.
Be Problem Oriented.
Create a Shared Mental Model.
Develop a Plan for the Day.
Don't Let Me Screw Up.
Lou Halamek, MD

Creating a shared mental model of the NICU patient during rounds

What are the patient's problems (prioritized)?
What are we going to do about these problems?
Diagnostic studies that need to be ordered?
Therapeutic interventions that need to be ordered?
What pending labs, x-rays, etc., do we need to follow up on?
Whom do we need to call?
Colleagues?
Family?
And who will be responsible for calling them?

Glossary of Crew Resource Management (CRM) Terms and Concepts

NOTE:
This glossary contains terms and concepts that we believe are crucial to your understanding of CRM. If a term is in this glossary, you must understand its significance. If you understand every term in the glossary, you have made the first step in understanding CRM concepts. Conversely if a term is not in the glossary, it is not crucial to your understanding of CRM.

3-Way Communication

Definition: a method to confirm understanding that proceeds as follows: the sender says a message, the receiver repeats what he or she understood using his or her own words, and the sender then agrees or disagrees with the receiver's statement. This process confirms that the receiver actually understood the sender's message.

In some professions and industries this method is called 2-Way Communication, Closed Loop Communication, or Readback.

Common Error: reading back the message verbatim or saying "copy"; this only lets the sender know the receiver heard the message but not if the receiver understood the message.

See Section 8.4.

ACTION - IMPACT - DESIRED BEHAVIOR (a-i-d OR A-I-D)

Definition: a method of debriefing where you state the action you observed, its impact on team performance, and the behavior you believe to be correct.
"a-i-d" refers to the specific action, impact, and desired behavior. Example: "You said X. I thought you meant Y. Next time, say Z.".

"A-I-D" refers to the generalized action, impact, and desired behavior. Example: "You used a term that my organization uses differently. That caused me to do the wrong step. Next time you should use the lexicon so that we are all using the same terms with the same definitions."

Selecting observable actions and behaviors takes the debrief out of the realm of opinions (e.g., "I thought you were complacent." "Am not!" "Are too!")

Common Error: debriefings that focus solely on the specific error and fix (a-i-d) and do not address the more general problem (A-I-D).

See Section 9.2.5.

ACTIVE LISTENING

Definition: a method to deepen understanding that involves attempting to discover what is going on in the sender's head and understand how what he or she said makes sense to him or her.

Active Listening requires processing and keeping an open mind to the outsider's perspective.

Active Listening lets you compare and check situation awareness and mental models. When you are actively listening, you are considering the possibility that your team member might have seen or heard something that you did not (different situation awareness), or that your team member's knowledge or previous experience provides a different comprehension or projection (different mental model).

Common Error: failing to carefully observe body language, and listen for changes in tone of voice, as well as questions and caveats that indicate whether or not your team member understands what you are saying.

See Section 8.4.

BEHAVIORALLY ANCHORED RATING SCALES (BARS)

Definition: a list of organizational/cultural/team agreed-upon Unacceptable, Acceptable, and Excellent behaviors for a set of CRM skills.

We propose that you use BARS as a quick reference for CRM behaviors. The goal is to remind you and your team what good CRM behaviors are, and how to do them. We suggest using BARS to pick:

1) 1-3 items that you need to discuss in your briefing; 2) 1-3 items that you

need to discuss in a mini-debriefing prior to starting the next phase of a task or shift; and 3) any skills that need to be debriefed at the end of the task or shift.

Common Error: failing to use BARS with the result that team members disagree as to whether they are doing good CRM.

See Appendix A.

BEST PRACTICES

Definition: research- and/or evidence-based behaviors that have been demonstrated to be the most effective implementation of a skill. Best practices for each CRM skill are covered in each specific CRM Skills chapter.

BRIEFING

Definition: a discussion, usually led by the team leader, performed prior to a task or shift where the team learns what it will be doing and how, from both a technical and CRM standpoint.

In our concept of CRM, the briefing may be the most important CRM tool that you have. If done properly, the briefing embeds CRM best practices. It can also help less experienced team members by helping build their situation awareness and mental models by discussing what is happening, what success looks like, what threats or errors are possible and how you plan to prevent, avoid, or mitigate them.

A briefing brings together the entry conditions, goals, risks, critical data, critical factors, etc. from the Problem Definition phase with the approved course of action that covers how each will be met. The briefing also includes each team member's roles, responsibilities, and tasks; coordination and communication plan; and possible contingencies.

Common Error: failing to discuss the CRM behaviors required to perform the task.

See Section 14.2.

CODIFIED DECISION MAKING (CDM)

Definition: decision making based on pre-made rules.

CDM often appears as a pre-made conditional statement: if the team sees X, then they shall do Y. The rules could be documented in an organization's philosophies, policies, procedures and practices days, weeks, or even years before the team shows up for their task or shift. The rules could also be decided by the team minutes or hours before the task during the team briefing. The main point is the decision has been made beforehand and team just has to decide to use it.

CDM is best for inexperienced decision makers in situations where the entry conditions are well known. Common Error: using CDM when the entry conditions are subtly different than presumed by the people who made the rule.

See Section 13.1.

COGNITIVE BIAS

Definition: a heuristic or cognitive shortcut which, due to context or framing, results in an incorrect situation assessment.

See Section 5.1.

COMMUNICATING

Definition: the CRM skill of determining how to pass information.

The important behaviors are delivering information clearly and concisely through protocols (the format and terminology of information to be delivered) and confirmation (3-way communication and active listening in an effort to understand).

NOTE: Communicating is different than Exchanging Information. Exchanging Information deals with determining what information to pass to whom and when. Both Communicating and Exchanging Information have their own unique demons and best practices.

Common Error: characterizing an error in Exchanging Information as an error in Communicating and applying the wrong remedial action.

See Chapter 8.

COMPREHENSION

Definition: a second level of situation awareness dealing with understanding the significance of what is happening (Endsley 1997, 207).

Common Error: not providing a team member enough time and cognitive resources to properly comprehend.

See Section 2.1.

COURSE OF ACTION

Definition: a plan to deal with a situation.

Common Error: starting Course of Action selection prior to fully defining the problem.

See Chapter 13.

CREW RESOURCE MANAGEMENT (CRM)

Definition: the Federal Aviation Administration (FAA) considers CRM as a team using all human, hardware, and software resources to be safe and effective (FAA 2004). This definition encompasses a broad approach to exclude nothing. This definition may be too difficult to understand and adopt in practice in healthcare.

Our definition emphasizes the team aspect. Our version of CRM is a way of managing all team interactions to improve performance and positively impact safety. In our CRM model, the core skills are your interpersonal skills of Exchanging Information, Communicating, Leading and Following, and Mutually Supporting.

Our version of CRM will give you definite behaviors to improve team performance and safety on your next task or shift.

Common Error: not developing an organizationally accepted CRM model, so different team members have different ideas on what the CRM skills are and how to do them.

CRITICAL DATA	Definition: any information that you need to determine what the situation is (or is not), whether a threat or error is materializing, or whether a course of action is working. Also called Essential Information. Common Error: not defining critical data during the Think phase of STAR and therefore, not properly monitoring the patient or task. See Section 12.4.
CRITICAL FACTORS	Definition: any criterion that must be achieved for a course of action to be successful (Success Criteria); prevents consideration of a particular course of action (Limiting Criteria); or would allow a course of action to be considered if it appeared (Enabling Criteria). Common Error: not defining critical factors during the Think phase of STAR and, therefore, executing a plan does not meet the team's goals. See Section 12.5.
CUS (CONCERNED, UNCOMFORTABLE, OR SAFETY)	Definition: a set of organizationally/culturally accepted terms to get a leader's attention to listen to a concern: I am Concerned! I am Uncomfortable! This is a Safety Issue!

Common Error: the organization not having or a team member not using the accepted terms, therefore, the team member's concerns are lost to a distracted or overwhelmed leader.

See Section 8.3.

DEBRIEFING

Definition: a meeting of the team after a task, event, or shift to discuss what happened and why in an effort to improve team and individual performance prior to the next task, event or shift.

Common Error: not conducting the right type of debriefing based on the experience of the team (i.e., conducting a leader-led debriefing for a team both technically and CRM experienced, where a self-discovery/self-correction debriefing is appropriate).

See Chapter 18.

DELIBERATE DECISION MAKING (DDM)

Definition: also called Analytical or Classical Decision Making; DDM requires you to list various possible courses of action, evaluate each course of action against various discriminating factors (determining possible benefits, costs, and risks for each course of action), and pick the course of action that scores the best.

Common Error: using DDM when it is not appropriate or selecting a poor set of discriminating factors.

See Section 13.3.

DEMONS	Definition: any factor that makes it difficult for a team to do CRM well. Demons specific to each CRM skill are covered in their respective CRM skill chapter.
EMBEDDING CREW RESOURCE MANAGEMENT	Definition: we use the term in two ways: 1) incorporating CRM into an organization, culture, or team's philosophies, practices, training, and procedures. 2) calling out specific CRM behaviors in the planning (see Section 13.2), briefing (see Section 13.3) and debriefing (see Section 13.4). Common Error: failing to embed CRM into the planning or briefing, assuming the team will automatically know what CRM behaviors to do, how, and when.
ERROR	Definition: any slip of attention, lapse of memory or mistake in recall of content knowledge, decision-making, technical skills, and CRM. An important difference between errors and threats is errors are made by the team, and the team has direct control on whether an error may occur. Threats are external to the team's actions: the team has no control as to whether a threat may materialize and just has to deal with any threat as it occurs.
EXCHANGING INFORMATION	Definition: the CRM skill of determining what information to pass to whom, and when. The what is based mainly on the status of the patient,

task, and environment. To whom is based on each team member's roles and responsibilities. The when is based on the schedule, any times-to-effect, and margin.

Everyone within a team will need information from another team member at some point. Exchanging Information is concerned with the transfer of elements of situation awareness and mental models between team members. Because no single team member can have access to all the information he or she needs at all times, the purpose of Exchanging Information is to fill gaps in individuals' situation awareness (what you think is happening) and mental models (why and how you think it is happening). The products of Exchanging Information are every member of the team having situation awareness and valid mental models.

NOTE: Exchanging Information is different than Communicating. Communicating deals with determining how to pass information. Both Communicating and Exchanging Information have their own unique demons and best practices.

Common Error: characterizing an error in Exchanging Information as an error in Communicating and applying the wrong remedial action.

See Chapter 3.

FACILITATED DEBRIEFING (FD) Definition: a type of debriefing of a team's technical and CRM actions and behaviors where the facilitator, ideally the team leader, asks a series of open-ended questions to enable the team to determine for themselves what they did right and wrong (i.e., self-discover), as well as why, and how to improve (i.e., self-correct). The team members do the majority of the talking, while the facilitator ensures that the debriefing covers all major areas and issues, interjects with probing questions or comments if required to guide the discussion, and ensures that the debriefing is efficient and effective (McDonnell, Jobe and Dismukes 1996).

NOTE: A FD differs from a leader-led or instructor-led debriefing where the leader or instructor tells the team members what they did wrong and how to improve (i.e., there is no self-discovery or self-correction).

A FD also differs from a debriefing where there is no facilitator, but the team decides for themselves what the issues were, and how to fix the (see Chapter 18).

Common Error: using the wrong level of facilitation for the experience of the team.

See Appendix B.

HANDOVER Definition: the transfer of situation awareness, mental models, plans, etc. from one individual/team to another.

We emphasize that a handover must cover situation awareness and mental models in all areas of Status-Team-Environment-Progress (STEP) and give the on-going team a chance to check their situation awareness and mental models.

Common Error: covering only one or two areas of STEP and only at Situation Awareness Level 1, a statement of perceptions.

See Chapter 4.

IM SAFE

Definition: a mnemonic device reminding a team to check for any adverse effects of Illness, Medication, Stress, Alcohol (and drugs), Fatigue and (not) Eaten (or hydrated).

We use IM SAFE as a checklist for the team to decide if they are physically and emotionally ready for the upcoming task/shift.

Common Error: minimizing the risks that adverse personal physiological and psychological states present to a situation.

See Section 5.1.

LEADING AND FOLLOWING

Definition: the CRM skills of leadership and followership. Everyone is both a leader and a follower at various times, and in various situations. Leading enables CRM by setting up psychological safety, articulating CRM expectations and then modeling and rewarding those behaviors. Following enables CRM by inquiring when a team member does not understand the leader or the situation, and then advocating and even asserting a position when they believe that safety is at risk.

As a consequence of Leading and Following behaviors, followers provide the leader with all the information and knowledge that he or she needs to make safe and effective decisions.

Common Error: failing to establish psychological safety, resulting in followers being reluctant to inquire, advocate or assert; the leader may then be deprived of all the information that he or she needs.

See Chapter 9.

LEVELS 1, 2, AND 3 SITUATION AWARENESS	Definition: Level 1 is Perception. Level 2 is Comprehension. Level 3 is Projection (Endsley 1997, 207). See Section 2.1.
MARGIN	Definition: there are 2 types of margin: present and in depth. Present margin is how much a critical data parameter (pressure, temperature, resource, etc.) can increase or decrease before something bad happens or before you must go to a contingency plan. Present margin is gone when you reach a trigger. Margin in depth is how many contingency plans you have. Margin in depth is gone when you run

out of contingency plans (i.e., you are all in).

Common Error: not determining both margins in the planning phase, discussing them in the briefing, monitoring them during execution or debriefing them at the end of a task or shift.

See Section 12.3.

MENTAL MODEL

Definition: How and why you believe something works (Rouse and Morris 1986).

A mental model allows you to turn what you see, hear, feel, taste, or smell into present and future consequences. Another way of saying that is what you see, hear, etc. (Perception, or Level 1 Situation Awareness) are inputs to your mental model and the outputs are your comprehension of present consequences (Level 2 Situation Awareness) as well as projection of future consequences (Level 3 Situation Awareness) (Endsley 1997, 207).

Different mental models are required to cover Status, Team, Environment and Progress (STEP). In healthcare,

- Status includes the Patient and Tasks;
- Team includes Teamwork and Team Members;
- Environment is the physical and organizational context in which the team works; and

- Progress includes the schedule, times-to-effect, and margins.

The authors believe in the concept of complementary mental models. Mental models are complementary when mental models of team members have the same task intersections and the same team interactions. Task intersections are how my tasks affect your tasks, and how your tasks affect my tasks. Team interactions are what I need to do or say for you to do your job, and what you need to do or say for me to do my job.

Common Error: failing to activate the correct/complete mental models; this can be remedied by a thorough briefing by the leader.

See Chapter 7.

MULTITASKING

Definition: when an individual attempts to do two or more tasks simultaneously, where all tasks are cognitively demanding (i.e., have not passed into automaticity).

Common Errors: placekeeping errors (missing or re-doing a step) or prospective memory errors (forgetting to do a task in the future).

See Section 5.2.

MUTUALLY SUPPORTING

Definition: the CRM skill whereby team members offer and accept physical, cognitive, psychological, and emotional support as well as providing

feedback on both technical and CRM behaviors.
The product of Mutually Supporting others is a reduction in the impacts of Performance Shaping Factors such as stress and fatigue, thereby supporting fewer errors and reduced risk, even in complex and extreme environments.

Common Error: losing situation awareness on the performance shaping factors that affect a team member resulting in failure to provide mutual support.

See Chapter 10.

NATURALISTIC DECISION MAKING (NDM)

Definition: decision making based on previous experience. NDM is the "been there, done that" means of decision making. NDM is how experienced people naturally make decisions. Highly experienced people have a repertoire of past experiences upon which to draw and can rapidly decide what to do based on what worked in the past. Experts recognize a situation and remember what they did last time.

Common Error: failing to recognize subtle differences in a situation from those previous experienced, resulting in an incorrect course of action that does not account for those differences.

See Section 13.2.

PERCEPTION

Definition: the first level of situation awareness dealing with seeing,

	hearing, feeling, tasting, or smelling what is happening (Endsley 1997, 207). Common Error: failing to provide a team member enough time and cognitive resources to properly perceive. See Section 2.1.
PERFORMANCE SHAPING FACTOR	Definition: any psychological, emotional, or physical stressor that affects performance. See Section 5.1
POWER OF AND	Definition: a belief that since no one person can have perfect situation awareness and mental models, it is possible that team members with different situation awareness and mental models may have different perspectives of the same situation. Integrating those diverse situation awareness and mental models ("And"-ing) will result in broader, deeper, more refined situation awareness and mental models. Common Error: refusing to believe that your mental model might be wrong or dismissing the ideas from the "new guy" or a subordinate. See Section 3.3.
PROBLEM DEFINITION	Definition: the first part of the Think portion of STAR where team members take their situation awareness and focuses it to determine if they have a problem and how best to define it.

Consider Problem Definition as developing situation awareness about the problem. Problem Definition makes sure that the team is solving the right problem. A Problem Definition is done if the team can answer these 6 questions:

1. Are there any quick response actions required?
2. How much time or margin do you or can you have?
3. What is the problem?
4. What are the critical factors?
5. What is your first goal?
6. How do you validate your Problem Definition?

Common Error: starting a Course of Action selection before the team can answer the six questions listed above.

See Chapter 12.

PROJECTION

Definition: third level of situation awareness dealing with predicting the significance (Level 2 Comprehension) of what is happening (Level 1 Perception) into the near future, usually to a critical point in time. (Endsley 1997, 207)

Common Error: failing to provide a team member enough time and cognitive resources to properly project.

See Section 2.1.

PSYCHOLOGICAL SAFETY	Definition: a condition where team members believe that they can admit to an error, ask a question, or advocate and assert a recommendation without fear of retribution. Without psychological safety, team members will not be willing to give a leader all the information that the leader needs to make sound decisions. Common Error: failing to establish psychological safety during the briefing, task, or debriefing. See Section 9.2.2.
SELF-DISCOVERY AND SELF-CORRECTION	Definition: a condition where the team habitually discusses among themselves what they did right and wrong and why, and then how they can improve. Self-discovery and self-correction are the goals of debriefings. Common Error: discussing team errors in an effort to diffuse responsibility and/or to avoid discussion of individual errors (rather than trying to fix errors in Exchanging Information, Communicating, Leading and Following, and Mutually Supporting). See Section 18.1.
SITUATION AWARENESS	Definition: per Mica Endsley, "the perception of the elements in the environment within a volume of time and space, comprehension of their meaning and the projection of their status in the near future." (Endsley 1997, 207) See Section 2.1.

SITUATION-BACKGROUND-ASSESSMENT-RECOMMENDATION (SBAR)	Definition: one of many handover formats designed to ensure that all required information in all areas is passed on. SBAR stands for Situation - Background - Assessment - Recommendation, where S is Level 1 Situation Awareness, B and A support Level 2 Situation Awareness, and R supports and allows comparison of Level 3 Situation Awareness. Common Error: failing to cover all areas of STEP, usually concentrating only on Status at only Level 1 Situation Awareness. See Section 4.1.
SITUATION MONITORING	Definition: "The process of continually scanning and assessing what is going on around you to maintain situation awareness" (TeamSTEPPS Pocket Guide 2020). By monitoring the situation, the team is trying to determine what is happening so that they can make informed choices about when, how, and why to act. The product of Situation Monitoring is Situation Awareness. See Section 2.1.
STANDARD OPERATING PROCEDURE (SOP)	Definition: an organizationally/culturally/team agreed-to set of instructions on how to accomplish a task. An SOP is essentially a codified mental model

which allows ad hoc teams to accomplish tasks without having to define each mental model in the briefing.

Common Error: applying a SOP in a situation that is subtly different than the situation presumed by those who developed the SOP.

STATUS-TEAM-ENVIRONMENT-PROGRESS (STEP)

Definition: we use a modified form of a TeamSTEPPS' mnemonic device, where STEP stands for Status (Patient and Task), Team (Teamwork and Team Members), Environment and Progress (Schedule, Times-to-Effect, and Margins).

Each letter represents one or more mental models required to have Total Situation Awareness.

Common Error: failing to consider fully all four areas of STEP.

See Section 2.4.

STOP-THINK-ACT-REVIEW (STAR)

Definition: STAR stands for Stop Think-Act-Review, or if you see something you did not expect, you:

- Stop to get over the startle effect, and manage workload and distractions
- Think to define the problem and determine a course of action
- Act to develop, and then execute, a plan
- Review at the end of every step, but also the end of every task and phase

	When faced with a situation during execution in which the team is not sure what is going on or what to do, they call for a STAR moment. Common Error: failing to take a few seconds, minutes, or hours (depending on the situation) to do a complete STAR. See Chapters 11-15.
STORY	Definition: a narrative of events that explains how the situation developed. A team must understand the possible ways that the situation might have unfolded or how they found themselves in the situation. Considering different stories is part of the Comprehension level of situation awareness. A story that explains all the present conditions (Level 1 Situation Awareness) is required to develop Total Situation Awareness. If a team is not sure of the background or context, alternate stories that would have brought you to the same place must be considered until critical data allows you to disregard them. Common Error: considering only one story as an explanation for a situation. See Section 12.4.
TEAMSTEPPS	Definition: "Team Strategies and Tools to Enhance Performance and Patient Safety," is a teamwork system developed jointly by the Department of Defense and the Agency for Healthcare Research and Quality to

improve institutional collaboration and communication relating to patient safety. Our CRM model uses elements of TeamSTEPPS.

THREAT

Definition: any event or condition external to the team that may adversely affect a team's performance. Threats are different than errors. Threats are external to the team's actions and the team has no control over whether a threat materializes, or not; the team simply has to deal with any threats as they occur. Errors, on the other hand, are made by the team and the team has direct control over whether an error may occur.

TIME-TO-EFFECT (TTE)

Definition: the length of time before a task needs to be performed or an adverse event occurs (also known as the "no kidding, drop dead, deadline"). TtE is part of the Progress Mental Model in STEP.

Common Error: failing to proactively determine (e.g., during a briefing) a TtE and neglecting to assign someone to monitor the time.

See Section 2.4.4.

TOTAL SITUATION AWARENESS

Definition: possessing situation awareness in all the levels and areas you must have, as enumerated in Status-Team-Environment-Progress (STEP). Total Situation Awareness can also be as Systems Thinking or Holistic Thinking, and STEP is the mnemonic to remind you what you must consider to be Systems or Holistic Thinking.

Common Error: failing to achieve situation awareness in all areas of STEP.

See Section 2.4.

References

Endsley, Mica R. "Toward a Theory of Situation Awareness in Dynamic Systems." Human Factors: The Journal of the Human Factors and Ergonomics Society 37, no. 1 (1995): 32–64. https://doi.org/10.1518/001872095779049543.

Endsley, Mica. "The Role of Situation Awareness in Naturalistic Decision Making." Essay. In Naturalistic Decision Making, 269–83. New York, NY: Psychology Press, 1997.

"Facilitating LOS Debriefings: A Training Manual." Accessed October 30, 2021. https://humansystems.arc.nasa.gov/flightcognition/Publications/Final_Training_TM.pdf.

Rouse, William B., and Nancy M. Morris. "On Looking into the Black Box: Prospects and Limits in the Search for Mental Models." Psychological Bulletin 100, no. 3 (1986): 349–63. https://doi.org/10.1037/0033-2909.100.3.349.

TeamSTEPPS: Pocket Guide: Strategies & Tools to Enhance Performance and Patient Safety. Bethesda, MD: U.S. Dept. of Health and Human Services, Agency for Healthcare Research and Quality, 2006.

"Crew Resource Management Training." U.S. Federal Aviation Administration, 2004. https://permanent.fdlp.gov/LPS109002/LPS109002/www.airweb.faa.gov/Regulatory_and_Guidance_Library/rgAdvisoryCircular.nsf/0/80038cf51aace53686256e24005cbb23/$FILE/AC120-51e.pdf. Report No. AC120-51E.

BIBLIOGRAPHY

"2020 NSI National Health Care Retention & RN Staffing Report." NSI Nursing Solutions. Accessed October 30, 2021. https://www.nsinursingsolutions.com/Documents/Library/NSI_National_Health_Care_Retention_Report.pdf.

Aeronautical Information Manual - aim. Accessed October 30, 2021. https://www.faa.gov/air_traffic/publications/atpubs/aim_html/index.html.

Anderson, Janet E., Alastair J. Ross, and Peter Jaye. "Modelling Resilience and Researching the Gap Between Work-as-Imagined and Work-as-Done." Essay. In Resilient Health Care: Reconciling Work-as Imagined and Work-as-Done 3, edited by Jeffrey Braithwaite, Erik Hollnagel, and Robert L. Wears, 3:133–41. London: CRC Press, 2015.

Austin, Matt, and Jordan Derk. "Lives Lost, Lives Saved: An Updated Comparative Analysis of Avoidable Deaths at Hospitals Graded by the Leapfrog Group." Armstrong Institute for Patient Safety and Quality, Johns Hopkins Medicine, 2019. https://www.hospitalsafetygrade.org/media/file/Lives-Saved-White-Paper-FINAL.pdf.

Banja, John. "The Normalization of Deviance in Healthcare Delivery." Business Horizons 53, no. 2 (2010): 139–48. https://doi.org/10.1016/j.bushor.2009.10.006.

Barnett, Jeffrey E., Ellen K. Baker, Nancy S. Elman, and Gary R. Schoener. "In Pursuit of Wellness: The Self-Care Imperative." Professional Psychology: Research and Practice 38, no. 6 (2007): 603–12. https://doi.org/10.1037/0735-7028.38.6.603.

Barshi, Immanuel. Multitasking Myth - Handling Complexity in Real-World Operations. Ashgate Publishing Group, 2009.

Borges, Anna. The More or Less Definitive Guide to Self-Care. New York: The Experiment, 2019.

Christianson, Marlys K, Kathleen M Sutcliffe, Melissa A Miller, and Theodore J Iwashyna. "Becoming a High Reliability Organization." Critical Care 15, no. 6 (2011): 314. https://doi.org/10.1186/cc10360.

Cohen, Marvin S., Jared T. Freeman, and Steve Wolf. "Metarecognition in Time-Stressed Decision Making: Recognizing, Critiquing, and

Correcting." Human Factors: The Journal of the Human Factors and Ergonomics Society 38, no. 2 (1996): 206–19. https://doi.org/10.1518/001872096779048020.

"Columbia Accident Investigation Board." NASA. NASA. Accessed October 30, 2021. https://history.nasa.gov/columbia/CAIB.html.

"Conflict in the Workplace by Monica A. Frank, Ph.D.." Excel At Life. Accessed October 30, 2021. https://www.excelatlife.com/articles/conflict_at_work.htm.

Cook-Cottone, Catherine P. Mindfulness and Yoga for Self-Regulation: A Primer for Mental Health Professionals. New York: Springer Publishing Company, 2015.

"Crew Resource Management Training." U.S. Federal Aviation Administration, 2004. https://permanent.fdlp.gov/LPS109002/LPS109002/www.airweb.faa.gov/Regulatory_and_Guidance_Library/rgAdvisoryCircular.nsf/0/80038cf51aace53686256e24005cbb23/$FILE/AC120-51e.pdf. Report No. AC120-51E.

"Critical Thinking Skills in Tactical Decision Making: A ..." Accessed October 30, 2021. https://www.researchgate.net/profile/Marvin-Cohen-2/publication/236030478_Critical_Thinking_Skills_in_Tactical_Decision_Making_A_Model_and_A_Training_Strategy/links/02e7e515e220e2e87f000000/Critical-Thinking-Skills-in-Tactical-Decision-Making-A-Model-and-A-Training-Strategy.pdf.

Darling, Marilyn, Charles Parry, and Joseph Moore. "Learning in the Thick of It." Harvard Business Review, August 1, 2005. https://hbr.org/2005/07/learning-in-the-thick-of-it.

de Vries, Eefje N., Maya A. Ramrattan, Susanne M. Smorenburg, Dirk J. Gouma, and Marja A. Boermeester. "The Incidence and Nature of In-Hospital Adverse Events: A Systematic Review." Quality & Safety in Health Care. U.S. National Library of Medicine. Accessed October 30, 2021. https://pubmed.ncbi.nlm.nih.gov/18519629/.

de Wit, Frank R., Lindred L. Greer, and Karen A. Jehn. "The Paradox of Intragroup Conflict: A Meta-Analysis." Journal of Applied Psychology 97, no. 2 (2012): 360–90. https://doi.org/10.1037/a0024844.

DeChurch, Leslie A., and Jessica R. Mesmer-Magnus. "The Cognitive Underpinnings of Effective Teamwork: A Meta-Analysis." Journal of Applied Psychology 95, no. 1 (2010): 32–53. https://doi.org/10.1037/a0017328.

"Deep Water: The Gulf Oil Disaster and the Future of Offshore Drilling." Govinfo. National Commission on the BP Deepwater Horizon Oil Spill and Offshore Drilling, 2011.

https://www.govinfo.gov/app/details/GPO-OILCOMMISSION.
Dekker, Sidney. Drift into Failure from Hunting Broken Components to Understanding Complex Systems. London: CRC Press, 2016.
Druskat, Vanessa Urch, and Anthony T. Pescosolido. "The Content of Effective Teamwork Mental Models in Self-Managing Teams: Ownership, Learning and Heedful Interrelating." Human Relations 55, no. 3 (2002): 283–314. https://doi.org/10.1177/0018726702553001.
"ECFR :: 14 CFR 121.542 -- Flight Crewmember Duties." Accessed October 28, 2021. https://www.ecfr.gov/current/title-14/chapter-I/subchapter-G/part-121/subpart-T/section-121.542.
Endsley, Mica R. "Situation Awareness." Handbook of Human Factors and Ergonomics, 2006, 528–42. https://doi.org/10.1002/0470048204.ch20.
Endsley, Mica R. "Toward a Theory of Situation Awareness in Dynamic Systems." Human Factors: The Journal of the Human Factors and Ergonomics Society 37, no. 1 (1995): 32–64. https://doi.org/10.1518/001872095779049543.
Endsley, Mica R., and Daniel J. Garland. Situation Awareness: Analysis and Measurement. Boca Raton: CRC Press, 2008.
Endsley, Mica, and Debra Jones. "Sources of Situation Awareness Errors in Aviation." Aviation, space, and environmental medicine. U.S. National Library of Medicine. Accessed October 30, 2021. https://pubmed.ncbi.nlm.nih.gov/8827130/.
Endsley, Mica, Betty Bolté, and Debra Jones. "SA Demons." Designing for Situation Awareness, 2003, 31–42. https://doi.org/10.1201/9780203485088.ch3.
Endsley, Mica. "The Role of Situation Awareness in Naturalistic Decision Making." Essay. In Naturalistic Decision Making, 269–83. New York, NY: Psychology Press, 1997.
"Facilitating Los Debriefings: A Training Manual." Accessed October 30, 2021. https://humansystems.arc.nasa.gov/flightcognition/Publications/Final_Training_TM.pdf.
Feldman, Robert S. Social Psychology: Theories, Research, and Applications. New York: McGraw-Hill, 1985.
Grenny, Joseph, Kerry Patterson, David Maxfield, Ron McMillan, and Al Switzler. Influencer: The New Science of Leading Change. New York, NY: McGraw-Hill, 2012.
Halamek, Louis P., Robert A.H. Cady, and Michael R. Sterling. "Using Briefing, Simulation and Debriefing to Improve Human and System Performance." Seminars in Perinatology 43, no. 8 (2019): 151178. https://doi.org/10.1053/j.semperi.2019.08.007.

Halamek, Louis P., Robert A.H. Cady, and Michael R. Sterling. "Using Briefing, Simulation and Debriefing to Improve Human and System Performance." Seminars in Perinatology 43, no. 8 (2019): 151178. https://doi.org/10.1053/j.semperi.2019.08.007.

Hefner, Jennifer L., Brian Hilligoss, Amy Knupp, Judy Bournique, John Sullivan, Eric Adkins, and Susan D. Moffatt-Bruce. "Cultural Transformation after Implementation of Crew Resource Management: Is It Really Possible?" American Journal of Medical Quality 32, no. 4 (2016): 384–90. https://doi.org/10.1177/1062860616655424.

Henricksen, Jared W., Catherine Altenburg, and Ron W. Reeder. "Operationalizing Healthcare Simulation Psychological Safety." Simulation in Healthcare: The Journal of the Society for Simulation in Healthcare 12, no. 5 (2017): 289–97. https://doi.org/10.1097/sih.0000000000000253.

Henricksen, Jared W., Catherine Altenburg, and Ron W. Reeder. "Operationalizing Healthcare Simulation Psychological Safety." Simulation in Healthcare: The Journal of the Society for Simulation in Healthcare 12, no. 5 (2017): 289–97. https://doi.org/10.1097/sih.0000000000000253.

Kahneman, Daniel. Thinking, Fast and Slow. New York: Farrar, Straus and Giroux, 2013.

Klein, Gary A. Decision Making in Action: Models and Methods. Norwood, NJ: Ablex, 1995.

Klein, Gary A., Roberta Calderwood, and Anne Clinton-Cirocco. "Rapid Decision Making on the Fire Ground." Proceedings of the Human Factors Society Annual Meeting 30, no. 6 (1986): 576–80. https://doi.org/10.1177/154193128603000616.

Klein, Gary, David Snowden, and Chew Pin. "Anticipatory Thinking - USDA," 2011. https://www.fs.usda.gov/rmrs/sites/default/files/Klein%20et%20al%20-%20Anticipatory%20Thinking.pdf.

Klein, Gary, David Snowden, and Chew Pin. "Anticipatory Thinking." Essay. In Informed by Knowledge: Expert Performance in Complex Situations; Based on Presentations from the 8th International Conference on Naturalistic Decision Making, edited by Ute M. Fischer and Kathleen L. Mosier, 235–44. New York, NY: Psychology Press, 2011.

Klein, Gary. "Performing a Project Premortem." IEEE Engineering Management Review 36, no. 2 (2008): 103–4. https://doi.org/10.1109/emr.2008.4534313.

Klein, Gary. Sources of Power: How People Make Decisions. Cambridge, MA: MIT Press, 1999.

Kotter, John P. Accelerate: Building Strategic Agility for a Faster Moving World. Boston, MA: Harvard Business Review Press, 2014.

Le Roy, Grégory. "Critical Decisions - Redeciding Cognitive Biases - Gary Klein (Sources of Power)." HEC Stories, February 5, 2021. https://hecstories.fr/en/redeciding-cognitive-biases-gary-klein-sources-of-power.

LeSage, Paul, Jeff T. Dyar, and Bruce E. Evans. Crew Resource Management Principles and Practice. Sudburry, MA: Jones and Bartlett Publ, 2011.

Marshall, Pam, and Rob Robson. "Preventing and Managing Conflict: Vital Pieces in the Patient Safety Puzzle." Healthcare Quarterly 8, no. sp (2005): 39–44. https://doi.org/10.12927/hcq..17660.

Mathieu, John E., Michael R. Kukenberger, Lauren D'Innocenzo, and Greg Reilly. "Modeling Reciprocal Team Cohesion–Performance Relationships, as Impacted by Shared Leadership and Members' Competence." Journal of Applied Psychology 100, no. 3 (2015): 713–34. https://doi.org/10.1037/a0038898.

McClelland, G, and MB Smith. "Just a Routine Operation: A Critical Discussion." Journal of Perioperative Practice 26, no. 5 (2016): 114–17. https://doi.org/10.1177/175045891602600504.

McCormick, Iain A., Frank H. Walkey, and Dianne E. Green. "Comparative Perceptions of Driver Ability— a Confirmation and Expansion." Accident Analysis & Prevention 18, no. 3 (1986): 205–8. https://doi.org/10.1016/0001-4575(86)90004-7.

McDonnell, Lori K., Kimberly K. Jobe, and R. Key Dismukes. Facilitating Los Debriefings: A Training Manual. Moffett Field, CA: National Aeronautics and Space Administration, Ames Research Center, 1997.

McPherson, James A., Rhonda L. Zeisig, and Kimberley A. Smith-Jentsch. "Team Dimensional Training: A Strategy for Guided Team Self-Correction." Essay. In Making Decisions Under Stress: Implications for Individual and Team Training, edited by Janis A. Cannon-Bowers and Eduardo Salas, 271–96. Washington, D.C.: American Psychological Association, 1998.

Meginniss, Anne, Frances Damian, and Francine Falvo. "Time out for Patient Safety." Journal of Emergency Nursing 38, no. 1 (2012): 51–53. https://doi.org/10.1016/j.jen.2011.04.007.

Moffatt-Bruce, Susan D., Jennifer L. Hefner, Hagop Mekhjian, John S. McAlearney, Tina Latimer, Chris Ellison, and Ann Scheck McAlearney. "What Is the Return on Investment for Implementation of a Crew

Resource Management Program at an Academic Medical Center?" American Journal of Medical Quality 32, no. 1 (2016): 5–11. https://doi.org/10.1177/1062860615608938.

Nagoski, Emily, and Amelia Nagoski. Burnout: The Secret to Unlocking the Stress Cycle. New York, NY: Ballantine Books, 2020.

Neff, Kristin D., Marissa C. Knox, Phoebe Long, and Krista Gregory. "Caring for Others without Losing Yourself: An Adaptation of the Mindful Self-Compassion Program for Healthcare Communities." Journal of Clinical Psychology 76, no. 9 (2020): 1543–62. https://doi.org/10.1002/jclp.23007.

"Online Resource - Resources for Pilots." FAA. Accessed October 30, 2021. https://preprod.faasafety.gov/gslac/onlineresources.aspx?categoryId=27&masterId=1.

"Online Resource - Resources for Pilots." FAA. Accessed October 30, 2021. https://preprod.faasafety.gov/gslac/onlineresources.aspx?categoryId=27&masterId=1.

O'Connor, Paul, Angela O'Dea, and Ivan Keogh. "Is Crew Resource Management Training Effective in Healthcare Settings?" Proceedings of the International Symposium on Human Factors and Ergonomics in Health Care 2, no. 1 (June 2012): 105–7. https://doi.org/10.1177/2327857913021020.

Parke, Bonny, and Barbara G. Kanki. "Best Practices in Shift Turnovers: Implications for Reducing Aviation Maintenance Turnover Errors as Revealed in ASRS Reports." The International Journal of Aviation Psychology 18, no. 1 (2008): 72–85. https://doi.org/10.1080/10508410701749464.

Patterson, Kerry, Ron McMillan, and Joseph Grenny. Crucial Conversations: Tools for Talking When Stakes Are High. New York etc.: McGraw-Hill, 2002.

Plant, Katherine L., and Neville A. Stanton. "The Process of Processing: Exploring the Validity of Neisser's Perceptual Cycle Model with Accounts from Critical Decision-Making in the Cockpit." Ergonomics 58, no. 6 (2014): 909–23. https://doi.org/10.1080/00140139.2014.991765.

quoteresearch, Author. "I Would Spend 55 Minutes Defining the Problem and Then Five Minutes Solving It." Quote Investigator, November 22, 2018. https://quoteinvestigator.com/2014/05/22/solve/.

quoteresearch, Author. "I Would Spend 55 Minutes Defining the Problem and Then Five Minutes Solving It." Quote Investigator, November 22, 2018. https://quoteinvestigator.com/2014/05/22/solve/.

Rouse, William B., and Nancy M. Morris. On Looking into the Black Box Prospects and Limits in the Search for Mental Models. S.l.: Distributed by ERIC Clearinghouse, 1985.

Rouse, William B., and Nancy M. Morris. "On Looking into the Black Box: Prospects and Limits in the Search for Mental Models." Psychological Bulletin 100, no. 3 (1986): 349–63. https://doi.org/10.1037/0033-2909.100.3.349.

Sawyer, T, D Loren, and L P Halamek. "Post-Event Debriefings during Neonatal Care: Why Are We Not Doing Them, and How Can We Start?" Journal of Perinatology 36, no. 6 (2016): 415–19. https://doi.org/10.1038/jp.2016.42.

Sawyer, Taylor Lee, and Shad Deering. "Adaptation of the US Army's after-Action Review for Simulation Debriefing in Healthcare." Simulation in Healthcare: The Journal of the Society for Simulation in Healthcare 8, no. 6 (2013): 388–97. https://doi.org/10.1097/sih.0b013e31829ac85c.

Scott, S D, L E Hirschinger, K R Cox, M McCoig, J Brandt, and L W Hall. "The Natural History of Recovery for the Healthcare Provider 'Second Victim' after Adverse Patient Events." Quality and Safety in Health Care 18, no. 5 (2009): 325–30. https://doi.org/10.1136/qshc.2009.032870.

"Secondary Navigation." Air Traffic Plans and Publications, June 24, 2021. https://www.faa.gov/air_traffic/publications/.

Skovholt, Thomas M., Tabitha L. Grier, and Matthew R. Hanson. "Career Counseling for Longevity: Self-Care and Burnout Prevention Strategies for Counselor Resilience." Journal of Career Development 27, no. 3 (2001): 167–76. https://doi.org/10.1177/089484530102700303.

Smith-Jentsch, Kimberley. "On Shifting from Autonomous to Interdependent Work." NASA Johnson Space Center, February 2014. https://www.researchgate.net/publication/292783480_On_Shifting_from_Autonomous_to_Interdependent_Work. NASA/TM-2015-218563

Stanton, N. A., R. Stewart, D. Harris, R. J. Houghton, C. Baber, R. McMaster, P. Salmon, et al. "Distributed Situation Awareness in Dynamic Systems: Theoretical Development and Application of an Ergonomics Methodology." Ergonomics 49, no. 12-13 (2006): 1288–1311. https://doi.org/10.1080/00140130600612762.

Taleb, Nassim. The Black Swan: The Impact of the Highly Improbable. New York. N.Y.: Random House, 2010.

Tannenbaum, Scott I., and Eduardo Salas. Teams That Work: The Seven Drivers of Team Effectiveness. New York, NY: Oxford University Press, 2021.

"Teach Teamwork." American Psychological Association. American Psychological Association. Accessed October 30, 2021. https://www.apa.org/education/k12/teach-teamwork.

TeamSTEPPS: Pocket Guide: Strategies & Tools to Enhance Performance and Patient Safety. Bethesda, MD: U.S. Dept. of Health and Human Services, Agency for Healthcare Research and Quality, 2006.

Tompkins, Mimi. "Facilitating a Critical Incident Stress Debriefing." Essay. In Facilitation and Debriefing in Aviation Training and Operations, edited by R. Key Dismukes, 93–104. Burlington, VT: Ashgate, 2000.

Vaughan, Diane. The Challenger Launch Decision: Risky Technology, Culture, and Deviance at NASA. Chicago: The University of Chicago Press, 2016.

Weick, Karl E., Kathleen M. Sutcliffe, and David Obstfeld. "Organizing and the Process of Sensemaking." Organization Science 16, no. 4 (2005): 409–21. https://doi.org/10.1287/orsc.1050.0133.

Weick, Karl, Kathleen Sutcliffe, and David Obstfeld. "Organizing for High Reliability: Processes of Collective Mindfulness." Essay. In Research in Organizational Behavior: An Annual Series of Analytical Essays and Critical Reviews, edited by Robert I. Sutton, Barry M. Staw, and Larry Cummings, 81–122. Greenwich, CT: JAI Press, 1999.

Zheng, Min, Jessecae K. Marsh, Jeffrey V. Nickerson, and Samantha Kleinberg. "How Causal Information Affects Decisions." Cognitive Research: Principles and Implications. Springer International Publishing, February 13, 2020. https://cognitiveresearchjournal.springeropen.com/articles/10.1186/s41235-020-0206-z.

Zheng, Min, Jessecae Marsh, Jeffrey Nickerson, and Samantha Kleinberg. "How Casual Information Affects Decisions." Essay. In Cognitive Research: Principles and Implications 5, Vol. 5. Springer, 2020.